PROFESSIONAL TRANSITIONS IN
NURSING

PROFESSIONAL TRANSITIONS IN NURSING

A GUIDE TO PRACTICE IN THE AUSTRALIAN HEALTHCARE SYSTEM

ALISTER HODGE + WAYNE VARNDELL

with Roianne West

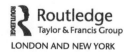

Routledge
Taylor & Francis Group

LONDON AND NEW YORK

First published 2018 by Allen & Unwin

Published 2020 by Routledge
2 Park Square, Milton Park, Abingdon, Oxon OX14 4RN
605 Third Avenue, New York, NY 10017

Routledge is an imprint of the Taylor & Francis Group, an informa business

A catalogue record for this book is available from the National Library of Australia

Internal design by Romina Panetta
Index by Puddingburn
Set in 11/14 pt Caslon 540 by Midland Typesetters, Australia

ISBN-13: 9781760293499 (pbk)

We dedicate this book first to our families and colleagues—without their tireless support these pages would still be blank; and second, to nurses beginning their journey in Australia—good luck!

Alister Hodge and Wayne Varndell

CONTENTS

FIGURES AND TABLES

Figures

Tables

AUTHORS

Alister N. Hodge

MN (Nurse Prac), MN (Emerg), PGCert (Crit Care), BN
Nurse Practitioner, Emergency
Clinical Lecturer, School of Nursing, The University of Sydney

Wayne F. Varndell

MN (Research), BSc (Hons), Nursing PGCert (Ed), GradDipHE (Nursing),
    PhD Candidate
Clinical Nurse Consultant, Emergency
Associate Lecturer, Faculty of Health, University of Technology Sydney
Associate Editor, *Australasian Emergency Nursing Journal*

with

Professor Roianne West

PhD, MMHN, RN, BN
Director, First Peoples Health Unit
Griffith Health Institute for the Development of Education and Scholarship
    (Health IDEAS)
First Peoples Health Unit I, Menzies Health Institute, Griffith University

PREFACE

Alister Hodge and Wayne Varndell work within the Australian health system as clinicians, Alister as an emergency nurse practitioner and Wayne as a clinical nurse consultant. Both authors have broad experience in the United Kingdom and Australia, primarily within the emergency specialty, in which they maintain the delivery of patient-centred, evidence-based care as a core priority. They share a key interest in supporting the professional development of clinical nurses and have extensive experience in education resource creation and delivery in both the hospital and the postgraduate setting.

The combined experience of the authors has enabled an understanding of the challenges facing new graduate and overseas nurses entering the Australian workforce for the first time. Few areas deal with the sudden impact of illness, trauma and societal change more than the acute health setting. Nurses today care for greater numbers of acutely ill patients with more complex conditions. The knowledge, skills and expertise needed for early detection of deterioration in, and subsequent resuscitation and stabilisation of, critically ill or injured patients in line with current best evidence and practice require a lifelong learning effort by nurses. While post-registration courses have been developed to assist nurses in mastering key areas of knowledge particular to different specialties, the essential first steps for nurse graduates in preparing to enter the workforce and for overseas-qualified Registered Nurses (RN) in continuing their careers in Australia are rarely discussed.

This book has been written to support a successful transition to the Australian health environment for the new graduate and the overseas nurse, by pinpointing need-to-know information that will help them adapt to the health environment and culture, provide safe patient care and understand professional obligations in clinical practice and ongoing development. This text aims to provide key information in an easily accessible format. Definitions of common terms are provided in the margins and there is a list of the meanings of common acronyms and abbreviations used within the health system. Introductory summaries are supplied at the start of each chapter, with review questions at the end.

Information has been organised in three sub-sections. **Part I, The Australian health system, professional standards and legislation,** provides information to support the graduate nurse entering the workforce, detailing the role's challenges, expectations, scope, boundaries and strategies. We discuss the Australian health system, professional practice requirements and medico-legal responsibilities of the RN in order to explain the context in which nurses practise. **Part II, Key clinical skills and practices,** provides essential information for day-to-day care delivery on the floor—the essentials underpinning safe clinical practice. **Part III, Gaining employment and career planning,** details how to manage the registration requirements of ongoing professional development and provides insight into career planning and ways to support clinical progression with relevant academic development. Importantly, it also provides vital information on the employment process, giving tips to support interview preparation for jobs and graduate programs.

ACKNOWLEDGEMENTS

This book would not have been possible without the efforts of multiple individuals. We wish first to thank the publisher Allen & Unwin for their early interest, encouragement and guidance, and our editors and reviewers—these pages have greatly benefited from their assistance, suggestions and feedback. Second, we wish to thank the many colleagues and mentors who have supported our development as clinicians and helped shape our career.

And third, but by no means less important, we thank our families and friends for their encouragement and support in completing this book.

Alister Hodge
Wayne Varndell

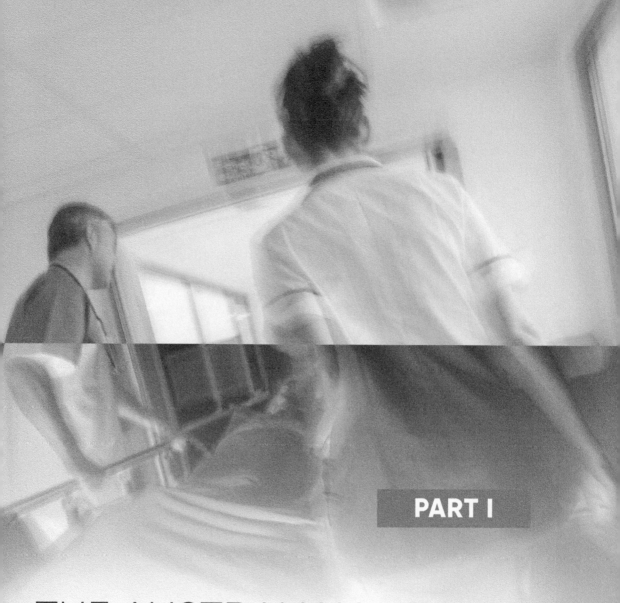

PART I

THE AUSTRALIAN HEALTH SYSTEM, PROFESSIONAL STANDARDS AND LEGISLATION

1 THE TRANSITION TO REGISTERED NURSE

Alister Hodge

In this chapter, you will develop an understanding of:

- challenges facing the new graduate nurse
- new graduate nurse scope of practice and role boundaries
- developing professional identity
- strategies to support your transition to the workplace
- adapting to shiftwork, sleep hygiene and maintaining a work–life balance
- managing personal stress.

CHALLENGES FACING THE NEW GRADUATE NURSE

As nurse graduates, the first year in the health workforce will involve a major transition from being a student to taking on the responsibilities of a Registered Nurse (RN). The authors' own experience as graduates, together with the experiences of the many nurses we have been privileged to support during their transition to practice, informs this book.

During transition, each graduate will experience different issues that may be challenging on a personal level—for example, learning how to manage fatigue on a rotating shift roster, and developing time-management skills on a busy ward. You will share many challenges with your fellow graduates, such as adjusting to a new workplace culture, interacting with complex technology and developing functional communication patterns. It can be a steep learning curve!

Registration as a nurse changes your world significantly. Adjusting to the cultural differences between university and hospital environments presents an initial challenge as you move from the familiar role of a student to that of an accountable, practising RN (Johnstone et al., 2008). You will exchange the defined support structures of a university for a constantly evolving clinical environment without the guarantee of mentorship or support (Phillips et al., 2014). In addition, you may experience a degree of stress due to uncertainty about your role and a lack of clearly defined responsibilities, making it difficult to know what is expected of you (Chang & Hancock, 2003).

All new graduates entering the acute care setting face the contemporary health challenges of rising patient **acuity**, shorter lengths of stay, complex technologies such as monitors and electronic documentation, compounded by an intimate exposure to end-of-life situations (Walker et al. 2013). Some work sites may have poor staffing ratios that contribute to heavy workloads, issues with skill mix and an increased likelihood of being asked to manage complex patients whose conditions stretch your knowledge and skill set. The pressure is such that research by Dyess and Sherman (2009) found some new graduate nurses were concerned they might not be able to provide safe care and concurrently meet the expectations of their employer.

acuity Relates to the intensity of nursing care required by the patient.

In the interests of delivering safe patient care, you must learn to effectively communicate with other members of staff, including doctors and allied health professionals. Failures in communication may result in important information being missed and increased patient risk. (Patterns of communication that help information transfer are discussed in depth in Chapter 6.) Although it may take some time for you to feel confident about expressing yourself—particularly with senior clinicians—it is a fundamental skill that will be required throughout the course of your nursing career. In addition to discussing clinical information, you may have to supervise and delegate aspects of care to Assistants in Nursing (AIN) and Enrolled Nurses (EN), who may be older and have more years of practice in the health workforce (Dyess & Sherman, 2009).

Early in your graduate year, you may encounter 'reality shock', finding major discrepancies between what you understood about nursing during your undergraduate education and your real-life experience of nursing in the clinical environment. In some cases, you may be forced to prioritise tasks that ensure basic patient safety at the expense of meaningful interactions, such as patient education regarding their illness and treatment that will allow the patient to become a true contributor to their own health. This conflict between what you are asked to do as an RN and what you were taught to consider as key priorities in your undergraduate degree may cause dissatisfaction and disillusionment, and in some cases results in graduates leaving the profession (Duchscher, 2009). This period of 'reality shock' usually occurs in the first four to six months of practice. Although the new graduate may lose their idealised version of the nurse's role, interestingly it often coincides with them starting to become more confident in their ability to undertake a more holistic role that is not purely limited to routine tasks (Missen et al., 2014).

For a profession that prides itself on 'caring' for patients, it is disappointing that bullying, victimisation and undermining by other staff has been found to be a common experience for new graduate nurses. Even when bullying is not overt, lacking support structures can leave you feeling that you are not part of the nursing team (Duchscher, 2009). Methods to combat bullying are discussed in detail in Chapter 6.

Aside from the challenges of care provision and interacting with the health team, you will experience many other life-changing events. For example, adjusting to a rotating roster inclusive of night shifts can lead to physical and mental exhaustion, and invariably places strain on family relationships by altering living arrangements and household patterns.

EXPECTATIONS OF THE NEW GRADUATE, SCOPE OF PRACTICE AND ROLE BOUNDARIES

Historically, nurse employers have frequently complained that new graduates are inadequately prepared for clinical practice, with many institutions having an unrealistic expectation that a new graduate can 'hit the ground running' at the practice level of a seasoned RN (Phillips et al., 2014). Much research has focused on a theory–practice gap and inadequate university preparation of students, but interestingly this complaint also existed when nurses were trained exclusively within hospitals (Haddad et al., 2013). The take-home message for you as a graduate is that no matter what the profession or training system may be, everyone faces a steep learning curve on entry to their chosen career.

When institutions, other staff and new graduates themselves have unrealistic expectations about their ability to perform at a high level immediately on entering the workforce, stress invariably results. This has significant wider implications for the nursing profession, which already suffers from staff shortages, as new graduates who experience high levels of stress are more likely to have increased rates of sick leave, poor work satisfaction and an increased likelihood of leaving nursing altogether (Chang & Hancock, 2003).

The university undergraduate qualification prepares the student to a beginner level of practice. Australian universities base degree curricula on the Nursing and Midwifery Board of Australia (NMBA) National Competency Standards for Registered Nurses (discussed in Chapter 4). The NMBA considers the RN to be a professional capable of critical thinking, who is able to accurately assess patient needs to provide evidence-based, holistic and collaborative health management across a range of settings. With the award of registration, the new graduate nurse is considered to be safe and competent at a novice level (Haddad et al., 2013). Being new to the clinical environment, you cannot be expected to have knowledge and understanding of situations with which you are coming into contact for the first time. Employers must be mindful that new graduates are entering a period of intensive learning that requires dedicated support.

A rational starting point for novice-level clinical practice is being able to provide safe patient care. It is also desirable that during the first year of employment, you consolidate the knowledge and skill base acquired during your degree, adapt to the health workplace culture, and achieve a balance between work and personal demands. To achieve these expectations, employers are beginning to note the importance of finding new graduates who already possess generic skills such as communication, problem-solving and enthusiasm (Walker et al., 2013). Four key attributes that demonstrate your work readiness are:

1 *social intelligence:* the ability to communicate with a range of people, work in teams, manage interpersonal conflict, and seek support when needed
2 *organisational acumen:* having knowledge of the ward, hospital policy and procedures, together with maturity and a willingness to engage in ongoing professional development
3 *work competence:* having basic clinical skills for patient management supported by sufficient theoretical knowledge to understand the basis of your practice, experience commensurate with a beginning practitioner, the confidence to use and implement the knowledge you have gained and an awareness of its limitations, and willingness to be responsible for your treatment decisions
4 *personal characteristics:* resilience and flexibility to cope with changing workplace demands and challenges, and the ability to manage your own stress to maintain a healthy work–life balance (Walker et al., 2013).

Initially, you will most likely question the scope of practice within which you are permitted to work. Simply put, the extent of any nurse's scope of practice is determined by their education, training and competence (NMBA, 2010). As all nurses are accountable for their own actions, this means you must consider whether you have the required knowledge to complete the task safely prior to completing a specific action. If the answer to this question is 'no', then you should not undertake the activity until the appropriate education and supervision are acquired. The extent of the nurse's scope of practice is then influenced in the clinical setting by the organisational policies, quality and risk-management framework and requirements of their site of employment (NMBA, 2010). This means that in some cases, despite having an adequate knowledge set to complete a task safely, the local policy states that the nurse is not permitted to undertake the named activity, or that the education will not be provided for a given task until the nurse has met a certain development milestone. In most cases, this is designed to protect the new nurse from a more onerous workload until they are comfortably proficient with the basic nursing care of their patients. One example involves the procedure of intravenous cannulation. In some emergency departments, new graduate nurses are not permitted to cannulate until they have completed four months of their placement. This allows the new graduate to concentrate on core nursing duties prior to taking on extended roles that may also be completed by the treating doctor.

DEVELOPING PROFESSIONAL IDENTITY

It is important for you to develop a positive professional identity. Professional identity is linked to, yet different from, your overall self-concept as an individual (who you think you are). It is a sense of self that is acquired from the role and work that you complete as a nurse, and is influenced by interactions with others as well as your position in society (Cowin et al., 2013). Developing a professional identity requires you to successfully combine your own values and personal attributes with those of the nursing profession. A positive professional identity has been noted as being important for staff retention, job satisfaction and patient care, and is also linked to increased resilience regarding pressures in the nursing role and improved self-efficacy (Cowin et al., 2013; Johnson et al., 2012; Madsen et al., 2009; McAllister et al., 2009).

Professional identity in nursing has evolved over recent decades. In the mid-20th century, nurses viewed themselves primarily as doctors' assistants; however, nurses today see themselves as active participants in the direction and delivery of care (Johnson et al., 2012). Changes in professional identity will continue throughout a nurse's career in response to changes in professional life, such as exposure to new technology in the clinical setting, and role modification and expansion.

Professional identity is developed through a process of socialisation that starts in the community, with students holding pre-existing beliefs about the nursing profession. Interestingly, it is thought that people choose a profession that they feel matches their own values and self-perception (Cowin et al., 2013; Johnson et al., 2012). Since the 1980s, nurse education has moved into the tertiary sector. The requirement of a degree qualification has been instrumental in changing community perceptions of nursing and achieving recognition as a profession. It is also critical to professional identity, as it is via formal education that the nurse now becomes a professional (Johnson et al., 2012). During their undergraduate degree, the student acquires a refined understanding of what it means to be a nurse in the contemporary health environment, developing a sense of the values, practices and purposes of the professional nursing role. It has also been suggested that having a greater understanding of the history of the nursing profession—where it came from, the contribution nurses have made to Australian health and society, how nursing culture and practice has evolved, and subsequently how these factors affect modern-day nursing and the health system—is critical to the development of the nurse's professional identity (Madsen et al., 2009, McAllister et al., 2009).

On entering the workforce, you may find that the professional identity you developed at university is challenged when your expectations don't correspond with your experience of completing the actual job. Poor experiences during transition to the workforce contribute to the development of a negative professional identity, where the nurse feels unsatisfied with their role. Negative professional identity is associated—understandably—with higher rates of attrition (Madsen et al., 2009). Nurse educators and preceptors in the clinical environment play a prominent role in the creation of positive professional identities in new graduates. As a new graduate nurse, you can seek help from your nurse educator and **preceptor**. They can help you to gain a clear understanding of your new role and expectations of practice, and can provide examples of accurate application of theory to clinical practice—both of which may positively affect professional identity. Taking the opportunity to forge good working relationships with the staff involved in your orientation program can foster a sense of belonging and relationships that will contribute to the shaping of a positive professional image (Johnson et al., 2012; Willetts & Clarke, 2014).

> **preceptor** A nurse who provides support and guidance to the new graduate as they transition to a new clinical area.

STRATEGIES TO SUPPORT TRANSITION

The way in which you are socialised and supported on entry to the workforce has a significant influence on your future views, expectations, satisfaction and likelihood of remaining within the profession (Haddad et al., 2013; Phillips et al., 2014). With this in mind, most acute care settings across Australia have implemented transition programs for new graduate nurses; however, there is great variation between the structures of individual programs and the level of support provided. A functional transition program can provide you with a positive experience by fostering a sense of belonging, improved clinical confidence and increased job satisfaction (Missen et al., 2014). It can also provide you with an opportunity to replace the support available in the university setting with appropriate structures for ongoing development, collegial support and mentorship in the workplace (Duchscher, 2009).

When you take on your role in the clinical environment, ask for clear explanations from the manager and educator about their expectations of your practice. This can help to prevent any ambiguity between what you and other staff believe is your role as a new graduate nurse while you adjust to the workplace. An appropriate workload is also very important. During your orientation, clarify with your educator what they believe is an appropriate workload and patient complexity for a new graduate nurse's scope of practice. It is also worthwhile to seek strategies ahead of time regarding how the educator and manager would like you to notify them in the event that future patient loads fall outside these suggested parameters, so that the situation can be rectified simply or appropriate support provided.

New graduates have reported finding supportive senior nurse structures and the provision of constructive criticism to be very helpful in making the transition to professional practice (Duchscher, 2009; Dyess & Sherman, 2009). Constructive criticism involves noting a feature of your care delivery or interpretation of clinical findings that needs improvement or correction. Although it may be difficult to be told that, despite your best efforts, your work can be improved upon, being open to such criticism is important for you to grow as a clinician and continually improve your practice. While you must be receptive to constructive criticism, also take note of compliments for a job well done and own them. It is an important work and life skill to accept and celebrate small everyday wins.

Nurse educators and preceptors are there to help you to adjust to the work environment with as little stress as possible. They will do their best to assist you, and may ask whether there are specific ways in which you feel they can provide additional support to you during this transition phase. Some examples of support that new graduates have found useful include having approachable clinical teachers to whom questions can be asked without fear of ridicule; being encouraged towards 'best practice'; having senior support at hand if a clinical situation deteriorates or a new graduate needs to ask a question; provision of constructive feedback in a timely manner; being given reassurance when the graduate is doing well; and having the option to debrief after a challenging experience (Johnstone et al., 2008).

As you become proficient in managing your workload safely, you will likely be expected to embrace a slow graduation of clinical responsibility and practice autonomy, with increasing exposure to more advanced clinical complexity over time. Seek out frequent constructive feedback, and make time to share experiences with new graduate and senior colleagues. Open lines of communication with your educators and managers help them to identify gaps in knowledge and practice that they can assist you to fill, and allow them to match your developing skill and knowledge base with appropriate patients who will keep you challenged without compromising safety. Discussing your experiences with new graduate colleagues can be helpful to reassure you that you are not alone on this challenging journey, and that others are likely experiencing similar things to you.

As a new graduate, you are by no means a passive player during your transition to the workplace. Actively seeking learning opportunities and approaching the clinical environment and staff interactions with a positive outlook will improve your experience. Also acknowledge that you are entering a difficult period of adjustment with significant challenges on numerous fronts, as self-awareness and realistic expectations have been linked to improved overall coping (Duchscher, 2009). Investigate the transition programs offered by different institutions to find out what support will be provided.

The creation of a multifaceted support network during the first year of practice is extremely important. It can be very helpful to maintain contact with friends from university. As a group, you are likely to be experiencing similar situations that you can share, explore and offer each other mutual support to manage. While in the clinical environment, developing a mentor relationship can be extremely beneficial. The mentor may be a clinical educator, nurse unit manager or an experienced nurse (Duchscher, 2009; Pigott, 2001). Chapter 7 discusses in detail the advantages of having a mentor, how to identify an appropriate mentor, and how to establish a mentor–mentee relationship and subsequently gain the most benefit from the connection.

Try to incorporate exercise into your week. Clinical work can often leave you feeling drained by the end of a shift; however, emotional weariness does not always equate to physical tiredness. Exercise can function as an effective de-stressor for the mind and body, and can be useful as a circuit breaker to disengage from thoughts of work and make the most of time at home or with friends. Not all exercise has to be strenuous to achieve the same outcome. Choose something that suits your level of fitness or need at the time, whether it be a run, yoga or a social team sport. Sometimes simply taking the dog for a walk is effective for breaking a negative series of thoughts while getting some fresh air.

ADAPTING TO SHIFTWORK, SLEEP HYGIENE AND WORK–LIFE BALANCE

When you enter the workforce, you will probably encounter your first experience of a rotating roster inclusive of day and night shifts. While rotating shift rosters have significant impacts upon all nurses, the effects are undoubtedly more stressful for new graduates. Shiftwork can have negative effects on physiological and psychological health, including fatigue, increased risk of accidental injury, poor performance, increased stress, decreased wellbeing and a raft of health issues (Tremaine et al., 2011). Two of the key difficulties that you may experience when you begin shiftwork include disturbed sleep patterns and challenges in achieving a work–life balance.

Sleep hygiene

Nurses experiencing shift patterns inclusive of night shifts commonly achieve less than the recommended hours of sleep per day, with midwives in one study routinely sleeping an average of just 6 hours. This resulted in the midwives reporting that they felt moderately to very mentally and physically exhausted on up to 50 per cent of their shifts and days off (Tremaine et al., 2011). Disturbed sleep patterns also lead to an increased risk of accidents and illnesses, higher rates of stress and lower levels of wellbeing, contributing to a greater risk for feelings of isolation from family and friends who don't work the same hours. Unsurprisingly, poor sleep is cited as a common reason for new graduate nurses leaving the profession (Simmons, 2012; West et al., 2007).

You can improve the amount and quality of sleep that you get by targeting sleep hygiene. Sleep hygiene refers to a number of different practices that contribute to improved quality of sleep. Unfortunately, the most important sleep hygiene measure involves maintaining a regular sleep pattern, something that is impossible while working a rotating roster inclusive of night shifts. Try to establish a regular bedtime routine that can be completed irrespective of the time of day when you need to go to sleep—for example, have a shower then read for 20 minutes to wind down prior to going to bed. Leave your phone in a different room to charge and set a 'do not disturb' so that it won't wake you with calls or notifications. Utilise days off to regain a few hours of lost sleep.

Bonnet and Arand (2017) identify some tips that may improve sleep amount and quality:

- Avoid napping where possible.
- Avoid stimulants such as caffeine after lunch.
- Avoid alcohol close to sleep time. (Although it may help the onset of sleep, the latter half of your sleep will likely be disrupted as the body begins to metabolise the alcohol, leading to arousal.)
- Take regular exercise to facilitate improved sleep once you hit your bed.
- Make your bed a place you associate with sleep by not watching television, using electronic devices or listening to the radio in bed.
- Make your bedroom as conducive to sleep as possible. (Being able to block light while sleeping in the day is important. If your blinds aren't enough, consider the use of a mask and earplugs to prevent disturbance by sudden noises.)
- Resolve worries or other concerns before going to bed.

Work–life balance

Shiftwork can at times leave you feeling that there is an imbalance between the demands of the workplace and time with family. Maintaining a healthy work–life balance requires you to constantly re-evaluate how you are dividing your time between work and other activities that you value. A lack of time away from work can contribute to 'burnout', referring to a state of mental and physical exhaustion that can lead to the worker becoming dissatisfied with and disconnected from work. Home life also has its own challenges, and may include relationship problems, monetary pressures, daily chores and children's activities. Achieving a work–life balance means bringing work and leisure time into balance in such a way that physical, emotional and mental health are maintained (Simmons, 2012).

As a profession, nursing has promoted a holistic approach to health for our patients. It is just as important for nurses to take similar actions to promote and take responsibility for their own wellbeing, satisfaction and happiness. Achieving a work–life balance requires a degree of self-awareness. Within the work arena, identify what it is about your job that you like and focus upon positive aspects that you find fulfilling or satisfying (Westwood, 2010). Examine what you do outside work. What things do you value and enjoy doing? Try not to equate leisure time with tuning out in front of the television, as enjoyment of leisure activities is improved when we are engaged and challenged in ways that stimulate our brain (Simmons, 2012). This may be spending time with family or friends, exercise or hobbies. Forward planning is often required to ensure that you make time for positive experiences outside of work that contribute to a balanced life.

Some suggestions for maintaining a healthy balance between work and life include:

- Work:
  - It is necessary, so make the most of it. Take pride in a job well done, focus on what you like about nursing.
  - Avoid complaining, find solutions and generate positive rather than negative energy.
  - Say 'no' when you can.
  - Leave work at work.
- Home:
  - Plan your week, using calendars and to-do lists.
  - Decrease pressure on yourself for non-essential chores such as errands and cleaning, or delegate to other family members.
  - Consider whether your children have too many extra-curricular activities.
  - Identify activities that ensure you have contact time with family and friends (Lewis, 2011).
- Self:
  - Focus on a healthy diet.
  - Improve sleep hygiene.
  - Incorporate exercise into a daily routine.
  - Take up a hobby.
  - During relaxation periods, spend time with friends or family.
  - Pursue development activities that will lead to opportunities in your desired career path (Simmons, 2012).
  - Plan holiday leave and, if possible, space regular leave throughout the year to give yourself something to look forward to, and time to recover (Lewis, 2011).

MANAGING PERSONAL STRESS

One of the leading causes of staff dissatisfaction is stress. Common stressors within the workplace for nurses include workload, interpersonal relationships, failure to meet self-expectations or the patient's needs, having minimal clinical experience, and taking on new roles and responsibilities (Billingsley et al., 2007; Hurley, 2007). Ongoing stress that is poorly managed has been linked to illness, decreased productivity, burnout and attrition, and increased sick leave (Harris, 2001; Woodrow, 2005).

Stress can be defined as the emotional and physical response experienced when an imbalance is perceived between demands placed on you and your ability to meet these demands at a time when coping is important (Brunero et al., 2006). Stress manifests in identifiable signs and symptoms, from minor symptoms such as altered sleep patterns through to life-threatening events like acute myocardial infarction. Ongoing stress may lead to a variety of illnesses such as depression, hypertension and anxiety (Harris, 2001). It is vital that you learn to identify your own signs and symptoms of stress prior to them harming health and wellbeing. Signs and symptoms of stress include:

- hypertension and tachycardia
- altered sleep patterns and pervasive tiredness
- shallow, rapid respirations
- muscular tension
- changes to appetite (loss of appetite, over-eating)
- dry mouth
- excessive sweating
- nausea
- greater use of alcohol and/or other drugs
- anxiety
- decreased ability to concentrate upon a task
- poor memory
- changes to mood: increased irritability and impatience, moodiness, feeling sad or upset
- feelings of helplessness in the face of even minor problems (Brunero et al., 2006).

Multiple avenues can be pursued to decrease your overall stress in the workplace. A beginning point is to tackle stressors that it is in your power to improve. For example, management of workload is a common challenge for new graduate nurses, so improving time management, and learning to prioritise and cope with competing demands, will help to minimise this stressor. Outside of work, improving sleep hygiene, healthy eating and physical exercise may improve your ability to cope with stressors in the clinical environment, while exercises such as deep breathing, muscle relaxation and stretching can be useful to help you unwind and relax (Billingsley et al., 2007).

Cognitive-behavioural interventions are another effective method for you to decrease stress. This technique aims to improve emotional self-management to help you change the things that are in your power to change, and accept those that you cannot. Cognitive-behavioural interventions target the thinking process, and seek to alter emotions and behaviours through changing the way an individual thinks about or views a situation. By altering thoughts that lead to negative feelings, the person can change the way they feel or perceive that situation (Brunero et al., 2006).

Negative thought patterns can increase stress and impact emotions. The first step to preventing negative thoughts from leading to a stress reaction is to identify these errors in thinking. Once damaging thought patterns have been identified, the automatic negative thought can be challenged and replaced with a realistic and rational option (Brunero et al., 2006).

Examples of negative thought patterns include:

- *Black and white thinking:* viewing situations in extremes—for example, success or failure.
- *Filtering:* positives are ignored with a focus only on the negatives.
- *Personalising:* automatically jumping to an incorrect conclusion that an occurrence is related to you—for example, 'They're laughing about me.'
- *Fortune-telling:* predicting the future in a negative light—for example, 'This will be another difficult shift.'
- *Mind-reading:* jumping to negative conclusions or making a guess about what someone else is thinking—for example, 'I didn't get picked for in-service because the educator doesn't like me' (Brunero et al., 2006).

Problem-focused and emotion-focused coping have been suggested as two strategies to manage stress. Problem-based coping involves doing something constructive about the event that is found to be difficult, such as framing the incident as a learning opportunity and seeking information. Emotion-focused coping involves attempting to decrease the negative emotional responses associated with stress, such as fear, embarrassment, anxiety and frustration, through strategies such as seeking company and debriefing (Pigott, 2001).

Most organisations have Employee Assistance Programs (EAP) that staff can access to help with stress or other issues that they feel are starting to affect their work and personal life. EAP is a work-based professional and confidential service for staff, to assist you to identify and resolve personal, health or work-related issues (Brunero et al., 2006).

Summary

In this chapter, we have looked at the challenges facing new graduate nurses as they enter the profession. We have noted that a Bachelor of Nursing degree prepares the new graduate to enter the workforce at a beginner level of practice, and that new graduate nurses will require support in their professional role to adjust and further their development. We saw that generic skills such as effective communication, problem-solving ability, self-awareness and enthusiasm can indicate a new graduate nurse's work readiness. We discussed the importance of developing a professional identity to improve your job satisfaction, patient care and resilience to pressure in your new role. We looked at strategies to support transition, including supportive senior nurse structures and constructive criticism. Finally, we examined adapting to challenges such as shiftwork, sleep deprivation and stress, and the importance of self-care.

Review questions

1.1   'Reality shock' refers to finding discrepancies between what you understood about nursing and your real-life experience of it in the clinical environment. True or false?

1.2   Challenges faced on starting work may include:
   a   Time management
   b   Adjusting to a new workplace culture
   c   Developing functional communication patterns
   d   All of the above

1.3   What is a rational expectation of practice for a new graduate nurse?
   a   That they hit the ground running, functioning at the same level of practice as a seasoned nurse
   b   That they need direct supervision during all nursing activities during the first three months
   c   That they are able to provide safe patient care

1.4   Key attributes that demonstrate work readiness include:
   a   Social intelligence
   b   Healthy social life

    c Organisational acumen
    d Basic clinical skills supported by a theoretical knowledge base
    e Resilience and flexibility

1.5   Constructive criticism is an example of bullying in the workplace. True or false?

1.6   Who should you seek to include within a multifaceted support network during your first year of practice?

1.7   What is a professional identity?

1.8   What are some useful strategies to improve sleep quality?
    a Avoid stimulants near bedtime
    b Have a small measure of alcohol to help fall asleep
    c Sleeping pills
    d Regular exercise
    e Establish a regular bedtime routine

1.9   Common stressors in the workplace include:
    a Workload
    b Interpersonal relationships
    c Your own expectations of performance
    d Taking on new roles and responsibilities.
    e All the above

2 THE AUSTRALIAN HEALTHCARE SYSTEM

Alister Hodge

> **In this chapter, you will develop an understanding of:**
>
> - the mixture of public and private services in the Australian healthcare system
> - the role of Medicare, the Medicare Benefits Schedule (MBS) and the Pharmaceutical Benefits Scheme (PBS)
> - the role of federal, state and local governments in health funding and delivery
> - the impact of politics on the formulation of health policy
> - the influence of the nursing profession on health policy
> - contemporary factors impacting professional nursing practice and care delivery.

PUBLIC HEALTHCARE

Australia has a combination of public and private services that work together to deliver healthcare, and is classified as a welfare-orientated healthcare system, similar to those of countries such as Germany, the United Kingdom and Canada (Gray, 2006). Welfare states tend to have governments that provide healthcare insurance for the vast majority of the population; however, they also commonly have a private sector contributing to healthcare for those who are able to pay (Gray, 2006).

The responsibility for public healthcare is spread across federal, state and local tiers of government, but the states hold the primary role of provision. The public healthcare system is supported by Medicare, which is a form of Commonwealth

Government-sponsored health insurance that funds hospitals and doctors. Medicare enables access to high-quality healthcare services for all Australian citizens, which are often free at the point of access.

Due to Medicare, all Australian citizens are able to access free comprehensive healthcare within public hospitals. Since 1984, the Commonwealth Government has committed to five-year agreements with each state to enable the Commonwealth to fund hospital services. The Commonwealth Government provides a capped contribution to the states to deliver hospital services, with the states left responsible for any increase in hospital budgets during the period of the agreement. State governments remain the main funders of public hospitals, and currently contribute 60 per cent of total expenditure. Public hospitals account for 66 per cent of hospital beds, are operated by the state or territory government and are supervised by hospital boards appointed by government or local health authorities. The public hospitals include psychiatric and specialised facilities as well as acute general hospitals (Duckett & Willcox, 2015).

In the community setting, Medicare undertakes a direct funding role in relation to consultations provided by a medical practitioner. Doctors are able to bill Medicare directly for the episode of care, a practice known as 'bulk billing'. Under 'bulk billing', the doctor accepts the Medicare rebate (payment) as full settlement of the account. The doctor can alternatively bill the patient for the consultation, with no upward limit of fees charged. It is then the patient's responsibility to subsequently obtain a rebate from Medicare for a percentage of the schedule fee. The difference between the Medicare rebate and the doctor's fee is termed a 'gap payment', and is paid by the patient.

For the majority of GP consultations, the Medicare rebate is 100 per cent of the Medicare Benefits Schedule (MBS) fee; however, for medical specialist services provided outside a hospital, the rebate is 85 per cent of the schedule fee. Nurse Practitioners working in private practice are also able to provide MBS services and bill Medicare for the treatment provided. The benefit payable for services provided by a Nurse Practitioner is 85 per cent of the schedule fee. If an individual or family requires multiple health services, their monetary outlay on health expenses may be high despite the Medicare benefit. Due to this, a Medicare Safety Net threshold exists. This means that once a threshold is reached—that is, gap payments exceed $430.90 in a calendar year—the Medicare benefit will be increased to 100 per cent of the schedule fee (Duckett & Willcox, 2015).

Medicare is made up of the MBS, the Pharmaceutical Benefits Scheme (PBS) and the National Health and Hospitals Network Agreement. The MBS pays for consultations by doctors and a number of procedures and tests, such as diagnostic imaging and pathology; the PBS provides subsidised medicines and the National Health and Hospitals Network Agreement outlines the funding of public hospitals between federal and state governments (COAG, 2010).

The PBS enables access to reasonably priced medicines for most treated medical conditions in Australia through subsidies to over 770 different medications (Duckett & Willcox, 2015). Patients within a concessional category, such as pensioners or war veterans, pay a smaller percentage of the medication cost compared with other members of the community, with the PBS paying the balance (Department of Health, 2013a).

PRIVATE HEALTHCARE

Approximately one-third of all Australian hospital beds are located in the private sector. Private hospitals are divided between 'not-for-profit' organisations such as religious orders, and the 'for-profit' sector of business. Private hospitals have expanded rapidly over the last three decades, with an increase of 15 per cent in the number of private hospitals between 1993 and 2000 (Gray, 2006). Private hospitals have largely specialised in elective surgery, while emergency services are delivered primarily by the public health system (Duckett, 2005).

Despite Medicare, it could be argued that the Australian healthcare system lies more at the private end of the international spectrum for health service provision. Over the last 30 years, a trend towards increased private provision of care and a shift of the funding burden back to the individual has occurred. Private health insurance was championed as an adjunct to the Medicare system by the Liberal–National (LNP) Coalition government led by John Howard between 1996 and 2007 (Gray, 2006), with approximately 43 per cent of all Australians having private health insurance by 2004 (Duckett, 2005). The government employed a number of 'carrot and stick' strategies to increase uptake of private health insurance by those people who normally would not have sought an insurance policy. In 1996, the LNP Coalition government introduced the Private Health Insurance (PHI) rebate as an incentive, meaning that for any private health insurance package bought, the government would pay 30 per cent of the total cost. On the other side, a Medicare Levy Surcharge (MLS) was established, compelling high income-earning citizens without private health insurance to pay an additional 1–1.5 per cent levy each financial year (Duckett, 2005). Lifetime Health Cover (LHC) is another government strategy to encourage young people to take out and maintain insurance cover. Under LHC, those who do not have health insurance by the age of 30 must pay an additional 2 per cent loading for every year aged above 30 that they did not have insurance (Private Health Insurance Ombudsman, 2017a). For example, under the LHC system, if you took out private health insurance for the first time at age 45, you would pay 30 per cent more than a person who took out health insurance at the age of 30.

The government has imposed some regulations upon the insurance industry to improve equity of access to private health insurance. Insurance companies have to charge everyone the same amount for the same premium, regardless of current health status or claim history. This system is called community rating, and aims to stop the chronically ill and elderly from being priced out of private health insurance (Private Health Insurance Ombudsman, 2017b). Community rating depends on healthy people buying insurance, thus subsidising people with active health complaints who are likely to claim more often. Uptake of insurance by those less likely to benefit from the outlay in cost is achieved by the previously discussed PHI rebate, MLS and LHC strategies.

NON-GOVERNMENT ORGANISATIONS

Non-Government Organisations (NGOs) play a significant role in health provision in the public and private health systems of Australia. NGOs are voluntarily formed organisations that are independent from the government, provide not-for-profit services and chiefly aim to better the circumstances of 'at need' populations (Ball & Dunn, 1995). NGOs frequently provide services considered non-viable for delivery by government or the for-profit sector (Cancer Council NSW, 2013). Due to their independence, they have at times been able to drive for change in government policy by advocating for issues that would not otherwise have been on a government's political agenda (Cancer Council NSW, 2013).

Examples of NGOs involved with Australian health service provision or research include:

- the Australian Red Cross Blood Service, which is funded by the federal and state governments to supply blood products within the public and private sector (Australian Red Cross, 2017)
- the National Aboriginal Community Controlled Health Organisation (NACCHO), which represents 142 Aboriginal Community Controlled Health Services throughout the nation on Aboriginal health issues (NACCHO, 2017)
- the Cancer Council, which targets cancer through research while providing patient support services and information (Cancer Council NSW, 2013)

- Headspace, the national youth mental health intiative, which provides early intervention mental health services for young persons between the ages of 12 and 25, and focuses on mental and physical health, alcohol and other drug services, and work and study support (Headspace, 2017).

COMMONWEALTH AND STATE ROLES: FUNDING AND RESPONSIBILITY FOR SERVICE

Health expenditure in Australia currently accounts for 9.7 per cent of Gross Domestic Product (GDP) (AIHW, 2014a). The funding of Medicare comes from a mix of taxation measures. Australians pay a 1.5–2 per cent Medicare levy on their income, although low-income thresholds exist below which people are excluded from paying a levy (Duckett & Willcox, 2015). People who do not hold private health insurance and earn over a defined threshold are required to pay an additional MLS of between 1 and 1.5 per cent of their income (Duckett, 2005). The remainder of Medicare funding comes from a range of taxes, such as income tax, goods and services tax (GST) and non-tax revenue.

The allocation of funding to hospitals has changed over the years. Australian public hospitals used to receive money under a funding model called 'cost-based funding'. Under this arrangement, the hospital is funded upon what it spent the previous year. Cost-based funding was criticised for failing to motivate and provide incentives for improvement in outputs of care, and over time has led to money being funnelled into metropolitan centres, contributing to a poor match between the needs of the rural population and available health resources. It also provided incentives for the hospital to spend money just to assure the following year's revenue (Eager, 2001).

Recently, there has been a move towards output-based funding. 'Outputs' or 'products' of the health system are typically patient care episodes for the treatment of a disease or injury. Episodes of care are given a Diagnosis Related Group (DRG) classification that determines the amount of money provided by the government. The DRG system classifies thousands of different diseases into a set number of DRGs, for which the cost of treatment tends to be similar. Case-mix refers to the varying types of DRGs, or 'mix' of patients managed by the hospital. Output-based funding has become known as case-mix funding, where the hospital is funded the same amount for each episode of care assigned to a particular DRG. Case-mix is created on the premise that the outputs of the system can be quantified and costed, and that each provider should be given the same amount of money to complete the same task. Case-mix funding aims to promote productive and technical efficiency by rewarding increased output and decreased costs.

POLITICS AND HEALTHCARE POLICY

Since the 1940s, healthcare policy has been a key topic debated between Australia's political parties. The main drivers for the ongoing disagreement are differing political ideology and conflicting stakeholder interests. Broadly, the main stakeholders include:

- consumers, who want to access high-quality health services at fair prices
- providers, who seek to maximise profits and wages
- governments, which want to maintain close control of expended monies (Gray, 1998).

Arguably, the greatest impact upon health policy over the past half-century has come from the Liberal–National Party (LNP) Coalition and the Australian Labor Party while forming government. Historically, the Coalition has pursued a liberal individualist view that calls for minimal government involvement in healthcare policy, and supports a major role for private medicine and private insurance in providing healthcare to the public (Palmer & Short, 2007). This is in direct opposition to the Labor Party, which advocates for a stronger government role in providing public healthcare, maintaining that in order to achieve equity in health-care access for all citizens regardless of socio-economic status, healthcare should be publicly financed (Gray, 1998). The ideological clash over healthcare delivery has resulted in an oscillation between public and private insurance systems that is unique among fellow OECD member countries. Of the smaller Australian political parties, The Australian Greens support a government role in ensuring universal access to health and dental care through a publicly funded health insurance system, funded from progressive taxation. In recent elections, some of the minor parties have enjoyed greater success, meaning their influence upon health policy debate may likewise increase in future years—especially within the Senate, where parties such as the Nick Xenophon Team (NXT), The Greens and Pauline Hanson's One Nation currently hold the balance of power.

The federal government first became involved with public healthcare in 1946 when the Chifley Labor government implemented a national pre-paid hospital system. Attempts at establishing a national health service were quashed by an uncompliant medical profession. The subsequent Menzies LNP Coalition government dismantled the prepaid hospital scheme, introducing subsidised private health insurance in the 1950s. The LNP Coalition insurance scheme encountered heavy criticism due to poor coverage, high patient charges and overall expense. In response, the 1975 Whitlam Labor government established a national health insurance scheme called Medibank. However, the subsequent Fraser Coalition government dismantled it and re-implemented a voluntary health insurance system. In 1983, the next Labor government, led by Bob Hawke, reinstated a national health insurance scheme under the title of Medicare (Gray, 1998).

Medicare is a 'redistributive policy' for health, whereby the cost of the universal health insurance is paid for by the greater community through taxation, to enable equity of access to health resources for all citizens. This means that people with scant monetary resources to pay for healthcare, such as the unemployed or low-income earners, are subsidised by citizens with higher wages. This type of redistributive policy is ideologically opposed by the LNP Coalition, which favours individualist principles that families should strive to be responsible for their own welfare (Palmer & Short, 2007).

Over the following 12 years, Medicare became accepted and trusted by the public, and LNP Coalition policies for the dismantling of the scheme were firmly rejected by the electorate in the 1993 elections. Although the Howard Coalition government elected in 1996 promised to maintain Medicare, since this time gradual erosion of the scheme has occurred, commencing with the abolition of the Commonwealth dental program (Gray, 1998). Further policy shifts towards greater involvement of the private sector in providing public health services have recently been flagged by the Coalition, encouraging the state governments to open up the delivery of health to the private sector (Australian Politics, 2015).

THE INFLUENCE OF THE NURSING PROFESSION ON HEALTH POLICY

Historically, nurses have had little input into state and national health policy. The reasons for this are multifactorial, including a lack of engagement by government during policy formation, and the expertise and knowledge of nurses not being valued or sought for consultation by policymakers (Lane & Cheek, 1997). Numerous theories abound regarding why nurses have had little influence in the policy arena, including:

- oppression/subordination as a profession
- absence of an identifiable leadership direction

- minimal experience in politics and policy creation
- failure of social scientists and economists to incorporate nurses in analysis during examination of the health workforce (Lane & Cheek, 1997).

Nursing's experience is in direct contrast to that of the medical profession, which arguably has the most powerful voice in the area of health and politics in Australia. Historically, medicine has enjoyed significant influence around health policy for multiple reasons. These include its knowledge base, maintenance of an apex placement in the hierarchy of the health professions, and community acceptance as an authority on health and illness (Lewis, 2005).

For the nursing profession to maintain professional autonomy, and some control over the direction of the profession and the role it performs in the changing health system, it needs to be equipped and willing to challenge the public health policy agenda that has often ignored issues directly impacting nursing practice. Not only is this important for the profession as a whole; it is also vital for the public that utilises healthcare services (Lane & Cheek, 1997).

The nursing profession can gain influence upon governmental health policy through nurse leader positions within the government structure and by the lobbying of professional nursing groups, unions and colleges. The role of 'chief nurse' now exists at both the state and federal levels, although it is relatively new at the federal level, being created for the first time in 2008. At both the state and federal levels, the chief nurse is a strong voice for the nursing workforce during policy development, acting as an adviser to the Minister for Health and the Department of Health and Ageing regarding a broad spectrum of nursing and midwifery issues (Keast, 2015).

The Australian Nursing and Midwifery Federation (ANMF) is the peak nursing union representing nurses' and midwives' interests to advance the political, professional and industrial standing of its members. There are various sub-branches of the ANMF at the state and territory levels. The ANMF is strongly in support of public provision of healthcare, as well as mechanisms to ensure equity of access to care through Medicare (ANMF, 2015).

The Australian College of Nursing (ACN) is a national professional nursing organisation that advocates for the nursing profession during policy development throughout the healthcare system as well as at state and federal levels of government (ACN, 2015). There are also numerous specialty colleges that represent the interests of their members at different levels of government. Examples include the College of Emergency Nursing, the Australian College of Critical Care Nurses and the Australian College of Mental Health Nurses.

CONTEMPORARY FACTORS IMPACTING ON PROFESSIONAL NURSING PRACTICE AND CARE DELIVERY

As a new graduate nurse entering the workforce, you have the potential for a varied and rewarding career in health. However, it must be acknowledged that today's nurses will also face some significant challenges as a result of changing community health needs and the resources available. These challenges include an ageing workforce, difficulties in recruiting new nurses, building a culture of lifelong learning to enable evidence-based practice (EBP), changing models of care in the clinical environment, unsafe workloads, increasing use of technology, and violence and bullying in the workplace (Jackson & Daly, 2004).

Over the past two decades, nursing practice has become increasingly complex and specialised, with more patient acuity in all sectors, coupled with new technology in a rapidly changing health environment. The increase in complexity reflects Australia's ageing population, with its growing chronic health issues, and places commensurate demands on the healthcare system and nurses who are coming in contact with higher numbers of acutely ill patients, an increased volume of hospital admissions and shorter lengths of stay (Haddad et al., 2013; Health Workforce Australia, 2013).

Australia's growing healthcare needs mean more nurses will be needed in the future, with Health Workforce Australia predicting a possible shortage of nurses by a staggering 110,000 by the year 2025 (Davidson et al., 2006; Haddad et al., 2013). Nurse shortages are even more evident in rural locations, where the local populations already experience inequity of health access compared with people in metropolitan settings. Unfortunately, the number of nurses in rural and remote locations in Australia has fallen, and of those remaining, fewer nurses hold midwifery or child health qualifications (Lenthall et al., 2011). Rectifying this situation is crucial to ensure that Australians living in these areas are able to access adequate health resources, and is also important to achieve the aims of the 'closing the gap' policy for Indigenous Australians living in rural and remote areas.

To meet the projected nursing shortfall, the federal government has increased funding for undergraduate RN education in all states. As such, larger numbers of new graduate nurses will become available. These new nurses require a broad theoretical knowledge base coupled with proficient clinical skills to enable them to deliver patient-centred care. The academic preparation of Australian students is of high quality; however, tertiary providers have reported difficulty in gaining appropriate placements for their students in many cases (Haddad et al., 2013).

This underlines the importance of achieving more meaningful clinical placements for student nurses to gain maximum advantage from these learning opportunities.

The support of graduates on leaving university provides a challenge for the healthcare system, to bridge the transition to practice in a way that not only enables the new graduate to provide high-quality care from the outset, but also increases the likelihood of retaining the nurse in the health system in the long term (Haddad et al., 2013).

Once new graduate nurses have successfully traversed the bridge to clinical practice, they will find that their learning journey has only just begun. The use of information technology (IT) in healthcare continues to escalate rapidly, with electronic documentation, internet, tele-health and bedside technology an everyday reality for RNs. State and federal governments support the increased use of IT to improve healthcare and, as frontline workers, nurses are at the forefront of use and interaction with a multitude of new technologies. Although increased usage of technology can provide benefits such as improved efficiency, safety and communication, some feel that the use of technology can impact the patient–carer relationship, and detract from the human component of nursing (Eley et al., 2009).

A culture of lifelong learning and professional development is now required of the RN in Australia, and is essential to allow nursing roles to continually evolve to meet the changing needs of the health environment. Nurses are taking on more diverse roles to meet the needs of patients within the acute and community settings, and will continue to do so. Nursing has recently begun to assume its rightful role at the table in health policy development at the state and federal levels. If the profession is to continue to have an active say about the future contribution of nurses, there is also a need for early identification and nurturing of future nurse leaders (Health Workforce Australia, 2013; Jackson & Daly, 2004).

Summary

This chapter has outlined the nature of the Australian healthcare system. We have noted that the system is based on a combination of public healthcare and private health insurance, and is classified as a welfare-orientated healthcare system. We have seen that public healthcare is provided at the federal, state and local government levels, but that states have primary responsibility for the provision of healthcare in public hospitals. We have discussed the role played by politics in the development of public healthcare schemes such as Medicare. We have also considered the contemporary challenges faced by nurses as a result of changing community health needs and the resources available.

Review questions

2.1   Australia has a mix of private and public healthcare provision. True or false?

2.2   Of the three levels of government, which retains the primary role of provision of healthcare?
   a   Federal
   b   State
   c   Local

2.3   To what does 'gap' payment refer?
   a   The cost the insurance company pays
   b   The remaining payment not covered by Medicare during a medical consultation that is usually paid by the patient
   c   Payment made to access private healthcare

2.4   What is Medicare?
   a   A form of government-sponsored health insurance
   b   A useful initiative launched by the Howard Liberal government in the early 1990s
   c   Provides access to healthcare for all

2.5   Medicare provides access for all Australian citizens, as well as citizens of countries with reciprocal healthcare agreements, to healthcare that is often free at the point of access. True or false?

2.6   All users must make a payment to access emergency care within the public hospital system. True or false?

2.7   What is the role of the Pharmaceutical Benefits Scheme?
    a   To enable access to reasonably priced medicines for the most treated medical conditions in Australia
    b   To license medication utilisation within the states
    c   To regulate prescribers of medications within Australia

2.8   The private hospital system accounts for approximately one-third of the hospital beds in Australia. True or false?

2.9   The private sector provides an equal delivery of emergency and mental health treatment as the public system. True or false?

2.10   Nurses form the largest percentage of the health workforce in Australia. True or false?

2.11   How is Medicare funded?
    a   1.5 per cent taxable income levy on all Australians
    b   GST revenue
    c   Income tax
    d   All of the above

2.12   How are hospitals commonly funded?
    a   Cost-based funding
    b   Case-mix or output-based funding

3 THE HEALTH WORKFORCE

Alister Hodge and Wayne Varndell

In this chapter, you will develop an understanding of:

- primary healthcare, secondary care and local hospital networks
- nursing and medical roles
- other common health roles
- advanced practice in nursing.

The health workforce in Australia is large, with registered health practitioners numbering nearly 660,000 people in 2016 (APHRA, 2016). Within this group, the largest percentage of the workforce comprises RNs (53%), with the next largest group being medical practitioners (16%) (APHRA, 2016).

HEALTHCARE DELIVERY: ORGANISATION AND STRUCTURES

Primary healthcare

Primary healthcare generally is the first point of contact for a patient entering the health system. It is usually delivered outside hospitals, and is provided most commonly by a general practitioner (GP); however, other primary care providers include Nurse Practitioners, dentists, RNs, Indigenous Health Workers, pharmacists and allied health professionals. Primary healthcare providers may be accessed through general practices, community health centres and other private practices, and through local government or non-government service settings such as Aboriginal Community Controlled Health Services.

Primary healthcare provides treatment for acute episodes of illness in the community and, where necessary, acts as a gateway to the wider health system, referring patients to specialists, hospitals and other primary care services for optimal patient management. Other activities performed in the primary healthcare setting include health promotion, prevention of unnecessary hospital admissions, early interventions and management of chronic illness (AIHW, 2014b). This is achieved by targeting key health and lifestyle conditions such as drug and alcohol services, oral health, sexual health, cardiovascular disease, asthma and diabetes. A high-functioning primary health service is desirable as strong primary health systems are associated with lower rates of hospital admission, greater efficiency, improved health outcomes and fewer health inequalities in the community (Standing Council on Health, 2013).

Primary Health Networks (PHNs) with general practice at the centre of the model were implemented in July 2015 to replace Medicare Locals as a means to fund and plan extra primary health services in communities across the country (AIHW, 2014a; Dutton, 2014). The implementation of PHNs was in response to a Coalition government-commissioned review of Medicare Locals. The PHNs have been altered to align more closely with existing state health networks in an attempt to reduce duplication and fragmentation of care, and reinforce general practice as the cornerstone of primary healthcare (AIHW, 2014a; Dutton, 2014; Horvath, 2014).

Secondary care

Secondary care is provided by a facility or specialist after referral by a primary health clinician (AIHW, 2014a). Acute care services are a branch of secondary care provided most commonly in a hospital. They deliver short-term care for serious episodes of illness or trauma that cannot be managed safely in the community (Merriam-Webster, 2007).

Local Hospital Networks

The establishment of Local Hospital Networks (LHNs) across the country is underway as a strategy to optimise delivery, coordination and access to secondary health services. LHNs consist of small groups of hospitals or a single hospital in an area, and link services within a region or through specialist networks across a territory or state (AIHW, 2014a). This ensures accepted referral patterns to access specialist services that may be only provided at a limited range of sites.

LHNs have also sought to devolve accountability for public hospital management and local service delivery to the local level. LHNs aim to provide a transparent approach to funding of public hospitals that is consistent nationwide, and also aim to improve engagement with local clinicians and the community to incorporate their views on quality and safety of care, and the day-to-day operation of hospitals (Department of Health and Human Services Tasmania, 2010). Some states use different terms for the LHN—for example, in New South Wales, LHNs are known as 'Local Health Districts'; in Queensland they are termed 'Hospital and Health Services'; in Tasmania they are called 'Tasmanian Health Organisations'; and in South Australia they are known as 'Local Health Networks'.

NURSING ROLES

Across the states and territories, the naming conventions, role descriptions and functions of nurse employment differ. Below is a summary of the main nursing roles and titles you may encounter. Each role provides care to patients in a number of ways.

Assistants in Nursing

Assistants in Nursing (AIN) are a much-valued part of the nursing workforce, and have played a role in the healthcare system for many years. Numerous terms are used among the states for AIN-type roles, which include Personal Care Assistant (PCA) and Nurse's Aide. Historically, AINs were located mainly within aged care facilities, as the necessary qualifications at the time were targeted towards aged care. However, there is now a national qualification, the Certificate III in Health Services Assistance, to train AINs for employment in the acute care setting. The AIN provides direct care to patients in accordance with the nursing care plan and under the supervision of an RN. Activities that the AIN may be allocated by the RN include showering, washing, mouth care, assistance with toileting, assistance with positioning, set-up and assistance with meals and fluids for low-risk patients, and application of anti-thrombotic stockings.

Enrolled Nurse

An Enrolled Nurse (EN) has completed a Certificate IV or Diploma of Nursing (Enrolled Nurse) and provides nursing care under the direction and supervision of an RN as part of the healthcare team. Although the scope of practice for an EN will vary with clinical setting and education, similar to RNs, ENs are responsible for maintaining their own professional development in order to maintain currency of essential knowledge, skills and attitudes to deliver safe, high-quality patient care (NMBA, 2016a). The scope of practice of an EN ranges from providing physical and emotional support to more complex activities such as wound care and administration of medication. The administration of medication by an EN requires further tertiary education and workplace assessment, as outlined within local policy. ENs who have completed the required NMBA units of study for administration of medication, but have not completed the additional required units of study for administration of intravenous medication, can administer medications by all routes except intravenously. However, ENs who have not completed intravenous medication education cannot check any intravenous medication including intravenous fluids (NMBA, 2016b).

The scope of practice of an EN will vary, but will be designed to support their workplace's requirements, such as:

vital signs Refers to clinical measurements that reflect the essential body functions; includes body temperature (T), heart rate (HR), respiratory rate (RR), peripheral oxygen saturation (SpO$_2$), blood pressure (BP) and pain.

- performing measurements and observations—for example, **vital signs**, urine testing, respiratory function tests and acquiring an electrocardiogram (ECG)
- performing treatments requested by a doctor or RN, such as wound care
- preparing for procedures—for example, pap smear, suturing and application of plaster casts
- administering medications once additional education has successfully been completed
- assisting patients with meals, showering, drinking and other essential nursing care.

Registered Nurse

An RN is registered and licensed under the appropriate *Nursing Act* to practise in Australia. Since 1992, education preparation for RNs has entered the tertiary sector, with RNs being required to complete a Bachelor of Nursing. Compared with an AIN or EN, an RN has greater autonomy, independence, accountability and responsibility, and undertakes a variety of highly specialised and complex roles, in-depth patient assessments and extended practices (NMBA, 2018a). RNs utilise evidence-based knowledge and complex nursing judgement to comprehensively assess and prioritise healthcare needs, and to develop, implement and evaluate a plan of care. Furthermore, they are accountable for ensuring that their care, and the care provided by others, is responsible, consistent with evidence, ethical and supported by appropriate standards. RNs work in a variety of clinical and non-clinical settings, depending on their educational preparation and practice experience, ranging from management and administration to education, research, advisory, regulatory and policy-development roles.

Midwife

A midwife is a degree-qualified clinician who works in partnership with women to provide support during pregnancy, childbirth, care of the newborn, and matters of sexual and reproductive health. Midwives practise in a range of settings, including the woman's home, the hospital, birthing centres and community health clinics. Midwives are educated and skilled to detect variations from the normal progress of pregnancy, labour and the post-partum period, including deterioration of a newborn; they refer to and work collaboratively with obstetricians and other medical specialists when a pregnant woman requires care outside their scope of practice (NMBA, 2018b).

New graduate nurses

New graduate nurses, sometimes called 'new-grads' or more recently 'transition nurses', are newly qualified RNs who are undertaking a 12-month induction in clinical practice. Graduate programs aim to facilitate clinical experience and confidence, mature nursing skills and abilities, and foster professional development (Levett-Jones & Fitzgerald, 2005). New graduate nurses remain accountable for the care they deliver, and have the same entitlements as a seasoned RN insofar as their scope of practice enables them to function safely. The new graduate or transition programs are often made up of two or three ward placements to broaden the new graduate's exposure to different clinical practice settings.

Clinical Nurse Specialist/Clinical Nurse

A Clinical Nurse Specialist (CNS) is an RN who has completed post-registration qualifications specialising in their context of practice—for example, a postgraduate certificate in oncology—and who utilises this higher level of clinical knowledge and skills to deliver complex nursing care in that specialised area of practice. A CNS actively contributes to the improvement of clinical practice in their workplace, actively contributes to their own specialist knowledge, and provides mentorship and support to the healthcare team (NSW Government, 2011).

Clinical Coach

The role of Clinical Coach in nursing and midwifery has recently emerged to advance the learning of clinical teams at the point of care and develop a learning culture, using concepts drawn from coaching in sport (Faithfull-Byrne et al., 2017). The Clinical Coach role is designed to provide additional support to clinical and nurse educators to complement real-time clinical education at the point-of-care.

Clinical Nurse Educator

A Clinical Nurse Educator (CNE) is an RN who holds relevant clinical experience and education qualifications to develop, deliver and evaluate clinical education programs at the workplace level. The responsibilities include:

- delivering nursing education in the workplace
- contributing to the development of the nursing workforce
- acting as a preceptor and mentoring new staff
- providing educational and clinical support in the workplace
- providing support for skills development in clinical procedures
- contributing to clinical policy development.

Nurse Educator

A Nurse Educator (NE) is an RN who holds relevant post-registration nursing clinical or education qualifications and is responsible for the design, development and delivery of nursing education courses at the workplace level, and tertiary-level programs at the public hospital, or the community-based service level (Australian Nurse Teachers' Society, 2010). The NE's role differs from that of the CNE as their primary responsibility is to design and develop education programs and courses.

Nurse Researcher

A Nurse Researcher works in hospitals, clinics and research laboratories to conduct or assist in research into nursing, healthcare delivery or specific health issues. A Nurse Researcher needs a wide range of skills, including management and organisational skills, teaching and mentoring, communication and a thorough understanding of the research process and data analytics. They lead or assist in designing and conducting research, undertake data collection and analysis, and publish results that ultimately inform evidence-based practice, patient outcomes, healthcare policy and delivery.

Clinical Nurse Consultant

A Clinical Nurse Consultant (CNC) is a role taken by an RN, often requiring masters level qualifications and three to seven years of full-time equivalent post-registration experience within a distinct specialty. The CNC provides clinical services and consultancy, leadership, research, specialist education and clinical services planning and management within that distinct specialty (Cashin et al., 2015).

Nurse Unit Manager

A Nurse Unit Manager (NUM) is an RN in charge of a ward, unit or group of wards in a public hospital or service. Responsibilities include coordination of patient services, nursing staff and ward management (e.g. implementation of hospital policies, rostering and allocation of staff).

Nurse Practitioner

Nurse Practitioners (NP) are advanced practice nurses who complete independent, autonomous assessment, diagnosis and management of patients within their care. The title 'Nurse Practitioner' is a protected title in Australia, and strict professional development and endorsement processes are enforced by Australian Health Practitioner Regulation Agency (AHPRA) (NMBA, 2014).

MEDICAL PRACTITIONERS

Interns/Junior Medical Officers

Across Australia, qualified medical practitioners are required to successfully undertake and complete at least one year of supervised practice, or internship. At this junior level, medical practitioners are undifferentiated, or unspecialised. During this time, interns or Junior Medical Officers (JMO) undertake rotations through many different specialties. While rotations will vary between hospitals and states, three core terms must be completed: a medical, surgical and emergency medicine placement (NSW JMO Forum, 2016).

Resident Medical Officers

Once interns have completed their one year of supervised practice successfully, they are eligible for full registration by the Medical Board of their state or territory. They are also licensed to engage in independent medical practice. As **provider numbers** are not issued to medical practitioners who have not completed postgraduate studies, virtually all doctors continue their training as a Resident Medical Officer (RMO) in a hospital, which lasts for two years (Central Coast Local Health Network & Northern Sydney Local Health Network, 2011).

> **provider number**
> A unique number that medical or endorsed nurse practitioners can acquire. It allows the clinician to make referrals for specialist services, requests for pathology or diagnostic imaging services, and their patients to claim Medicare rebates for the services provided.

Registrar

A registrar is a medical practitioner who is undertaking an accredited course of study leading to a higher medical qualification. Specialist training differs considerably between specialist colleges. In some specialist college training programs, a trainee may continue as an RMO at the early stages of their training while other trainees may begin at registrar level. While working in hospitals or other healthcare environments, registrars also prepare for examinations for admission into specialist medical colleges (Australian Medical Association, 2016).

Specialist/Consultant

Registrars who successfully complete the entry requirements of their specialist college program become 'Fellows' of that college. They are now classed as a 'specialist', and are also known as consultants within their area of specialist practice (Australian Medical Association, 2016). Specialists may also have managerial and administrative duties—for example, rostering—including responsibility for the quality of care and practices within a given department or healthcare team.

OTHER COMMON HEALTH PROFESSIONAL ROLES

Physiotherapist

Physiotherapists are degree-qualified healthcare professionals who use movement, exercise, education and manual therapy to target health/injury recovery, injury prevention and rehabilitation. The physiotherapy spectrum extends from health promotion to acute care, rehabilitation and chronic disease management (Australian Physiotherapy Association, 2017). Physiotherapists work within a variety of settings, including both private and public hospitals, private clinics, community health services and residential aged care facilities.

Occupational therapist

Occupational therapists are degree-qualified healthcare professionals who focus on assessing and enabling people to participate in the activities of daily life. This is achieved by improving the patient's ability to complete the task/occupation, or by modifying the environment to better support the client being able to complete their occupational engagement (Occupational Therapy Australia, 2017). Occupational therapists work in a variety of settings, often as part of a healthcare team. These include healthcare services, rehabilitation units, schools and education facilities, and in public and private practice.

Dietitian

Dietitians are degree-qualified healthcare professionals able to provide a broad range of evidence-based services related to public health nutrition, individual dietary counselling, medical nutrition therapy and food service management (DAA, 2017).

Pharmacist

Pharmacists are degree-qualified healthcare professionals that prepare or supervise the dispensing of medicines. Pharmacists may provide patient advice regarding how to take medications in the safest and most effective manner for the treatment of common conditions, and may advise other health clinicians regarding appropriate medication selection, dosage, drug interactions, potential side-effects and therapeutic effects (Pharmaceutical Society of Australia, 2017).

Speech Pathologist

Speech Pathologists are degree-qualified healthcare professionals who diagnose and treat communication disorders, including problems with speaking, reading, listening, understanding language, stuttering, using voice and swallowing (Speech Pathology Australia, 2017).

Social Worker

Social Workers are degree-qualified healthcare professionals who have a focus on assisting to improve patient wellbeing while identifying and addressing external factors that may negatively impact wellbeing. Social workers work in numerous environments and may take on roles such as casework, advocacy and counselling (AASW, 2017). Social workers can help with problems such as homelessness, domestic violence, alcohol and drug addiction, sexual assault and child abuse. They can also help people who have suffered a major crisis or are going through a bereavement.

ABORIGINAL AND TORRES STRAIT ISLANDER HEALTH WORKERS

Aboriginal and Torres Strait Islander Health Workers (ATSIHWs) play an important role in improving the health outcomes of Aboriginal and Torres Strait Islander people, and providing clinical and primary care for individuals, families and community groups. ATSIHWs undertake a variety of roles, such as mental health worker, hospital liaison officer, healthy living worker, sexual health worker, and maternal and perinatal health worker (NATSIHWA, 2016). ATSIHWs are employed within numerous settings, from Aboriginal Community-Controlled Health Organisations and the public sector to general practices and NGOs. An ATSIHW must be registered with AHPRA, and have completed a Certificate IV in Aboriginal and/or Torres Strait Islander Healthcare Practice (Aboriginal Health Council of South Australia, 2016). The title 'Aboriginal and Torres Strait Islander Health Worker' is protected under section 113 of the National Law.

'ADVANCED PRACTICE' IN NURSING: WHAT IS IT?

Advanced practice nursing roles have been developed in response to increased demand on the health service, shortages of nurses and doctors, and patient and government expectations of more efficient access to care (Hudson & Marshall, 2008). Rapid evolution of new nursing roles has, however, created confusion inter-professionally and within nursing itself regarding titles, scope of practice, role boundaries and educational requirements. Terms used to describe advanced practice roles vary not only between countries, but also within state and health services (Hudson & Marshall, 2008) (see Table 3.1).

Table 3.1 Advanced practice nursing roles by region

Country	Title
North America	Nurse Practitioner, Clinical Nurse Specialist, Advanced Practice Nurse
United Kingdom	Nurse Practitioner, Nurse Consultant, Clinical Nurse Specialist
Australia	Nurse Practitioner, Transitional Nurse Practitioner, Clinical Nurse Consultant, Clinical Nurse Specialist, Advanced Practice Nurse

There is ongoing disagreement concerning nursing titles that reflect 'advanced practice'. Some have argued that the term 'advanced practice' should be restricted to specific titles such as Nurse Practitioner (NP), or Clinical Nurse Consultant and Specialist (CNC, CNS), while others see 'advanced practice' as a term that can be used generically to describe high performance within nursing—for example, the ability to use knowledge and skills along with research evidence and academic thinking (Mantzoukas & Watkinson, 2006). Oberle and Allen (2001) suggest that advanced practice needs a theoretical knowledge base to support critical thinking and problem-solving in the clinical environment. This description is supported by the Nursing and Midwifery Board (NMBA, 2014), which states that advanced nursing practice is demonstrated by the application of knowledge, leadership, research and education into the nurse–patient relationship whilst treating patients with complex care requirements. Tightening of definitions supporting the term 'advanced' in relation to nursing is vital to decrease confusion about the scope of different nursing roles.

Summary

In this chapter, we have considered the nature of healthcare delivery in Australia. We have noted that primary healthcare is a patient's first port of call for healthcare, and is generally provided by a GP or other community health worker, while secondary healthcare is provided by a facility or specialist after referral by a primary health clinician. We defined the various roles in healthcare, including the range of nursing roles, medical officers, allied health professionals and ATSIHWs. Finally, we considered what is involved in advanced nursing practice.

Review questions

3.1 Primary healthcare can only be provided by a GP. True or false?

3.2 Where is primary healthcare usually provided?
a In the community   b In hospitals

3.3 Who has the primary responsibility for funding of primary healthcare?
a State government
b Federal government

3.4 A key activity of primary healthcare lies within health promotion and the prevention of unnecessary hospital admissions. True or false?

3.5 The purpose of LHNs is to:
a Optimise delivery, coordination and access to secondary health services
b Make access to specialist doctors cheaper
c Improve engagement with local clinicians and community to incorporate their views upon quality and safety of care

3.6 Common activities with which an AIN may help include:
a Showering
b Hygiene
c Vital signs
d Assistance with positioning

3.7 To be able to administer medications, an EN must first complete further tertiary education and workplace assessment. True or false?

3.8 In Australia, what nursing roles are considered 'advanced practice'?
a Registered Nurse
b Nurse Practitioner
c Clinical Nurse Consultant

3.9 Place in level of seniority, from junior to senior:
a Resident Medical Officer
b Registrar
c Intern
d Staff specialist

3.10 The largest component of the health workforce comprises:
a Doctors
b Registered Nurses and midwives
c Allied health workers
d Administrators

4 PROFESSIONAL PRACTICE

Alister Hodge and Wayne Varndell

In this chapter, you will develop an understanding of:

- national competency standards
- professional Codes of Conduct
- the Code of Ethics for nurses
- leadership in nursing and coping with change
- quality and safety of care
- specialty nursing clinical practice standards
- the Australian Nursing and Midwifery Federation
- registration standards for overseas-qualified RNs and midwives.

FIT TO PRACTISE

The health, welfare and protection of the public are paramount concerns of society and government. To ensure that nurses and midwives reflect the integrity of their profession in Australia, they must demonstrate a fitness to practise. This relates to the ability of the nurse and midwife to practise without restriction and within the Code of Professional Conduct (NMBA, 2018a, 2018b) and the Code of Ethics (NMBA, 2013a, 2013b). Fitness to practise is assumed if the nurse has successfully completed a recognised undergraduate degree in Australia and a year of clinical placement. For overseas-qualified nurses, further evidence must be provided. Fitness to practise can be demonstrated through evidence obtained from the authority that registered the nurse. This evidence must verify that:

- there are no previous proven disciplinary proceedings or criminal convictions sufficient to prohibit practice in Australia

- there are no restrictions resulting from physical or mental incapacity
- there are no physical or mental impediments that would disqualify practising as a nurse or midwife in Australia.

NATIONAL COMPETENCY STANDARDS FOR THE REGISTERED NURSE

The Nursing and Midwifery Board of Australia (NMBA) has produced national standards that are an integral component of the regulatory framework, to assist nurses (NMBA, 2016c) and midwives (NMBA, 2006) to deliver safe and competent care. These standards have now been reviewed to ensure congruency with state and territory nursing regulatory authorities.

The competencies that form the NMBA National Competency Standards for registered nurses (NMBA, 2016c) are organised into seven domains:

1 *critical thinking and analysis*—questioning and reflecting upon experiences, decisions and actions; weighing up opinions and examining evidence for and against an action or decision
2 *engaging in therapeutic and professional relationships*—providing care and assistance based on mutual trust, respect and equality while maintaining professional boundaries with patients and members of the healthcare team
3 *maintaining the capability for practice*—investing in lifelong learning and professional development to sustain and grow clinically and academically
4 *comprehensively conducting assessments*—the ability to conduct an accurate and thorough health assessment; appropriate utilisation of physical assessment skills (e.g. observation, inspection, palpation, auscultation), history-taking and interpretation of findings
5 *developing a plan for nursing practice*—the ability to formulate and evaluate a patient-focused plan of care based upon assessment findings
6 *providing safe, appropriate and responsive quality nursing practice*—the ability to provide care that is safe, evidence based and goal orientated; that appropriately delegates to others; and that identifies and minimises harm to self and others
7 *evaluating outcomes to inform nursing practice*—monitors and evaluates outcomes of care, and communicates effectively with the patient, healthcare team and employer to optimise patient care quality and safety.

The competencies that make up the National Competency Standards for midwifery (NMBA, 2006) are organised into four domains:

1 *legal and professional practice*—the ability to practise safely; invests in lifelong learning and ongoing professional development to maintain clinical, academic and practice skills and knowledge; recognises and advocates for the woman's right to receive accurate information
2 *midwifery knowledge and practice*—maintains and develops knowledge, skills and practice; operates according to role and scope of practice; able to assess the needs of women and newborns by conducting an accurate and thorough health assessment, history-taking and interpretation of findings
3 *midwifery as primary healthcare*—practises within a woman-centred, primary healthcare framework across multiple settings; provides information to optimise women's health, their newborn and family; and prepares women for pregnancy
4 *reflective and ethical practice*—questions and analyses experiences and decisions, and critically evaluates evidence for and against an action or decision; engages in critical reflection (see Chapter 11).

Each domain has been extensively defined and detailed by a team of expert nursing and midwifery consultants, and is based on the latest evidence-based practice to ensure safe patient care. Dual-qualified nurses and midwives would have to meet both standards.

PROFESSIONAL CODE OF CONDUCT

Professional conduct refers to the way a person behaves while acting in a professional capacity. The Code of Professional Conduct for Nurses in Australia sets out the minimum standards for practice that a professional person is expected to uphold both within and outside the professional domains to ensure the 'good standing' of the nursing profession. It also informs the community of the standards of professional conduct to be expected from nurses in Australia, and provides consumer, regulatory and employing/professional bodies with a basis for evaluating the professional conduct of nurses. The Code of Professional Conduct for Nurses in Australia (NMBA, 2018a, p. 4) lists seven principles, which set out the requirements, expected professional behaviour and conduct for all nurses:

1 *legal compliance*—nurses practise ethically and adhere to their professional responsibilities under National Law and other laws (e.g. drugs and poisons legislation)
2 *person-centred practice*—nurses provide safe, ethical, quality care in partnership with the person that is evidence-based, and foster shared decision-making

3 *cultural practice and respectful relationships*—nurses engage with people as individuals and value the inherent worth and dignity of every individual in a culturally safe and respectful way
4 *professional behaviour*—nurses' behaviour and actions embody integrity, honesty, respect and compassion
5 *teaching, supervising and assessing*—nurses commit to teaching, supervising and assessing students and other nurses, creating opportunities for nursing students and other nurses to learn and develop
6 *research in health*—nurses recognise the vital role of research in informing evidence-based professional nursing, which is necessary for continuing advancements that promote optimal nursing care
7 *health and wellbeing*—nurses maintain their physical and mental health, protect and advance the health and wellbeing of people, colleagues and the broader community.

CODE OF ETHICS FOR NURSES IN AUSTRALIA

Nursing is a complex, dynamic, social process that is built on a relationship between the nurse, the patient, their family, community and culture, and the clinical organisation (Duffy, 2013). The very nature of the nurse–patient relationship, in which respect, confidence and privacy play important roles, demands that nurses consider the ethical nature of their actions (Chaloner, 2007).

According to the International Council of Nurses (2012), nursing involves four critical responsibilities: (1) the promotion of health; (2) the prevention of illness; (3) the restoration of health; and (4) the alleviation of suffering. Ethics is concerned with the actions, effects and value of those actions (Rumbold, 1999), and knowing what is the right way to proceed or what should be done in a given situation (Winch, 2007). Nurses at all levels and in all areas of practice, experience a range of ethical issues during the course of their day-to-day work (Johnstone et al., 2004). It is therefore important for all nurses to be aware of the ethical frameworks, values and beliefs that shape nursing care.

The Code of Ethics for Nurses in Australia (NMBA, 2013a) has been developed to assist in channelling the nursing profession's commitment to respect, protect and uphold the fundamental rights of people who are both recipients and providers of nursing and healthcare. This Code of Ethics has been guided by standards and principles set forth in the United Nations Universal Declaration of Human Rights (1948) and International Covenant of Economic, Social and Cultural Rights (1966); the World Health Organization's Constitution (1946) and its publication series entitled Health and Human Rights (2017); and the

United Nations Development Programme *Human Development Report 2004: Cultural liberty in today's diverse world* (Fukuda-Parr, 2004). The Code of Ethics for Nurses in Australia consists of eight statements (NMBA, 2013a, p. 1):

1   Nurses value quality nursing care for all people.
2   Nurses value respect and kindness for self and others.
3   Nurses value the diversity of people.
4   Nurses value access to quality nursing and healthcare for all people.
5   Nurses value informed decision-making.
6   Nurses value a culture of safety in nursing and healthcare.
7   Nurses value ethical management of information.
8   Nurses value a socially, economically and ecologically sustainable environment promoting health and wellbeing.

Nurses—undergraduate or registered—are strongly encouraged to critically analyse their clinical, managerial, educational or research practice using the above statements as a guide, to ensure it upholds the values of protecting human rights, liberties, equality and dignity.

LEADERSHIP AND WORKING WITH STAFF

association A linear and predictive relationship between two variables that move in relation to each other.

Leadership style is positively **associated** with higher levels of quality patient care and staff morale, and is a highly sought after and valued commodity (Northouse, 2015). Many factors lead to better team performance, but one of the most significant and most widely researched factors is that of team leadership. Leadership is commonly attributed to and expected of people who are in management and administrative nursing positions. While this is certainly true, all nurses must develop leadership skills in order to be effective at delivering high-quality patient care, as knowledge of clinical practice and patient care skills alone are not sufficient in today's clinical environment. Non-clinical skills such as facilitating, mentoring, communicating and negotiating are key leadership skills. How teams are directed in achieving goals is important. Both managers and leaders need to envision the future and lead the way towards a productive and efficient workplace with satisfied staff.

The terms 'manager' and 'leader' are often used interchangeably, yet they are not synonymous. While this does not mean that an individual cannot claim both manager and leader tasks, the term 'manager' is considered separate from 'leader'.

A manager has an assigned position within an organisation, and is generally much more task orientated, with formal power and definite responsibilities ensuring that the day-to-day business is carried out. A manager also has specific duties with formal reporting lines, control over processes, decision-making and resource allocation, including regarding the work of others (Kotter & Rathgeber, 2016). Conversely, a leader does not have delegated authority, as a leader's 'power' is derived informally from the group and the building and sustaining of relationships. Leaders use a process of persuasion, empathy and person-centredness to motivate others to take action towards achieving a goal or change.

For complex organisations to function properly, both managers and leaders are necessary. However, how they lead is pivotal to the way patients and staff experience the organisation and clinical environment. Leadership comes in many guises and is difficult to define. Several leadership types and theories have emerged that are relevant to leadership in nursing.

Great man theory

The great man (or woman) theory argues that one is simply born a great leader with innate qualities relating to intelligence and personality suitable for all situations. The theory emerged during the 19th century, and was based on the behaviours of great military figures of the time, and popularised by Thomas Carlyle. Authoritative positions during the 1800s were predominantly held by men, and typically were passed from father to son. Women were rarely afforded the opportunity to occupy positions of authority—hence the name of the theory. While leaders may appear to hold unique leadership qualities and abilities, leadership is not bound to a person's gender, genetics or social status. There is no empirical evidence to support the great man theory, yet it does provide a starting point to explore and understand which qualities or traits are desirable in leaders (Marquis & Huston, 2009). Leaders can and do emerge from unexpected sources, and can be grown given the necessary knowledge and skills (Northouse, 2015). As Herbert Spencer (1820–1903) argued, leaders are both a product of their environment and the society in which they work and live, and in turn affect the environment and society themselves.

Situational leader

A situational or contingency leader is a leader by virtue of their skills and ability in a particular situation. For example, in a cardiac arrest, the person with the most experience and training in advanced life support would, by virtue of their abilities, lead the resuscitation of the patient. However, while the leader would direct the action needing to be taken, situational leadership is unidirectional and task-relevant, and may not be flexible enough to sustain action and teamwork as the context and dynamics of the situation change (Reynolds & Rogers, 2003).

Transactional leadership

Leadership within the clinical workplace has traditionally been about trans-actional leadership (Cook & Leathard, 2004). A transactional leader is concerned with fulfilling daily goals, and relies on the power of their organisational position and formal authority to reward and reprove performance. While a transactional leadership style can work well with frontline supervision of low-skilled workers, it can limit independent and creative thinking by staff to examine ways to improve care and service delivery. Nurses frequently experience organisational and clinical practice change, especially when moving into more senior roles within the organisation. To cope with the rapid change, nurses need to advance to more team-based models of leadership, which foster innovative and creative thinking in the workforce (Faugier & Woolnough, 2003; Smith, 2011).

Transformational leadership

Transformational leadership hinges on a high level of engagement between leaders and followers that focuses on team building, and is a radical departure from previously discussed theories centred on hierarchical, command-and-control styles of leadership that previously have dominated healthcare. This style of leadership involves emotions, motives, ethics and effective communication, and incorporates both charismatic and visionary leadership to influence followers to achieve more than is usually expected of them (Northouse, 2015). Further, trans-formational leaders generate an environment whereby boundaries can shift, and creativity and innovation can emerge (Robbins & Davidhizar, 2007; Smith, 2011). Common attributes of a transformational leader include:

- *individualised consideration*—listening to the follower's concerns and needs, acting as a mentor or coach to the follower
- *intellectual stimulation*—challenging assumptions, nurturing and developing followers to be innovative and to think creatively
- *inspirational motivation*—the ability to clearly articulate a vision that engages and inspires followers to strive towards achieving future goals

- *idealised influence*—role modelling, which provides a standard for high ethical behaviour, instils pride, gains respect and trust (Johnstone et al., 2004), and is linked to charisma (Gellis, 2001).

The ability to establish a vision and support/motivate adaptation to change has led transformational leadership to be increasingly promoted in health organisations, where change and service improvement occur frequently (Brewer et al., 2016; Fischer, 2016; Jooste, 2004). However, in a series of studies exploring clinical leaders' attributes and characteristics, some attributes of transformational leadership—specifically creativity and vision—were not rated highly by nurses or nurse leaders (Stanley, 2006a, 2006b, 2006c). Further, the organisation's need or the transformational leaders' desire for employees to adapt, and the culture in which this occurs, may dominate individual creativity, thus hindering innovation and empowerment (Murphy, 2005; Rafferty, 1993).

Servant leadership

Servant leadership is a paradox, in that it runs contrary to the commonly held notion put forward in leadership theories and style that leaders lead and followers (servants) follow. Originating from the writings of Greenleaf (1977), servant-leaders serve the needs of the followers by first empowering them to achieve their potential, and second, inspire and mature them to lead; organisational concerns are peripheral. Nurses are frequently at the forefront of care delivery, managing competing demands, diverse consumer needs and the limitations of the structures in which they work. Despite the multitude of performance targets, standards and resource challenges, at the core of nursing is the patient and community. Servant leadership assists nurse leaders to frame their decisions and actions with the patient and community in mind: respecting and valuing people, advocating and expressing a human face in an often sterile, impersonal environment, and treating individuals as ends rather than means (Waterman, 2011). Effective servant leadership characteristics include: active listening, empathy, healing and negotiation, emotional intelligence, self-awareness by viewing situations from a holistic perspective, persuasion, nurturing personal growth, foresight, stewardship, and growth of people and building communities (Spears, 2010).

The servant leadership style is based on mutual trust and empowerment of followers, which may best be suited to moving groups forward in organisations of multidisciplinary teams. Since its original inception, Greenleaf's servant leadership theory has been built upon by several leadership scholars. The outputs, which range from the development of theoretical concepts and constructs to identifying servant-leader characteristics, have been summarised by van Dierendonck (2011). Servant leadership overlaps with several other leadership theories, but the most notable is transformational leadership. Transformational leadership and servant leadership have many similarities: person-centredness, valuing followers, listening, mentoring and empowering followers. However, there are two distinct differences between transformational and servant leadership styles: first, servant leadership focuses on humility, authenticity and interpersonal acceptance, elements that are not present in transformational leadership; and second, the focus of the servant-leader is the follower and the follower's needs. While transformational leaders and servant leaders both show concern for their followers, the overriding focus of the servant-leader is on service to the followers, whereas the transformational leader has a greater concern with getting followers to engage with and support organisational objectives (Stone et al., 2004).

Authentic leadership

Authentic, or congruent, leadership occurs when the activities, actions and deeds of the leader are matched and driven by their values and beliefs about practice— in this case, nursing and clinical practice (Stanley, 2008). It is through sustained conviction to following shared values, beliefs and principles that authentic leaders gain followers. Authentic leaders have five distinguishing characteristics:

1 *purpose*—understanding their own purposes and passions as a result of continual self-reflection and self-awareness
2 *values*—purpose and passion are congruent with their beliefs and actions (deeds)
3 *heart*—leaders care for themselves and the people they lead; they are compassionate
4 *relationships*—the leader is focused on building relationships and establishing connections with others
5 *self-discipline*—they maintain a balance between their personal and professional lives (Marquis & Huston, 2009).

Authentic leadership can provide a broad guideline for new graduate nurses transitioning into clinical practice, helping you develop greater self-awareness, your own moral perspective reflected in ethical decision-making and behaviour, and balanced and objective processing of information.

In a rapidly changing healthcare system, leadership plays an important part in helping organisations to meet their future goals. Nurse leaders have a unique role to play in increasing patient safety and quality of care because of the high level of contact and diverse range of interactions nurses have with patients (Riley, 2009). All nurses need to acquire leadership skills to facilitate practice change and workforce development. Across all theories of leadership, key attributes and characteristics of clinical leaders include being approachable and open; honesty; actively displaying and holding to values and beliefs; being an effective communicator; objectivity; being a good relationship-builder; presenting a positive clinical role model; being empowering; being visible; and being clinically competent. The effectiveness of the clinical team and the quality of teamwork are linked to the behaviours and practices of leaders (Wong et al., 2013).

Positive workplace environments and effective teamwork do not simply occur; they are built and sustained by strong leadership (Duffield et al., 2011; Malloy & Penprase, 2010). Positive work environments empower team members by giving them autonomy and accountability within their scope of practice, as well as support, resources and opportunities for individual and team growth. The extent to which nurses experience their workplace as empowering is linked to the behaviours and practices of leaders—particularly when the style of leadership is transformational (Laschinger et al., 2013) or servant leadership (Wong & Cummings, 2007). These styles tend to support nurses' self-efficacy and sense of competence in the workplace (Salanova et al., 2011; Wong & Cummings, 2007; Wong et al., 2013). Nurses who feel valued and recognised for their contributions by management are more likely to be satisfied at work (Sveinsdóttir et al., 2016).

COPING WITH CHANGE

Leadership is connected with coping with change, as frequent change in the workplace means that existing systems and hierarchies are more often challenged. Frequent change has become a necessary feature of the health environment, as practice evolves in line with best evidence. Therefore, the ability to embrace and cope with change is an essential skill to develop.

Coping refers to the way we interpret and manage stressful events. It is impossible to avoid change; however, each individual has the power to choose how they interact with the change-management process. Maintaining openness towards change, through viewing the process as an opportunity to learn and mature as a clinician, enables you to become part of the process and take ownership of the situation. Focusing on the positives that the change process will achieve, rather than dwelling on perceived negatives, can also help you to feel better about the overall situation.

Negative coping behaviours commonly employ avoidance as a strategy. For example, you may choose to miss an education session regarding a practice change or show up late. Avoidance may provide some short-term relief and escape from the inevitable change; however, it usually ends up making the process more difficult than it needed to be through lost opportunities to prepare.

Maintain a level of self-awareness regarding how the change process is affecting you personally. Early identification of stress symptoms related to change allows you to enact stress-management strategies before symptoms become more serious.

CHANGE MANAGEMENT IN HEALTHCARE

Healthcare has a rapidly evolving evidence base to support best practice. Therefore, to continue delivering high-quality care to patients in line with the current evidence, changes in clinical practice and models of care must also occur. Knowledge of common change-management processes will enable you to contribute more effectively during these times of practice evolution.

Achieving change in the clinical setting is often difficult, particularly when the change involves altering work processes that have become entrenched over many years. Factors that are critical to success in any change process include stakeholder involvement, functional leadership, time and flexibility, appropriate resources and incentives for participants, and clear communication pathways (Allen & Stevens, 2007). Generally, clinicians are more receptive to change if adequate time and resources have been applied to prepare them properly, and they can clearly see that the alteration in practice aligns with core professional aims such as an improvement to patient care, or a greater ability to complete their work.

A key barrier to change implementation common to many health change initiatives involves a failure to engage clinicians. If the staff member does not feel that the suggested change will achieve better outcomes for their patients, or has serious concerns about the rationale for change, timeframe and implementation plan, they are unlikely to support the initiative (Callaly & Arya, 2005; McMurray et al., 2010). Sensibly, a key means to overcome resistance to change is to ensure that the benefits associated with a given change clearly outweigh the negatives.

Many different change-management methodologies have been used in both the business and health environments. Three common approaches that you may come across in nursing include action research, practice development and clinical redesign methodology. Each employs a similar cyclical process to guide, implement and evaluate the success of changes made.

Action research

Action research involves an ongoing cycle of five stages:

1 *Diagnosis:* The problem stimulating the change process is clearly identified and defined.
2 *Planning:* An action to solve the problem is designed.
3 *Implementation:* The chosen action is implemented.
4 *Evaluation:* The consequences of the implemented action are examined.
5 *Reassessment:* The cycle is brought back to the first step to reassess the situation in its entirety to see whether the problem still exists, and whether the cycle needs to start once more (Sullivan et al., 2013).

Practice development

Practice development has been embraced as a vehicle to achieve practice improvement by nurses in numerous services across Australia. Similarities can arguably be found with action research through the four phases of a typical practice development change project:

1 *Orientation:* Clearly articulate the context and setting within which the change will take place. Identify precedents for the proposed change, and likely benefits of or barriers to implementation.
2 *Preparation for change:* Stakeholders in the project develop a set of goals, and agree on a change method and implementation strategy, as well as criteria for evaluation.
3 *Process of change:* The agreed change strategy is implemented.
4 *Evaluation and comparative analysis:* The project is evaluated against the nominated criteria and staff feedback is sought. Next a repeat analysis of data from Phase 1 occurs to complete a pre- and post-implementation data comparison (Hodge et al., 2011).

Redesign methodology

Redesign methodology, developed by the NSW Agency for Clinical Innovation, has developed a five-step process that can be applied to most change management, from alterations to clinical practice through to the design and implementation of new models of care.

1 *Project initiation:* During this initial phase, an opportunity or need for change is identified. An adequate amount of evidence must be acquired to demonstrate

the need for change, and what positives can be achieved through altering this area of practice. This evidence must be of sufficient depth to convince project sponsors and key stakeholders that change is warranted. Once an executive sponsor has been obtained, a working group and overall project manager/lead must be identified. The working group of key stakeholders, such as clinicians, managers and consumers, is brought together. The working group will contribute to the diagnostic phase and solution design. The working group should also ideally help create the project aim—a clear statement about what the project will achieve—and outline objectives that must be met in order to achieve the aim (Agency for Clinical Innovation, 2013).

2   *Diagnostic:* To truly understand what needs to be done to improve a given situation, a clear understanding must be acquired of the current state of play. During the diagnostic phase, further analysis will build on that gained during Phase 1. Data will likely be gained from multiple sources such as process mapping, complaints, reports, interviews with staff and patients, and analysis of patient data. A literature review will identify current best practice in the area of change, and may provide insight into potential solutions. Once the diagnostic work has been completed, a list of issues requiring resolution should be summarised and subsequently prioritised in relation to their impact upon achieving the project's aim (Agency for Clinical Innovation, 2013).

3   *Solution design:* During this phase, solutions are developed by the working group to address the issues identified during diagnosis. Once a shortlist of solutions is created, each option should be tested where possible via a small pilot project, or table-top exercises to identify the option most likely to be successful. Next, an evaluation framework for the chosen solutions and overall project must be created to assess whether the objectives have been met, and to evaluate the effectiveness and sustainability of the changes implemented. Ensure that endorsement is achieved for the identified solutions through a consultative process with key stakeholders outside the working group (Agency for Clinical Innovation, 2013).

4   *Implementation:* Preparation is key to the success of this phase. Ensure that the executive sponsor for the project is still supportive. An implementation plan should be developed for the introduction of changes. Staff who will be affected by the incoming change must be informed of the project, and gain a clear understanding of why change is required, what the project seeks to achieve and what their role will be. Once staff engagement is achieved, the change to practice is implemented (Agency for Clinical Innovation, 2013).

5   *Evaluation and sustainability:* During this phase, the evaluation framework developed during solution design is implemented. This ensures that monitoring occurs alongside implementation to identify the success of the changes.

It is recommended that regular feedback be sought from staff affected by the change to maintain engagement and enthusiasm. Early identification of problems allows intervention to make the project as successful as possible. At the end of the project a summative evaluation takes place regarding whether the project has met its objectives and overall aim (Agency for Clinical Innovation, 2013). Sustainability is a key phase of any project. After an initial period of enthusiasm, efforts may stall with a reversion to previous habits that require less mental engagement in the short term. The working party and project lead must work to maintain staff commitment and consolidate wins through frequent feedback to staff until the change becomes part of everyday culture (Callaly & Arya, 2005).

The following is an example of redesign methodology in action:

1 *Project initiation:* A nurse notes that family members are often left alone and poorly supported during a patient resuscitation event, and realises that this is an opportunity to improve practice. The nurse generates evidence that change is needed by completing a brief literature review of 'Family Presence in Resuscitation', noting the benefits and risks involved in having family members present, and finds that the benefits clearly outweigh the risks if the process is undertaken appropriately. The nurse discusses the suggested change with her manager in an informal meeting, and presents the initial findings of her literature review. The manager agrees to be the executive sponsor for the project. The nurse forms a working group with interested stakeholders who will be affected by the project—for example, Registered Nurse/registrar/staff specialist/Nurse Unit Manager/social worker. The working party agrees upon a project aim—for example, to enable family presence during resuscitation—and objectives that must be met to achieve the aim—for example, develop guidelines for the safe/appropriate facilitation of family presence during resuscitation.

2 *Diagnostic:* The working party completes different aspects of data acquisition to build on the initial literature search completed in phase 1. A more in-depth literature review is completed to identify current best practice in application of family presence during resuscitation. A process map is completed to clarify what current practice is for the management of family members during a resuscitation. Focus groups are held with key areas of staff, such as nurses, doctors and allied health professionals, to identify staff opinions/concerns/possible solutions to aid the design phase.

3 *Solution design:* A guideline for the application of family presence in resuscitation is written by the working group. The guideline is presented to stakeholders

outside the working group, and endorsement of its final composition is gained. Ethics approval is gained from the local Health Research Ethics Committee.

4 *Implementation:* Staff education sessions take place so that all clinicians who will be affected by the new practice are aware of how to enact the guideline and support family members adequately during a resuscitation without impeding care for the patient. Once all staff have been educated, and any final concerns worked through, the guideline is made active and family members are offered the opportunity to remain with their loved one while resuscitation takes place.

5 *Evaluation and sustainability:* Evaluation is carried out—in this case via focus groups and questionnaires with staff involved—to confirm whether the project has met the core aim of providing safe family presence during resuscitation. Family members who have been involved are invited to provide feedback regarding their experience through structured phone interviews. The working party contributes to the writing of a paper to submit for publication, thereby sharing the knowledge gained with the wider clinical community. Periodic in-services/feedback sessions are held with staff regarding family presence to ensure that the practice becomes embedded as usual practice and therefore achieves sustainability.

QUALITY AND PATIENT SAFETY IN HEALTHCARE

Australia has a healthcare system that rates well internationally on quality and safety, while servicing the health needs of the majority of the population. The two terms 'quality' and 'safety' are mentioned frequently in discussion of health; however, they are rarely defined. Quality in the context of health can be defined broadly as reflecting the extent to which the service achieves a desired outcome. The Australian Commission on Safety and Quality in Health Care (ACSQHC, 2015) proposes that quality is closely related to patient care effectiveness, appropriateness, accessibility and responsiveness. Safety in the health system refers to the degree to which possible risk, harm and unintended results are avoided or minimised (Mitchell, 2008). Thus safety is the foundation upon which all other aspects of quality care are built.

At the federal level, in 2006 the Liberal Minister for Health, Tony Abbott, created the Australian Commission on Safety and Quality in Health Care (ACSQHC) to coordinate improvement in healthcare quality and safety across Australia. The ACSQHC strategic plan focuses on four priority areas (ACSQHC, 2014):

* *patient safety*—keeping patients and consumers safe by designing and implementing systems to monitor and prevent harm

- *partnering with patients, consumers and communities*—proactive engagement and partnership with patients, consumers and communities in designing health-care services and their governance
- *quality, value and cost*—designing productive health services and systems that meet the needs of patients, consumers and communities while minimising waste
- *supporting health professionals to deliver safe care of optimal quality*—developing integrated systems to enable clinicians to drive safety and quality improvements locally, and provide access to guidance and tools to inform safe clinical practice.

At the state level, health departments have implemented programs to monitor and manage clinical incidents and risks, and improve clinical quality in public health organizations. An example of one such state quality program is the NSW Patient Safety and Clinical Quality Program, instituted by the NSW Labor government in 2005. This program has sought to improve patient safety and quality in the public health service through:

- implementation of an Incident Information Management System
- systematic management of incidents and risks
- implementation of Clinical Governance Units in each area health service
- establishment of the Clinical Excellence Commission
- initiation of a Quality Assessment Program for all public health organisations (NSW Health, 2005a).

NATIONAL SAFETY AND QUALITY HEALTH SERVICE (NSQHS) STANDARDS

The National Safety and Quality Health Service Standards were developed by ACSQHC (2012) and updated in 2017 following consultation with clinicians, health service managers, technical and safety and quality experts, and consumers (ACSQHC, 2017). The first edition of the NSQHS Standards contained ten standards that were developed primarily for use in the acute care sector. The second edition of the Standards now addresses safety and quality issues in mental health and cognitive impairment, health literacy, end-of-life care and Aboriginal and Torres Strait Islander health detailed across eight standards:

1 *Clinical governance:* implementation of safe, high-quality systems to optimise care and prevent harm to patients, consumers and communities.
2 *Partnering with consumers:* designing and building quality healthcare systems and strategies focused on the needs of the service consumer.

3 *Preventing and controlling healthcare-associated infections:* implementing systems and evidence-based approaches to prevent infection of patients, consumers and staff, and to identify and manage infections effectively when they occur.

4 *Medication safety:* developing and implementing systems, evidence-based procedures and strategies to ensure clinicians safely prescribe, dispense and administer appropriate medicines to informed patients.

5 *Comprehensive care:* implementation of integrated systems, rigorous practices and strategies to assess for, prevent and minimise the risk of harm to patients.

6 *Communicating for safety:* implementation of effective communication processes and strategies between patients, carers, clinicians and across the health service organisation.

7 *Blood management:* implementation of systems and evidence-based procedures and strategies to optimise the use of blood and blood products, including correctly identifying the patient and matching their identity and needs with the correct treatment or procedure from collection, testing, storage and administration.

8 *Recognising and responding to clinical deterioration in acute healthcare:* embedding systems and processes into practice to recognise and respond effectively to patients when their physical, mental or cognitive health deteriorates.

Within each standard, a nationally consistent statement about the level of care patients can expect from health service organisations, core actions regarding the systems and strategies to be implemented in order to achieve the standard and its intended outcomes are described. While the standards might appear to be targeted towards the organisational level, they greatly inform the level of safety and quality expected at the bedside when delivering care. We will now look at each standard in more detail.

Standard 1: Clinical governance

Clinical governance is a system through which organisations are accountable for continually improving the quality and safety of their services, by creating and maintaining an environment in which excellence in clinical care can grow (Brennan & Flynn, 2013; Scally & Donaldson, 1998). Clinical governance first emerged in the late 1990s in response to the Bristol Royal Infirmary Inquiry in the United Kingdom (Department of Health (UK), 2001), and has since been adopted in a range of countries, including Australia (Travaglia et al., 2011). Clinical governance structures within health organisations typically comprise several interacting key elements (see Figure 4.1):

- auditing (observing and comparing nursing practice with evidence-based standards) and observing patient outcomes
- clinical effectiveness and resource management
- practice standards and research
- continuing professional development and training
- risk management
- service user and staff experience
- culture and leadership (Bohmer, 2010; Goodall, 2011; Phillips et al., 2010).

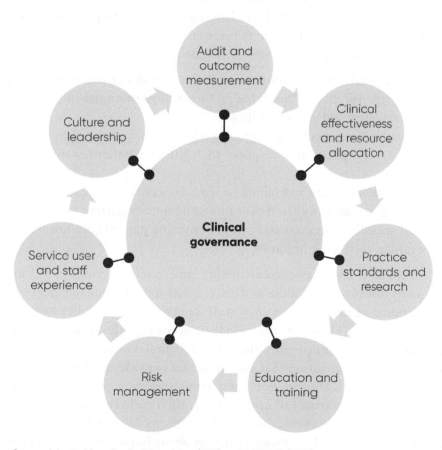

Source: Adapted from Scally & Donaldson (1998) and ACSQHC (2009).

Figure 4.1 Clinical governance framework

The key objectives of a clinical governance framework are to ensure that patients receive safe and effective care, protect the public from harm and improve the quality of healthcare. The importance of leadership, workplace culture and collaboration with patients, consumers and clinicians to develop processes, policies, standards and protocols to guide clinician decision-making and practice are essential to effective clinical governance. Leadership at all levels of the health organisation is vital to maximise the safety and effectiveness of care, reduce harm and ensure the workforce has the right qualifications, skills, expertise and supervision in order to deliver effective care in an environment that promotes safety and patient- and evidence-driven quality healthcare (ACSQHC, 2017).

The lack of effective governance and a poor workplace culture were identified as a leading cause of poor patient safety, outcomes and quality of care in the 2013 Mid Staffordshire NHS Foundation Trust Public Inquiry (Francis, 2013). The inquiry discovered systematic failures of care, leadership, transparency and accountability at multiple levels, which included:

- poor staff attitudes towards protecting patients from harm and unsafe care
- diffused responsibility for resolving problems, organisational culture of obviating responsibility and accountability
- widespread willingness to tolerate poor standards of patient care
- a failure to recognise and respond to legitimate patient, career and staff complaints
- communication failures and failure to share concerns or issues
- organisational goals prioritised over providing quality patient care
- financial spending directed away from delivering patient care towards achieving organisational recognition.

To continually improve clinical quality and safety requires a culture and environment that supports, values and develops its staff, and encourages consumer (patient) input, placing patient and staff safety as the number one priority.

evidence-based practice The process of making conscientious and judicious clinical decisions based upon proven evidence, combined with clinical experience and patient expectations.

However, individual healthcare professionals also need to continuously develop their professional practice standards; ensuring that their practice is **evidence-based** and aligned with the roles and responsibilities outlined within their contract of employment, their code of professional practice and their education and training (Travaglia et al., 2011).

Risk management is about improving the safety of care and proactively or reactively reducing injury to patients, consumers, staff and visitors by identifying, assessing, prioritising and ensuring action is taken to eliminate or minimise harm to others (Card et al., 2014). Auditing activities involved in the delivery of care form a large part of risk management. Clinical audit is integral to refining clinical practice and improving the quality and safety of care by observing and comparing practice with evidence-based standards. Auditing is a process that first begins with describing the issue of concern, setting standards or outcomes to be achieved based on a critical review of best evidence, observation of practice and data capture, and implementing change based upon the analysis of the data obtained to achieve the standard/outcome set (Benjamin, 2008). Further audits may be undertaken to evaluate the impact and success of the changes implemented (Figure 4.2).

One of the first clinicians said to have undertaken a clinical audit was Florence Nightingale, who sought to improve patient survival following surgery. Following the auditing of ward cleanliness and the management of surgical instruments, Florence Nightingale implemented strict sanitary routines and hygiene standards (hand-washing, doffing of overcoats prior to surgery, cleaning of medical equipment), which reduced patient mortality from 60 per cent to 42.7 per cent (Spiegelhalter, 1999). Continued auditing of sanitary and hygiene practices, and ensuring that only clean fresh water was used, together with introducing fresh

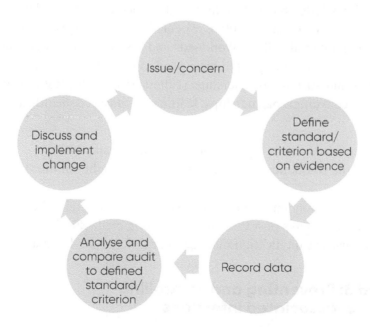

Figure 4.2 Clinical audit cycle

fruit and vegetables into patients' diets, further decreased patient mortality to 2.2 per cent, and reduced length of stay in hospital from 49 to 24 days (Gill & Gill 2005; Paton et al., 2015; Stanley, 2007).

Standard 2: Partnering with consumers

There is a growing recognition and acceptance of the need to embrace patient-centred care approaches in the development, implementation, measurement and evaluation of healthcare (Kitson et al., 2013). Dissatisfaction among consumers regarding their experience of healthcare has been the major catalyst in changing the delivery of care from a throughput-driven process to being more explicitly focused on the needs of the consumer (Batalden et al., 2016). This shift in focus has led clinicians and leaders of healthcare organisations to work in partnership with consumers to redesign and improve the effectiveness and quality of care delivery, and to communicate with patients and consumers in a way that supports effective partnerships, engagement and understanding (i.e. health literacy) (Bailey et al., 2015). Partnerships allow for diverse thinking and values to be shared, and have become the cornerstone of quality of care improvement (Doyle et al., 2013). At the organisational level, incorporating patient and consumer experiences and experiential knowledge has led to improved service design and delivery (Bate & Robert, 2006; Crawford et al., 2002), especially chronic disease services (Doyle et al., 2013; Pomey et al., 2015). Workloads and resources have been shared, new service models created and people motivated to contribute at every level, which in turn drives and sustains partnerships (Elliott et al., 2016; Rathert et al., 2013). Examples of consumer partnerships leading to positive healthcare outcomes include:

- cardiovascular disease symptom control (Arnetz et al., 2010)
- improving the frequency of physical activity and quality of life (Hanssen et al., 2007)
- reducing admission rates following myocardial infarction, heart failure and pneumonia at 30 days post discharge (Boulding et al., 2011)
- improving patient medication management (Nicholson Thomas et al., 2017).

Standard 3: Preventing and controlling healthcare-associated infections

Healthcare-associated infections (HAI) are the most common complications for consumers in hospital each year, and at least half of these infections are preventable (Russo et al., 2015). Historically called a 'nosocomial' infection, meaning 'hospital acquired', the term 'healthcare' is now used in recognition that today, much healthcare occurs outside a hospital. Many HAIs result in significant **morbidity** and **mortality**. It is estimated that in Europe and North America, 12–32 per cent of HAI are bloodstream infections causing death. In Australia, while the exact figure is unknown, it has been suggested that 175,000 HAIs occur annually (Russo et al., 2015). At present, there is no national HAI surveillance system in Australia.

> **healthcare-associated infection (HAI)** An infection that occurs as a result of a healthcare intervention.
> **morbidity** Refers to how often a disease occurs within a population.
> **mortality** Refers to the incidence of death in a population.

Local healthcare organisations must have systems in place to minimise and prevent patients from acquiring HAIs, and to effectively manage infections when they occur by using evidence-based strategies (ACSQHC, 2017). Strategies to prevent and manage infections include:

- audits to identify gaps in practice
- monitoring of high-risk practices (e.g. handling of infective agents)
- hand hygiene
- staff training in the use of personal protective equipment
- procedures for cleaning and decontamination of equipment (if not single use), and the healthcare environment (e.g. ward, theatres) in accordance with current best evidence-based practice
- the use of antimicrobial therapies (antibiotics, antivirals, etc.) as appropriate and where such use is evidence-based.

Further, patients who have acquired a HAI must be immediately identified and receive the appropriate management and treatment, including providing information to those affected, including family members and consumers.

Standard 4: Medication safety

Medicines are the most common treatment used in healthcare, and as a result are associated with a higher incidence of error and adverse events. Many of these events are costly and potentially avoidable. Medication-related adult presentations to the emergency department account for 3.3 to 7.2 per cent of attendees (AIHW, 2015a). Approximately 230,000 hospital admissions per year are associated with medication-related issues, with the cost estimated to be $1.2 billion per year (Roughead et al., 2016).

The risks associated with medication are most often errors in delivery, where the wrong medication is prescribed or used, or the correct medication is used inappropriately. These risks are known as adverse drug or medicine events, and often concern high-risk medications. High-risk medications can be remembered by the acronym A PINCH: Antibiotics, Potassium, Insulin, Narcotics, Chemotherapy, Heparin. Safe use of medication involves obtaining an accurate medication history, including any known allergies, selecting and reviewing currently prescribed medication based upon best evidence, documenting and communicating a clear medication management plan, and dispensing and administering medicines to informed patients and carers.

Confusion between drug names is increasingly associated with medication errors (Emmerton et al., 2015). Misreading medication names that look alike, or mishearing medication names that sound alike, have been attributed to up to 25 per cent of medication errors (Committee on Identifying and Preventing Medication Errors, 2007). Confusion between 'lookalike, sound-alike' medication names (e.g. Diprivan (propofol, an anaesthetic) and Ditropan (an anticholinergic/antispasmodic agent)) have also led to patient death. In one study, 5 per cent of deaths were attributed to brand name confusion and 4 per cent to generic name confusion (Garcia et al. 2017). Various approaches have been made to decrease confusion: tall-man lettering (amLODIPine, aMILoride); use of generic prescribing using international non-proprietary names so patients and clinicians can relate to one name only (Duerden & Hughes, 2010); harmonising Australian medicine names with international names (see Appendix 2); and redesigning medication package labelling (Garcia et al., 2017).

A further major cause of medication errors concerns the use of abbreviations, terminology and dose expressions when prescribing (Cheragi et al., 2013). A large study conducted at an urban US teaching hospital found that over one in four (29%) prescriptions contained dangerous abbreviations prone to misinterpretation (Garbutt et al., 2005). To improve medication safety in relation to medication prescribing, recommendations have been put forward to improve consistent prescribing terminology, including acceptable terminology and dose expression (ACSQHC, 2011, pp. 1–8):

1 Do not use jargon; use plain English (e.g. do not use 'Pink lady' when referring to the combination of lignocaine syrup and an antacid, Mylanta™).
2 Write in full; do not abbreviate, or use Latin phrases.
3 Print all text—especially drug names.
4 Use generic drug names. If a specific brand of medication is required, this should be printed in brackets following the generic drug name (e.g. 'Telmisartan (Micardis)').

5 Write drug names in full (e.g. use carbamazepine not CBZ).

6 Do not use chemical names or symbols, as these may be easily mistaken for other agents (e.g. HCl (hydrochloric acid or hydrochloride) may be mistaken for KCl (potassium chloride)).

7 Dose:
  – Use words or Hindu-Arabic numbers (e.g. 1, 2, 3) instead of Roman numerals (e.g. I, II, III, which could be misinterpreted as 1, 11 or 111).
  – Use metric units only (e.g. g, mg, mL).
  – For doses less than 1, write a zero in front of a decimal point (e.g. use 0.5 mg not .5 mg, as this may be mistaken for 5 mg).
  – Do not use trailing zeros (e.g. do not use 2.0 mg as this may be mistaken for 20 mg).
  – Oral liquid preparations must be expressed in weight as well as volume (e.g. 'Methadone syrup 20 mg (4 mL) once daily only').

8 Avoid using fractions.

9 Do not use symbols such as < or >; instead write instructions in full (e.g. 'less than' or 'more than').

10 Avoid acronyms or abbreviations for medical terms and procedure names on orders or prescriptions.

The national **Medication Management Plan** (MMP) is a standardised form for documenting medicines taken prior to presentation at the hospital and for reconciling patients' medicines. It has been designed for use by nursing, medical, pharmacy and allied health staff to improve the accuracy of information recorded on admission, and to be available to the clinician responsible for therapeutic decision-making. The form contains checklists to assist staff in obtaining a comprehensive medication history, identifying medication risks for the patient and determining which patients would benefit from a home medicines review post discharge (ACSQHC, 2013a).

Standard 5: Comprehensive care

Care is a social process, the result of complex interactions between the care provider (e.g. nurse, physician), the health organisation (e.g. clinic, **Nurse Navigator**) and care receiver (e.g. patient, community) that direct actions and responses

Medication Management Plan
A national, standardised chart used by nursing, medical, pharmacy and allied health staff to improve the accuracy of medication documentation and administration.

Nurse Navigators
Registered nurses who have an in-depth understanding of the health system, including disease-specific knowledge, who engage, guide and support patients with complex health conditions that require a high degree of comprehensive, clinical care.

and are fundamental to quality, comprehensive care (Grimmer et al., 2015). Comprehensive care is an approach that identifies, plans and coordinates health-care in partnership with patients and consumers around their physical, mental and cognitive needs, and evolves across the lifespan, including end-of-life (ACSQHC, 2017). Leadership, teamwork and collaboration with patients and consumers is the pivot of contemporary healthcare policy—one that has the potential to signif-icantly improve the safety and quality of care (Figure 4.3).

Features associated with effective and efficient comprehensive care include:

cognitive This term relates to the conscious processes of perception, imagining, memory, judgement, reasoning and communication. Cognitive impairment may be related to infections (e.g. sepsis), vitamin deficiency, medications or dementia.

- actively engaging patients, carers and families as partners in care planning to conduct a comprehensive assessment of the patient's health conditions, treatments, preferences, goals and potential risks (Naylor et al., 2013)
- evidence-based care planning and monitoring to meet the patient's physical, mental and **cognitive**-related needs and preferences, and continuous interactive education and coaching of patients, carers and families to engage and recognise problems early to avoid loss of symptom control, emergency visits and hospitalisations (Berry-Millett & Bodenheimer, 2009)

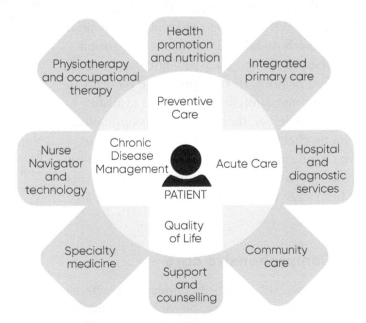

Figure 4.3 Comprehensive care model

- promoting and optimising the central role of the patients', carers' and family members' active engagement in care (Levine et al., 2010)
- timely, two-way communication among all the professionals engaged in a patient's care, especially during transitions from the hospital (Naylor et al., 2013)
- assessing and addressing health inequities, especially for populations known to be at higher risk of hospitalisation, including Aboriginal and Torres Strait Islander people (AIHW, 2015c), frail elderly people, people living in rural and remote locations (AIHW 2016), people from culturally and linguistically diverse backgrounds, and people of low socio-economic status and health literacy (Berkman et al., 2011).

Gaps in safety and quality are frequently reported as failures in implementing evidence-based strategies and practices to prevent and minimise the risk of harm, such as pressure injury and falls.

Pressure injury is considered one of the most common causes of **iatrogenic** harm to patients (State Government of Victoria, 2006), with an estimated treatment cost of A\$983 million per annum (Nguyen et al., 2015). Pressure injuries are localised areas of damage to the skin and/or underlying tissues caused by unrelieved pressure or friction. They commonly develop over bony prominences; however, they can develop anywhere on the body (Figure 4.4).

> **iatrogenic** Refers to an illness, injury or negative patient outcome caused by clinician activity or treatment.

Pressure areas are associated with prolonged immobility (such as prolonged bed rest) as well as poor nutrition, poor skin integrity and a lack of available oxygen to the tissues. Pressure areas are generally preventable. Patients should be screened on presentation and pressure-prevention strategies must be implemented when clinically indicated. Patients and carers should also be informed of the risks, prevention strategies and management of pressure injuries (ACSQHC, 2017).

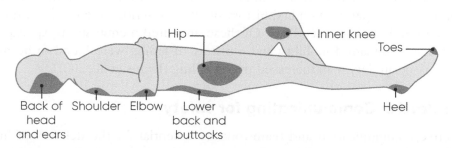

Figure 4.4 Common sites for the development of pressure sores

The estimated number of hospitalised injury cases due to falls in people aged 65 and over in 2009–10 was 83,768, up 7 per cent (n=5162) from the previous year (Bradley, 2012). Fall-related hospitalisations account for one in every ten days spent in hospital (1.3 million patient days over a year) of the same consumer age group, with an average hospital length of stay of 15.5 days. The cost to the Australian health system due to fall-related injuries is considerable, with a conservative estimate of $648.2 million. According to the Australian Institute of Health and Welfare (Bradley, 2014), women accounted for the majority (n=58,171; 69%) of fall-related injuries and hospitalisations. Typically, fall-related injury cases resulted in injuries to the hip and femur, with the majority (n=17,666; 21.1%) of these being hip fractures. Almost 70 per cent of hospitalised falls in 2009–10 occurred either at home or at an aged care facility, with falls due to slipping, tripping and stumbling being the most common circumstance (n=27,347; 32.6%).

In terms of morbidity and mortality, almost 25 per cent of persons aged 65 and over who suffer a fall-related hip fracture will die. Of those who survive, about one-third do not reach their pre-fracture level of functioning within a year post-fracture, and those who do recover tend to take around six months to return to their pre-fracture level of functioning (Bertram et al., 2011; LeBlanc et al., 2011). The impact of falling extends beyond the physical damage. A fall can result in loss of confidence, increased hesitancy and tentativeness, leading to loss of mobility, activity and independence. The risk of falling increases in people with impaired vision, poor balance, muscle weakness or reduced bone density, and those affected by certain medications.

falls risk screen Refers to a brief process to estimate the level of falls risk of a patient.

Identifying patients at risk of falls begins with assessment. A **falls risk screen** is a brief estimation of a person's risk of falling, usually classifying people as being either at low risk or increased risk. A falls risk assessment is a more detailed process that is used to identify underlying risk factors and the development of a detailed care plan to reduce risk. Falls risk assessment tools commonly consist of several key items: impaired mental status, impaired mobility, history of falls, prescribed medications, special toileting needs and advanced age. Of these, impaired mental status, special toileting needs, impaired mobility and a history of falling were found to be more closely associated with an increased risk of falling (Evans et al., 2001).

Standard 6: Communicating for safety

Effective communication and teamwork are essential for the delivery of high-quality, safe patient care. The delivery of care involves numerous people with varying levels of educational and occupational training, from doctors, nurses and allied health professionals, to the patient, their carers and family. However, ineffective communication among the healthcare team is one of the leading causes of errors and patient harm (Wong et al., 2008; Jorm et al., 2009). When health care professionals are not communicating effectively, patient safety is at risk for several reasons: lack of critical information, misinterpretation of information, and overlooked changes in status. It is vital that systems and processes are in place at times when effective communication and documentation are critical to patient safety, such as procedure matching and clinical handover.

Correctly identifying patients whenever care is provided and correctly matching patients to their intended treatment are essential to providing and receiving safe care. However, it does not always happen. Tragically, procedures have been performed on the wrong person, the wrong part of the patient's body, and medication administration errors have been made (WHO, 2007). Healthcare workers, administrators and technicians perform identification procedures so routinely that it is often seen as unimportant until errors are made. At least three patient identifiers must be used when providing care or therapies, and when confirming and transferring care responsibilities. Approved patient identifiers include name (family and given names), date of birth, gender, address and medical record number (ACSQHC, 2017).

Clinical handover is the 'transfer of professional responsibility and accountability for some or all aspects of care for a patient to another person or professional group on a temporary or permanent basis' (National Patient Safety Agency, 2004, p. 7). It involves the transfer of patient information, between individuals or groups. Relevant information includes:

- assessment findings
- any requests from the patient
- plans of care and changes in management.

Handover is an important part of clinical care. A breakdown in the transfer of information or communication can contribute to serious adverse events (Pascoe et al., 2014). Poor handovers can lead to a waste of resources, delays in diagnosis, treatment and care, repetition of tests, missed results, incorrect treatment and medication errors (Thomas et al., 2013). The information that is transferred between healthcare organisations should include all relevant data, be accurate and occur in a timely manner. Nurses provide care to patients on a 24-hour basis, so effective shift-to-shift communication is crucial. Clinical handover systems and processes can be implemented that include patients and carers (Nagpal et al., 2010), such as ISBAR (see Table 6.1 in Chapter 6).

Standard 7: Blood management

The donation and clinical use of blood and blood products has changed considerably over the last few decades. Ever-increasing regulatory controls, similar to those in the manufacturing of pharmaceuticals (i.e. medications), ensures that all aspects of blood collection, processing and storage are undertaken to the highest possible standard to safeguard patients and clinicians. The incorporation of pre-donation risk assessments, improved detection of pathogens that can be transmitted through blood, and development of technologies to enhance the quality of blood and blood products, have led to a substantial reduction in potential risks and complications associated with blood transfusion (Green et al., 2015). However, the transfusion of blood and blood products is not without risk, and can lead to complications and adverse outcomes for patients. Blood and blood products include fresh blood components, red blood cells, platelets, fresh and frozen plasma, cryoprecipitate and cryo-depleted plasma. Blood products also include plasma derivatives and recombinant products such as albumin, immunoglobulins and clotting factors.

The main areas that jeopardise safe transfusion are incorrect identification of the patient, leading to blood collection from the wrong patient; incorrectly labelling blood sample tubes; and no bedside verification that the blood being collected or administered is from or to the correct patient (Bolger & Moss, 2015). This standard requires that governance systems and procedures be put in place to ensure safe and appropriate prescribing and clinical use of blood and blood products, including receiving, storing, transporting and monitoring wastage of blood and blood products (ACSQHC, 2017). Further, systems and strategies must be implemented to ensure that the clinical workforce accurately records a patient's blood and blood product transfusion history and indications for use, and that patients and carers are informed of the risks and benefits of using blood and/or blood products and optional alternatives when a plan of treatment is developed.

Standard 8: Recognising and responding to clinical deterioration in acute healthcare

Evidence shows that the warning signs of clinical deterioration are not always identified, delaying treatment and resulting in adverse outcomes for the consumer (Jacques et al., 2006). Common factors associated with medical staff failing to observe a patient's deterioration include:

- a lack of monitoring of vital signs relevant to the patient's condition

- not understanding early and late changes (warning signs) in vital signs that could signal deterioration
- diffused responsibility and lack of awareness of the systems and processes in place for responding to deterioration
- a lack of knowledge and skills to manage patients who are deteriorating
- a failure to communicate clinical concerns
- low staffing levels (Ball et al., 2013).

More than 100 different early-warning systems have been developed (Churpek et al., 2013). Questions have been raised about the accuracy, sensitivity, specificity and utility of scoring algorithms and variation in physiologic parameters and thresholds as part of early-warning systems in relation to improving patient outcomes (Cuthbertson et al., 2007). However, there is strong evidence that implementing and embedding early-warning systems lowers cardiopulmonary arrest events, thereby lowering patient mortality and improving patient safety (Mathukia et al., 2015; Smith et al., 2014).

RISK MANAGEMENT, MONITORING AND REPORTING MECHANISMS

The potential, or risk, for harm to patients must be considered throughout the entire healthcare process. Risk management refers to the process of identification, analysis, evaluation and implementation of strategies to **mitigate** the identified risk, and ongoing monitoring and review (Sun et al., 2011). The goals of successful risk management include (ACHS, 2013):

> **mitigate** To lessen or make less severe.

- reducing the possibility of harmful events to patients, consumers, staff and service
- reducing the risk of injury, disease or death to patients, consumers, staff due to services provided by the organisation
- improving patient outcomes
- managing resources judiciously and competently.

Any activity within a health organisation that involves risk to a patient or staff member must be managed. All health organisations are required to maintain a register of organisational risks, and implement a functional system for the identification and management of risk. The risk-management policy should clearly state (ACHS, 2013):

- who is responsible for reporting a risk and taking action
- what information must be reported
- how risks, the assessment findings and the management plan are reported to clinicians and relevant departments of the health organisation
- how information is to be stored and accessed
- what tools and processes are to be utilised—for example, risk registers.

SPECIALTY NURSING CLINICAL PRACTICE STANDARDS

Specialist nursing standards and competencies have been developed in an ad hoc manner by special interest groups and colleges in Australia. Unlike specialty medical education, there has been no recognised accreditation structure for nursing specialty education and/or professional development programs until recently. In Australia, the interests of specialty practice in nursing and midwifery, as with other disciplines, is often represented by organisations and colleges. An increasing trend is for such groups to develop position statements, policies and competency standards that reflect their view of best practice in relation to their practice arena. The scope of such documents may include standards (however titled) related to professional practice, educational preparation and clinical practice.

Specialty nursing and midwifery associations that provide such resources include:

- the Discharge Planning Association Inc.
- the Australian College of Critical Care Nursing
- the Australian College of Children and Young People's Nurses
- the Australian Nurse Teachers' Society
- the College of Emergency Nursing of Australasia
- the Congress of Aboriginal and Torres Strait Islander Nurses and Midwives
- the Council of Remote Area Nurses of Australia
- Drug and Alcohol Nurses of Australasia
- the Australasian College for Infection Prevention and Control Association
- the National Enrolled Nurse Association
- Coalition of National Nursing & Midwifery Organisations
- the NSW Midwives Association Inc.
- the New South Wales Nursing and Midwives Association
- the Australian College of Operating Room Nurses
- the Professional Association of Nurses in Developmental Disability Areas (Australia) Inc.

- the Renal Society of Australasia
- the Australian Wound Management Association.

THE AUSTRALIAN NURSING AND MIDWIFERY FEDERATION

The Australian Nursing and Midwifery Federation of Australia (ANMF) is the national union for nurses and midwives. The main focus of the ANMF is to provide representation for its members in industrial, professional and political matters relating to nursing and midwifery. The ANMF also seeks to provide leadership in the areas of social welfare and social justice.

Core objectives of the union are to:

- promote, protect and support nursing and midwifery to ensure the health requirements of the Australian community are met
- ensure the industrial and professional interests of nurses and midwives are represented in Australia, and that workplace safety standards are adequate
- contribute to the health of the Australian community while positively influencing social welfare and social justice policy (ANMF, 2013a).

The ANMF is represented at the state level by sub-branches:

- *Victoria:* Australian Nursing & Midwifery Federation Victorian Branch
- *New South Wales:* NSW Nurses and Midwives Association
- *Queensland:* Queensland Nurses Union
- *South Australia:* Australian Nursing and Midwifery Federation (SA Branch)
- *Tasmania:* Australian Nursing and Midwifery Federation Tasmanian Branch
- *ACT:* Australian Nursing and Midwifery Federation Australian Capital Territory
- *Northern Territory:* Australian Nursing and Midwifery Federation Northern Territory
- *Western Australia:* Australian Nursing and Midwifery Federation Western Australia Branch.

The sub-branches also actively represent the professional, educational and industrial welfare of nurses working at all levels, whether public or private, in their respective states. Being a member of your relevant ANMF branch gives you:

- access to confidential advice and assistance
- the benefit of a legal safety net—legal representation
- professional development opportunities

- occupational health and safety advice
- access to scholarships, and
- superannuation protection and advice (NSWNMA, 2017).

REGISTRATION STANDARDS FOR OVERSEAS-QUALIFIED REGISTERED NURSES AND MIDWIVES

Australia is a diverse country that welcomes professionals from all across the globe. To enable overseas nurses and/or midwives to be recognised and registered to practise in Australia, the Australian Nursing & Midwifery Accreditation Council (ANMAC) has developed standards for the assessment of internationally qualified nurses and midwives for registration and migration (ANMAC, 2010, 2012, 2013), which are available online. ANMAC uses five criteria to determine suitability for migration to Australia:

1 The applicant establishes their identity.
2 The applicant meets the English language proficiency test for nursing and midwifery professions.
3 The applicant is assessed as meeting current Australian nursing and midwifery education standards.
4 The applicant proves their recency of nursing or midwifery practice.
5 The applicant demonstrates that they are 'fit to practise' nursing and/or midwifery in Australia.

These criteria have also been ratified and approved by the Nursing and Midwifery Board of Australia (NMBA, 2015a), and are referred to as core assessment criteria.

Establishing identity

To ensure that the person applying for registration is the person named and referred to in the supporting documents, the applicant must provide:

- photographic evidence that they are the person seeking registration (e.g. passport)
- the most up-to-date documents attesting to current professional registrations, or eligibility with a recognised international nursing and midwifery regulatory authority
- submitted evidence that matches the name stated on verified qualifications. If a name change has occurred, evidence of that name change needs to be

provided—for example, a marriage certificate or change of name certificate (ANMAC, 2010).

English language proficiency

All internationally qualified applicants must demonstrate English language proficiency. Proficiency can be demonstrated by providing evidence of completing five years of full-time tertiary and secondary education; tertiary and vocational education; combined tertiary, secondary and vocational education; or tertiary education taught in English (NMBA, 2015b) from one or more recognised countries, as outlined in section 49(1) of the Health Practitioner Regulation National Law (in force in each state and territory). This is also to include a minimum of two years of full-time study in an equivalent pre-registration nursing or midwifery program of study by the recognised nursing/midwifery regulatory body in any of the recognised countries: Australia, Canada, New Zealand, Republic of Ireland, South Africa, United Kingdom or United States of America.

Alternatively, applicants can demonstrate proficiency in the English language by completing the International English Language Testing System (IELTS) academic module, Occupational English Test (OET), Pearson Test of English (PTE) or Test of English as a Foreign Language (TOEFL). A minimum overall score of 7 and a minimum score of 7 in each of the four components (listening, reading, writing and speaking) is required to pass the IELTS test. With regard to the OET examination, applicants must score a minimum of B in listening, reading, writing and speaking. In the PTE English language test, applicants are required to achieve a minimum score of 65 in each communication skill. Applicants sitting the TOEFL test must achieve a minimum total score of 94 and obtain a minimum score in each section: 24 listening; 24 reading; 27 writing; and 23 speaking. ANMAC only accepts test results from one test sitting or a maximum of two test sittings in a six-month period; however, there are further restrictions depending upon what English language test has been taken. ANMAC accepts test results that are up to two years old.

The Nursing and Midwifery Board of Australia may grant an exemption where the applicant applies for limited registration in specialist circumstances, such as:

- to perform a demonstration in clinical techniques
- to undertake research that involves limited or no patient contact
- to undertake a period of postgraduate study or supervised training while working in an appropriately supported environment, which will ensure patient safety is not compromised.

The following are some useful information sites:

- www.ielts.org
- http://occupationalenglishtest.org
- http://pearsonpte.com
- www.ets.org/toefl/ibt/about.

Education standards

For registration as a registered nurse within Australia, the minimum qualification must be a university-based Bachelor degree, equivalent to six semesters of full-time study. An exception to this is where an applicant has completed a postgraduate nursing qualification in addition to a previous non-nursing/midwifery Bachelor degree. The nursing qualification is assessed against set NMBA-approved accreditation standards. Where appropriate, the NMBA may recommend that the international candidate undertake a bridging course, to meet missed standards (Table 4.1).

Table 4.1 Education providers for nursing

Education provider	Website
Australian universities	http://myuniversity.gov.au
TAFE NSW	www.tafensw.edu.au
TAFE Queensland	www.tafe.qld.gov.au
TAFE South Australia	www.tafe.sa.edu.au
TAFE Victoria	www.tafe.vic.gov.au
TAFE Western Australia	www.tafe.wa.edu.au
NSW Health	www.health.nsw.gov.au
Wodonga TAFE	www.wodongatafe.edu.au

RECENCY OF PRACTICE

It is recognised that nurses may take extended periods of time away from practice, to fulfil other pursuits such as a different career, raise children or care for family members. To ensure proficiency in nursing practice, nurses and midwives seeking registration, endorsement of registration or renewal of registration must demonstrate that they have maintained an adequate connection with, and recent practice in, nursing since qualifying for or obtaining registration. To meet the recency of practice requirements, you need to be able to demonstrate that you have practised for the equivalent of 450 hours in nursing over the past five years (NMBA, 2016d). This is the same for midwives. Dual-qualified nurses and midwives would need to be able to demonstrate 450 hours in nursing *and* midwifery in the past five years to meet the recency of practice requirements.

If you have not worked sufficient hours over the past five years to meet the recency of practice requirements, you will need to contact your local AHPRA office to get advice about your individual circumstances. Options may include successfully completing a supervised practice as approved by the NMBA, or a re-entry to practice program approved by the NMBA (2016d).

Summary

In this chapter, we have examined the requirements to practise as a nurse in Australia. We have noted that nurses must demonstrate 'fitness to practise' and that they must meet national competency standards for the registered nurse produced by the NMBA. We also outlined the Code of Professional Conduct for Nurses and the Code of Ethics. We next considered the importance of leadership for nurses and various leadership styles, as well as how leadership relates to coping with change. The importance of patient safety and the National Safety and Quality Health Service Standards were outlined, together with the principles of risk management, monitoring and reporting. We looked at specialty nursing clinical practice, the role of the ANMF and registration standards for overseas nurses. We concluded by considering recency of practice.

Review questions

4.1   Which board in Australia regulates nursing registration?
    a   AHPRA
    b   NMB
    c   DOH
    d   Your employer's nursing services board

4.2 How many standards form the National Competency Standards for Registered Nurses?
   a 3
   b 4
   c 5
   d 7

4.3 With regard to recency of practice, in what way can you demonstrate this annually?
   a Practise for the equivalent of 450 hours in nursing over the past five years
   b Pay your registration fees on time
   c Undertake further learning by completing a post-registration course

4.4 Which of the following sets out the minimum standards of professional conduct that nurses must demonstrate in their practice?
   a The Code of Professional Conduct for Nurses
   b The *Nursing Act 1980*
   c The *Healthcare Worker Act 2010*

4.5 The Code of Ethics for Nurses in Australia (2013a) outlines eight value statements. Which of the following is NOT a value statement?
   a Value the quality of nursing care for all people
   b Value informed consent
   c Value a culture of safety
   d Value evidence above patient choice

4.6 Which of the following schedules are likely to be encountered in private or public hospitals (you can answer with more than one response)?
   a Schedule 4
   b Schedule 4D
   c Schedule 8
   d Schedule 1

4.7 What level of educational qualification is required to become registered as a Registered Nurse in Australia?
   a Degree
   b Diploma
   c Certificate

5 NURSING AND THE LAW

Alister Hodge and Wayne Varndell

In this chapter, you will develop an understanding of:

- accountability and responsibility
- legal responsibilities for at-risk groups
- consent
- duty of care
- the mental health acts
- guardianship legislation
- medication and poisons legislation
- ethics in nursing.

ACCOUNTABILITY AND RESPONSIBILITY IN CLINICAL PRACTICE

Accountability means that 'nurses answer to the people in their care, the nursing regulatory authority, their employers and the public. Nurses are accountable for their decisions, actions, behaviours and the responsibilities that are inherent in their nursing roles including documentation' (NMBA, 2016e, p. 3). Accountability is an essential component of professional nursing practice and vital for patient safety, so it cannot be delegated. However, in order to be held accountable, there are some preconditions that need to be met: ability, responsibility, authority and autonomy (Burkhardt & Nathaniel, 2013).

Ability means that nurses are competent to carry out their role, and is dependent upon them having sufficient knowledge and skills to fulfil the requirements of that role or practice. The ANMAC, as the independent accrediting authority established under the Health Practitioner Regulation National Law for the nursing and midwifery professions in Australia, is responsible for ensuring that educational programs leading to registration and endorsement of nurses and midwives in Australia meet the NMBA approved standards for accreditation (Staunton & Chiarella, 2013). However, it is also the individual nurse's obligation, and that of the employing health organisation, to maintain competence and to have a contemporary knowledge and skill base in order to provide best-practice nursing care (NMBA, 2013d; ANMF, 2013a). Thus there are both collective and individual obligations within nursing to ensure that the workforce practises in a safe and competent manner.

Responsibility means an activity a person undertakes or is given to undertake and for which they are answerable (Batey & Lewis, 1982; Dohmann, 2009). As a result, nurses accept responsibility as part of their role for interventions that fall within an accepted scope of practice. Initial interventions that are accepted as falling within a nursing scope of practice are taught during pre-registration educational programs. As part of acquiring clinical experience, student nurses are required to assess, plan, implement and evaluate interventions under the supervision of a qualified Registered Nurse.

Supervision is an important concept to understand. Supervision encompasses elements of direct and indirect guidance. It is a formal process of professional support and learning that enables a practitioner (supervisee) to develop knowledge, skills and expertise. Direct supervision refers to when the supervisor takes direct and principal responsibility for the provision of nursing care and treatment of patients provided by a supervisee under the continual observance of the supervisor. Indirect supervision refers to when the supervisor, although present in the workplace, does not constantly observe the activities of the supervisee when undertaking nursing care and treatment. This level of supervision often occurs when the supervisee has significantly demonstrated growth and competence.

Within this context, while the student nurse is responsible for their actions relating to the intervention, the supervising qualified Registered Nurse is professionally accountable for the outcome, and must take reasonable steps to ensure that the intervention delegated does not compromise the safety or quality of care (ANMAC, 2010). The supervising qualified Registered Nurse must therefore ensure that the student is adequately prepared to undertake the intervention in a proficient manner, that the intervention being delegated is appropriate, that they are prepared to supervise the student, and that the patient is adequately informed and gives consent to the planned intervention. As nurses seek to expand their scopes of practice, the level of responsibility increases. However, it is a common misconception that doctors are ultimately responsible for the actions and therefore practice of nurses (Cashin et al., 2009). This belief continues to limit the expansion of nursing as well as other healthcare roles and scopes of practice. Nurses ultimately are responsible for their actions and omissions, and the quality and safety of care they provide (Kerridge et al., 2005).

Authority can be defined as sanctioned or legitimate power delegated to a nurse that allows the nurse to make decisions, and to perform role-related functions (Blanchfield & Biordi, 1996). The term 'authority' as opposed to 'power' has long been preferred, as for some power connotes negative images (Heineken, 1982). Authority is derived from several sources—for example, authority of expert knowledge and authority of position (Batey & Lewis, 1982). Authority of expert knowledge refers to specialist education and experience, such as completing an approved masters level qualification and sufficient advanced practice experience in order to be endorsed on the Register of Practitioners as a Nurse Practitioner (NMBA, 2014). Nurses authorised to practise as a Nurse Practitioner have additional authority tied to their position, such as the authority to assess, investigate, diagnose, admit, discharge and prescribe medications. This differs greatly from the authority held by a Clinical Nurse Specialist.

Autonomy can be defined as the freedom to independently carry out responsibilities without close supervision, and is closely linked to authority (Blanchfield & Biordi, 1996). For example, if nurses are authorised to make decisions and to act as judged necessary, nurses require autonomy to independently implement their responsibilities (Skår, 2010). The question of autonomy in nursing practice is still problematic. Autonomy is often regarded as being synonymous with independence and a lack of external control (Cushin et al., 2009). Autonomy in nursing, however, is about the right to practise in line with professional codes, standards and sound evidence. A nurse's autonomy is dependent upon the employer, the patient, society and government agencies and policies supporting the nurse's capacity for independent judgement; this can be defined as relational autonomy. Nurses, together with other healthcare providers, thus do not have absolute or unchecked autonomy; indeed, this would be undesirable and unethical, as healthcare providers must always practise with due care and awareness for the patient and the role played by other members of the healthcare team.

LEGAL RESPONSIBILITIES FOR AT-RISK GROUPS: ELDER ABUSE, CHILD ABUSE AND DOMESTIC VIOLENCE

Elder abuse

Elder abuse refers to any act within a relationship that contains an expectation of trust, which causes harm or distress to the older person. Abuse may take the form of neglect, or physical, financial, sexual, psychological or social abuse; however, the most common forms of elder abuse involve financial abuse and neglect (ANMF, 2014; Starr, 2010).

Elder abuse has only been recognised as a problem since the 1980s, and poor knowledge regarding what constitutes elder abuse has likely contributed to under-reporting or a lack of recognition. Elder abuse may occur in the community, residential care or hospital setting, and can be perpetrated by any person in close contact with the victim, such as a family member, friend or employed carer. It is thought to occur in up to 5 per cent of the population over 65 years of age (Kurrle, 2004).

Elder abuse is now recognised as a crime, with compulsory reporting of elder abuse introduced in the *Aged Care Act 2007* by the Commonwealth Government for all healthcare professionals (ANMF, 2014). The *Aged Care Act 2007* defines elder abuse that requires reporting as 'unlawful sexual contact, unreasonable use of force, or assault' (Starr, 2010).

Child abuse

Child abuse and neglect include 'all forms of physical and emotional ill-treatment, sexual abuse, neglect, and exploitation that results in actual or potential harm to the child's health, development or dignity in the context of a relationship of responsibility, trust or power' (ANMF, 2013b, p. 1). Nurses have a duty of care to children and their families, and an obligation in all states and territories to report reasonable suspicions that a child has been abused or neglected. They also play a key role in the prevention of future harm (ANMF, 2013b; Mathews et al., 2006; Simpson, 2014).

Child protection falls under state law, leading to some differences in terminology in the relevant legislation used between states. Penalties exist in each state for a failure of nurses to report an episode of child abuse. Most commonly, this is a monetary fine; however, in the Australian Capital Territory there is the possibility of up to six months' imprisonment. Provided the report of suspected child abuse is made in good faith, a nurse is granted immunity from legal liability in all states. This means that should abuse subsequently be found not to have taken place, the notifier is immune from legal action by the child's parents or guardian. The notifier's identity is also protected in all states (Mathews et al., 2006).

Domestic violence

Domestic violence is a major societal issue in Australia, as it is in many countries globally. In Australia, it is thought that one in three women will be a victim of physical or sexual assault in their lifetime (Hooker et al., 2012). Domestic violence can be defined as 'violent, abusive or intimidating behaviour carried out by an adult against a partner or former partner to control and dominate that person. Domestic violence causes fear, physical and/or psychological harm. It is most often violent, abusive, or intimidating behaviour by a man against a woman' (NSW Health, 2011a, p. 2). It can take the form of physical abuse, emotional/psychological/verbal abuse, sexual abuse, and social or economic abuse. Children and adolescents living with domestic violence are seriously affected by these events, so it is also considered a form of child abuse (Moylan et al., 2010).

People subjected to domestic violence often have frequent contact with health services, but the issue is rarely identified (NSW Health, 2011a). This prolongs the isolation of the person at risk, and results in a missed opportunity for intervention and prevention of further injury or, in some cases, death. People subjected to domestic violence will rarely initiate a discussion about their experience of violence unless specifically asked about it (NSW Health, 2011a), meaning that the responsibility lies with the clinician to actively seek information. Although there is no mandated reporting mechanism for domestic violence, as there is for child or elder abuse, a number of states have introduced formalised screening for domestic violence in specialty areas such as antenatal, early childhood health, mental health and drug and alcohol services (NSW Health, 2011a). Remember, in episodes of domestic violence where there are reasonable grounds to suspect that a child is at risk of harm, you are still mandated to report the risk of child safety to the relevant state authority (Boursnell & Prosser, 2010).

If an episode of domestic violence has been identified, a referral should be made to a social worker. In the advent of serious injuries (e.g. a gunshot wound, stabbing or broken bones), or where it is known that the assailant is armed or has made further threats, then the incident should also be reported to the police (Boursnell & Prosser, 2010).

CONSENT TO TREATMENT

The issue of consent is complex but fundamental to the provision of healthcare. The patient's right to choose who touches them and when, which professional advice to accept or reject, and what information is shared is protected by the ethical principle of autonomy (Avery, 2017), and reflected in local and international codes of nursing conduct (NMBA, 2013d; International Council of Nurses, 2012). Every adult must be assumed to have the capacity to make decisions unless it is proven otherwise. However, while most patients can make independent decisions regarding what treatment to accept, this is not always the case. Patients with reduced or absent capacity to make a decision may have to rely on healthcare professionals to make decisions on their behalf. Therefore, all healthcare professionals should be active patient advocates and be respectful of patient autonomy, ensuring that treatment delivered is in the patient's best interests.

Consent is defined and informed by several forms of legislation that govern the principles surrounding seeking, informing, obtaining and recording a person's approval to undertake a proposed course of action. Key legislation includes:

- state guardianship legislative acts (see Table 5.2)
- state child protection legislative acts
  - *Children and Young People Act 2008* (ACT)
  - *Children and Young Persons (Care and Protection) Act 1998* (NSW)
  - *Care and Protection of Children Act 2007* (NT)
  - *Child Protection Act 1999* (Qld)
  - *Children's Protection Act 1993* (SA)
  - *Children, Young Persons and their Families Act 1997* (Tas)
  - *Children, Youth and Families Act 2005* (Vic)
  - *Children and Community Services Act 2004* (WA)
- state mental health legislative acts (see Table 5.1)
- the *Family Law Act 1975* (Cth)
- state human tissue and transplant legislative acts
  - *Transplantation and Anatomy Act 1978* (ACT)
  - *Human Tissue Act 1983* (NSW)
  - *Human Tissue Transplant Act 1979* (NT)
  - *Transplantation and Anatomy Act 1979* (Qld)
  - *Transplantation and Anatomy Act 1983* (SA)
  - *Human Tissue Act 1982* (Vic)
  - *Human Tissue Act 1985* (Tas)
  - *Human Tissue and Transplant Act 1982* (WA)
- the *Australian Charter of Healthcare Rights* (ACSQHC, 2007).

The word 'consent' derives from the Latin word *consensere*, meaning 'to agree'; thus consent is an agreement between two parties, and requires a level of understanding (Staunton & Chiarella, 2013). Generally, no procedure or treatment may be undertaken without the consent of the patient if the patient is a competent adult. Adequately informing patients and obtaining consent regarding a procedure or treatment is both a specific legal requirement and an accepted part of good nursing practice. The absence of valid consent would render an otherwise legitimate act a crime, and could result in legal action for **assault** and/or **battery** against a clinician who performs the procedure or intervention.

Consent is not transferable to another practitioner, as the agreement for the procedure or treatment to take place (or contract) exists between the practitioner who requested permission and the patient who gave their consent. If a different healthcare practitioner proposes to undertake the procedure, then consent must be re-obtained. Additionally, consent is not expandable to other forms of treatment or procedures apart from what the patient has specifically granted. For example, if a patient has given valid consent to receive packed red blood cells, it does not mean that the practitioner can administer cryoprecipitate as well. Consent must also be acquired again prior to any subsequent episodes of the same intervention.

> **assault** A threat of bodily harm coupled with an apparent, present ability to cause the harm.
> **battery** The actual infliction of unlawful force or offensive contact with the 'person' of another—for example, touching a person's body.

Providing consent

Consent to treatment may be given in different forms: **implied consent**, verbal consent and written consent. Implied consent is most often used as a method of consenting to a minor procedure of 'common knowledge' (Staunton & Chiarella, 2013). Common knowledge refers to information that an average person would know and understand about the intended procedure (Westrick, 2013). An example of implied consent would be a nurse telling a patient that they need to take a blood sample from the patient, and the patient rolling up their sleeve and extending their arm out towards the nurse while pointing to the best place to locate a suitable vein. In this instance, the nurse has not specifically asked for the patient's consent to take the blood sample, but the patient's actions indicate that they understand the nature of the procedure and agree to it. While many clinical interactions with patients may occur based on implied consent—that is, the patient cooperates with you as you would expect from someone with knowledge of the procedure—it is entirely possible to over-estimate the level of the patient's understanding. The patient may be only partially aware of what is about to happen, or may continue to comply out of duress (e.g. pain, embarrassment, anxiety) or fear of reprisal. It is good practice to explore your patient's understanding of the intended procedure, likely outcome or possible complications,

> **implied consent** Consent that is not expressly granted by a person, but rather implicitly granted by their actions or inactions.

as it provides the opportunity to correct mistaken beliefs or partial accuracies (Wallace, 2014).

Verbal consent is the most common form of consent that occurs within the context of day-to-day nursing practice. Verbal consent is as valid as written consent, although verifying the validity by which consent was made is difficult (Staunton & Chiarella, 2013). Procedures requiring only verbal consent *must* be documented in detail in the patient's healthcare record. Documentation should reflect the four elements required for validating consent: (1) evidence of the patient's mental capacity to consent; (2) evidence that the patient has received the relevant information to make a decision; (3) specific consent for the procedure being given; and (4) no coercion or duress of the patient involved. Validating consent is discussed in further detail below.

Written consent is the most difficult to establish, as it is impossible to cover every outcome of the procedure. This style of consent often clashes with the third element in validating consent: being specific. For simpler procedures—for example, inserting an indwelling catheter—verbal or implied consent would be better.

Written consent is generally nothing more than documentary evidence of what has already been consented to verbally by the patient. Except for situations outlined within guardianship legislation, the law generally does not require consent or the provision of information, including warnings about material risks, to be documented in writing. Therefore, there is no legal principle that states that consent forms need to exist or be completed prior to commencing treatment, although there are now situations where written consent is required by policy. For example, in New South Wales written consent is required for the following procedures:

i   All operations or procedures requiring general, spinal, epidural, or regional anaesthesia or intravenous sedation;
ii Any invasive procedure or treatment where there are known significant risks or complications;
iii Blood transfusions or the administration of blood products;
iv Approved experimental treatment, unless there are sound reasons for doing otherwise (NSW Health, 2005b).

Consent obtained in writing can assist clinicians in any subsequent legal proceedings to demonstrate that treatment has been discussed with the patient and that consent has been obtained. However, written consent does not automatically guarantee that the consent obtained is valid.

Valid consent

As stated above, for consent to be valid, four elements *must* be present: (1) the patient must have the mental capacity to consent; (2) the individual must be supplied with the relevant information as far as practicable to make a decision; (3) consent must be specific and cover what is actually done; and (4) the patient must come to a decision without **coercion or duress**, and without deception (Staunton & Chiarella, 2013).

> **coercion or duress**
> Refers to a situation whereby an individual performs an act as a result of violence, threat or other pressure against them.

Any form of deception, however well intentioned, would invalidate consent. Some examples follow:

- A patient is admitted for drainage of an empyaema, and gives a past medical history of sharing needles with other intravenous drug users. During treatment, the admitting nurse receives a needle-stick injury while administering medication to the patient. The nurse, concerned about the possibility of being exposed to Hepatitis C and HIV, obtains consent to take a blood sample to test for anaemia, but also tests for hepatitis C and HIV serology without informing the patient.
- A patient is admitted with worsening pneumonia unresponsive to oral anti-biotics. The patient has a past medical history of bipolar disorder. During the morning medication round, the patient refuses to take prescribed antipsychotic medications, claiming they are contributing to a feeling of lethargy, but requests paracetamol to help reduce joint aches. The nurse then conceals the antipsychotic medication by dissolving it in the patient's water, which he drinks to swallow the paracetamol.

Capacity

Capacity is a key component in patient consent. Capacity refers to an individual's ability to understand the information provided, retain that information, be able to weigh up the benefits and informed risks, and communicate their decision adequately and without coercion (Avery, 2017). Every adult must be assumed to have the capacity to make decisions unless it is proven otherwise, even if their decision appears unwise or is contrary to professional advice. You cannot decide that someone lacks capacity based upon age, appearance, condition or behaviour alone. A person's capacity to make decisions may also be transient and situation specific. This means that a patient who cannot make decisions on some issues at a particular time may be able to make decisions on other issues or at other times (Staunton

& Chiarella, 2013). For example, a person with mild to moderate dementia may demonstrate capacity at certain times, and be able to make informed decisions in some areas, such as in relation to care and finance. Therefore, the capacity of a patient warrants continual assessment.

If the patient is found to be unable to complete any one of the four main elements of valid consent discussed above, valid consent cannot be obtained. It should also be emphasised that just because a person has a mental health disorder, this does not automatically mean that they are incapable of making a valid decision.

Example

Dave, a 69-year-old man, has been admitted to a ward from the emergency department with chronic cellulitis of the right lower leg and a low-grade fever. Dave has stated that he does not want any further treatment with intravenous antibiotics or surgical intervention and wants transport to take him back home. A case conference is held with Dave, his treating physician and the nurse in charge of the shift. During the discussion, the treating physician asks Dave to describe his current health, and what the priorities of care are for him. Dave can describe his past medical history, which includes diabetes, hypertension, obesity and chronic lower leg oedema. Dave goes on to describe the growing frequency with which he is brought into hospital due to recurring cellulitis. Dave states that he wants to return home as he cannot sleep and doesn't like being in hospital. The nurse in charge asks Dave to describe what the outcome could be if the infection was not treated. In response, Dave acknowledges that the infection might get worse to the point of needing amputation or even result in his death. The treating physician confirms Dave's assessment of his current health and likely outcome if the leg infection is not treated. In exploring other ways to provide treatment for the leg cellulitis, it is suggested to Dave that intravenous antibiotics could be provided at his home if he is willing to allow community nurses to visit. Dave likes this option; however, the treating physician asks whether Dave would be willing to stay in hospital for just one more day to allow for the results of blood tests to be considered, referrals to be completed and the community nursing team to attend the ward to develop a treatment plan. Dave stresses that he cannot stay one more night and wants to go home. The physician outlines the risks of leaving without knowing the full extent of the infection and whether the community nursing team would be able to attend for his next dose of intravenous antibiotics. Dave is adamant that he wants to go home.

- Has Dave demonstrated capacity sufficiently?
- How would you manage this issue?

Informed decision-making

Informed decision-making refers to the information or advice given to the patient to enable them to make a balanced judgement prior to any action being undertaken. The information provided must encompass the nature of the procedure and its purpose. A clinician competent to undertake the intervention should discuss potential complications and their management.

When is consent not required?

If a person is incapable of giving consent with respect to their treatment, substitute consent is required. A person responsible for the patient's wellbeing, as described in state and territory guardianship legislation, can give consent (see Table 5.2). Treatment that is considered urgent to save a person's life can be carried out without the consent of the patient if the patient is determined not to be competent to refuse medical advice. Non-urgent or minor treatment may still be provided if:

- there is no person responsible for the patient, or
- that person cannot be contacted, or
- that person does not wish to make a decision regarding treatment.

However, the clinician providing the treatment must document that the treatment was necessary to promote the patient's health and wellbeing, and that the patient has not made known their objection to the carrying out of the treatment (Batey & Lewis, 1982).

Doctrine of necessity

When a patient requires urgent, time-critical treatment, and is so incapacitated as to be incapable of providing valid consent (e.g. the patient is unconscious), you may have to initiate treatment that you believe is reasonable and necessary in the circumstances, under the common law 'doctrine of necessity' (Forrester & Griffiths, 2014). Doctrine of necessity is also known as 'doctrine of emergency'; however, the necessity principle is separate from the emergency principle, and has wider applications (Wallace, 2014). Doctrine of necessity essentially provides a defence to an action (e.g. inserting an intravenous cannula, or creating an artificial airway) that could otherwise be defined as assault and battery (Avery, 2017). However, as stated, the 'necessity' and the 'emergency' are two separate conditions that have to be satisfied before such a defence is justifiable (Staunton & Chiarella, 2013). To apply this justification, there must be a necessity to act when it is not practicable to communicate with the patient. While the term 'emergency' is not defined within common law, it has been described in case law as a treatment necessary 'to save life' or to 'prevent serious injury to their health' (*Murry v McMurchy* [1949] DLR (BC SC)). Further, the circumstances must indicate that the treatment is necessary and not merely convenient, and that the action that is taken is based upon evidence-based practice (*T v T* [1988] FamD 2 WLR 189).

DUTY OF CARE

Wherever there is a nurse–patient relationship, a duty of care will exist (Burkhardt & Nathaniel, 2013). However, a duty of care is not owed universally, and the existence of a duty of care must be proven. The legal test as to whether a duty of care exists was laid down in the case of *Donoghue v Stevenson* ([1932] AC 562 at 619). Lord Atkin stated that reasonable care should be taken to avoid acts or omissions that could foreseeably lead to injury or harm to those who are closely and directly affected by an individual's actions. Therefore, a duty of care can be said to exist if you can see that your actions are reasonably likely to cause harm to another person.

To ascertain whether a breach of duty has occurred, the 'reasonable man' test is applied (*Blyth v Birmingham Waterworks Co* [1856] 11 Exch 781). The reasonable man test compares the actions of the person under examination with that of another person, under the same circumstances. If it is considered that in the same circumstances a reasonable person would have acted in the same way, then it can be said that the action taken was reasonable and that there has been no breach of duty of care.

THE MENTAL HEALTH LEGISLATION

Mental healthcare in Australia is provided by a combination of specialised public mental health services and mental health professionals. Services are regulated by the relevant state or territory mental health legislation. In Australia, general practitioners are more frequently consulted by people with an ongoing mental health illness (70.8%), compared with psychologists (37.7%) and psychiatrists (22.7%). Almost half of the Australian population (45.5%) experiences mental illness at some point in their lifetime. Hospital admissions account for 2.6 per cent of the services used for mental health problems (ABS, 2007).

To work effectively with individuals experiencing mental health problems, nurses require a sound understanding of mental health legislation (Elder et al., 2009). Australia has developed national strategies, policies and standards in line with World Health Organization (WHO) principles, which are access, equity, effectiveness and efficiency. Together they enable healthcare professions to actively engage in caring for those experiencing mental illnesses. Each Australian state and territory has mental health legislation designed to protect individuals experiencing mental illness from inappropriate treatment; direct the provision of mental healthcare and the facilities in which it is provided; and instruct the practice of mental health professionals in principles of treatment and care (Table 5.1).

The term 'mentally ill person' means that the person has one or a number of symptoms set out in the mental health legislation, and as a consequence presents a risk of serious harm to themselves or others. These symptoms include hallucinations, delusions, serious thought disorder, serious mood disorder or sustained irrational behaviour suggesting the presence of one of these symptoms. A 'mentally disordered person' is a person whose behaviour is so irrational that they place themselves or someone else at risk of serious physical harm. People may also be admitted to a hospital following apprehension by the police if found

Table 5.1 Mental health legislation by jurisdiction

Jurisdiction	Legislation
Australian Capital Territory	*Mental Health Act 2015*
New South Wales	*Mental Health Act 2007*
Northern Territory	*Mental Health and Related Services Act 2004*
Queensland	*Mental Health Act 2000*
South Australia	*Mental Health Act 2009*
Tasmania	*Mental Health Act 2013*
Victoria	*Mental Health Act 2014*
Western Australia	*Mental Health Act 2014*

committing a criminal offence or engaging in self-harming behaviour. A person cannot be regarded as either mentally ill or disordered based upon the presence or lack of religious beliefs, personal philosophy or sexual preference/orientation; past or current involvement in sexual promiscuity, immoral or illegal conduct; or because the person has a development disability, takes or has taken alcohol or any other drug; or engages in anti-social behaviour.

Australian mental health legislation details the basis of admission and treatment of persons experiencing mental illness, the detention and review processes concerning persons held involuntarily, and the rights of persons being treated for mental health problems. The rights of clients experiencing mental illness include:

- the right to dignity, privacy and confidentiality of all information about their care
- the right to live and work in the community
- protection of minors and others deemed not able to give informed consent

voluntary client
An individual who voluntarily complies with treatment or action.

- the right to treatment as a **voluntary client** wherever possible by those specifically qualified to provide such care in approved mental health facilities
- the right to receive appropriate medical treatment, including medication, prescribed by mental health professionals, but never as punishment or for the convenience of others
- the right that no treatment will be provided without informed consent other than when held as an **involuntary client**

involuntary client
Refers to treatment or action undertaken against someone's will, to ensure their safety and that of others.

- the right that chemical or physical restraint or seclusion will not be used unless as a last resort to prevent imminent harm to the client or others
- the right that involuntary admission will only occur if authorised by a suitably qualified mental health professional, and that the person is suffering mental illness, and the treatment of that illness occurs within an approved mental health facility (Department of Health, 2012).

Subsequent amendments to mental health legalisation have incorporated the need to consider clients' perspectives and the provision for appropriate and timely response to complaints concerning care received during treatment. Where clients were previously detained forcibly, a larger proportion of clients are now more likely to receive care in the community. Australian mental health legislation allows for this context of care by using community-based treatment orders.

Community Treatment Orders (CTOs) were originally developed and introduced as a response to the coercive nature of involuntary hospitalisation. CTOs focused upon protecting the civil rights and liberties of clients who might otherwise have been admitted to hospital involuntarily. Today, CTOs within Australasian jurisdictions aim to increase engagement with services, and to prevent relapse (Power, 1999). While it is generally ordered by a psychiatrist, the necessary program of supportive care is almost exclusively provided by nurses (Davidson, 2005). Although requirements vary, as a general rule clients must attend treatment or face the possibility of re-hospitalisation. All CTOs are subject to judicial review and appeal processes. A guardianship order may be made and/or maintained over a person, irrespective of whether or not they are being held under the mental health legislation. The degree and application of guardianship are limited by the guardianship order or the relevant mental health legislation.

Difference between mental health legislation and guardianship legislation

Mental health legislation provides for involuntary detention of people with mental illness in special cases where, for example, there is a risk of serious physical harm to the person or to others, owing to the individual being mentally ill or thought disordered. Cases may often be urgent, and the scheme for involuntary admission allows for compulsory detention, containment and even treatment without any form of hearing until after the event. Mental health legislation can only be enacted upon a person thought to be mentally ill or thought disordered, and for the explicit purposes of detaining, assessing, treating and managing a person's mental illness or thought disorder. Mental health legislation cannot compel a person, whether mentally ill or thought disordered, to accept detention, assessment, treatment or management for any non-mental health-related condition—for example, cellulitis.

Guardianship legislation is the key regulatory mechanism for protecting a person's health, welfare, freedom and interests, that seeks to balance the rights of an adult with impaired decision-making capacity so they can be as independent as possible and receive appropriate support where needed. Following a judicial review, if a person lacks capacity to make reasoned decisions, a separate individual can be appointed to advocate and make decisions in the best interest on behalf of the person named in the order. The appointed guardian can give consent for treatment or other actions to occur, albeit within the limits stated in the guardianship order. The Guardianship Tribunal's focus is not on balancing public interest with private rights; rather, its sole concern is with the welfare, interests and rights of the person with the disability.

GUARDIANSHIP LEGISLATION

Guardianship legislation has been written with the express purpose of establishing protection for those within our community who are vulnerable to neglect, abuse and/or exploitation. The legislation applies to patients over the age of 18 who are found to be incapable of consenting to treatment, and who meet the criteria as specified within the legislation. Most people can make personal and lifestyle choices and decisions. However, when this is not possible, decision-making may be supported by family or friends. Sometimes a person who is unable (due to incapacity) to make a decision may not have anyone who can help, or their family or friends may disagree about the matter. In the event where such a decision must be made, a tribunal may consider it in the best interests of the person to appoint a guardian to make these decisions on their behalf. Common responsibilities of guardians concerning the treatment of persons under guardianship include:

- being as least restrictive as possible
- encourage the person to live a normal life in the community
- respecting and incorporating the person's views and beliefs where possible
- preserving family relationships, and cultural and linguistic environments
- where possible, encouraging the person to be self-reliant in matters relating to their personal, domestic and financial affairs
- protecting the person from neglect, abuse and exploitation.

Each Australian state and territory has guardianship legislation designed to protect the health of young persons, adults with disabilities and the elderly, and includes authority to make decisions on behalf of a person regarding accommodation, healthcare, end-of-life healthcare, medical and dental treatment, and access to services (Table 5.2).

MEDICATION AND POISONS LEGISLATION

Each state and territory has its own legislation regulating the manufacturing, distribution, supply, storage, prescribing and administration of medicines and poisons (Table 5.3), which is informed by the Poisons Standard (Australian Government, 2017). The Poisons Standard promotes uniform scheduling on drugs deemed hazardous to health or highly addictive (e.g. poisons, methamphetamine) to protect people's health and welfare, and regulates the practices regarding the intent and amount of active ingredient permissible under each schedule, as well as storage, handling, labelling, packaging, distribution and administration of drugs. Within

Table 5.2 Guardianship legislation by jurisdiction

Jurisdiction	Legislation
Australian Capital Territory	*Guardianship and Management of Property Act 1991*
New South Wales	*Guardianship Act 1987*
Northern Territory	*Guardianship of Adults Act 2016*
Queensland	*Guardianship and Administration Act 2000* *Powers of Attorney Act 1998*
South Australia	*Guardianship and Administration Act 1993* *Consent to Medical Treatment and Palliative Care Act 1995*
Tasmania	*Guardianship and Administration Act 1995*
Victoria	*Guardianship and Administration Act 1986*
Western Australia	*Guardianship and Administration Act 1990*

Table 5.3 Medicines, poisons and therapeutic legislation by jurisdiction

Jurisdiction	Legislation
Australian Capital Territory	*Medicines, Poisons and Therapeutic Goods Act 2008*
New South Wales	*Poisons and Therapeutic Goods Regulation 2008*
Northern Territory	*Medicines, Poisons and Therapeutic Goods Act 2012*
Queensland	*Health (Drugs and Poisons) Regulation 1996*
South Australia	*The Controlled Substances Act 1984 and Controlled Substances (Poisons) Regulations 2011*
Tasmania	*Poisons Regulations Act 2008*
Victoria	*Drugs, Poisons and Controlled Substances Act 1981*
Western Australia	*Poisons Regulations 1965*

the medication and poisons legislation relating to human healthcare, regulations relating to the access, storage, use and provision of medication are divided into eight Schedules:

- *Schedule 1:* Substances that pose extreme danger to life. This schedule is currently not used.

- *Schedule 2 (Pharmacy Medicine):* Lists substances that, while posing a danger to health if misused or carelessly handled, should be available to the public for therapeutic use or other purposes without undue restriction. Medicines belonging to this Schedule are labelled 'pharmacy medicine'.
- *Schedule 3 (Pharmacist Only Medicine):* Concerns substances that are for therapeutic use. Some of these drugs may be dispensed in cases of life-threatening emergency without the need of a prescription (e.g. salbutamol, adrenaline). Medicines belonging to this Schedule are labelled 'pharmacy only medicine'.
- *Schedule 4 (Restricted Substances):* Also referred to as 'Prescription only medi-cation' or 'POM'. These require a prescription from an authorised healthcare provider, such as a physician or Nurse Practitioner, to obtain and use. Exceptions can be made in some states and territories. For example, in New South Wales a nurse working in an isolated area can provide Schedule 4 and 8 medications under certain conditions. Substances that may be abused and are likely to cause dependency are listed in Appendix D of the *Poisons and Therapeutic Goods Regulation* (Schedule 4 Appendix D, or 'S4D'). Unauthorised possession of an Appendix D substance is a criminal offence.
- *Schedules 5 and 6:* List substances that, while of a dangerous nature, can be commonly used and readily available to the public in specific containers with appropriate labelling.
- *Schedule 7 (Special Precautions):* Concerns substances that mainly require special precautions—for example, arsenic (a highly poisonous substance that is now used in the preservation of wood).
- *Schedule 8 (Drugs of Addiction):* Lists substances that are addictive or have the potential to be addictive. However, those substances commonly known to be highly addictive, such as heroin, do not appear under Schedule 8, as they are typically controlled under criminal law.

Not every schedule affects the handling of medication in public or private hospitals. Principally, accountable medications such as Schedule 4 (Restricted Substances), Schedule 4 Appendix D ('S4D', Substances of Restricted Possession) and Schedule 8 ('S8', Drugs of Addiction) are the most commonly regulated med-ications dispensed in private and public hospitals. The handling of restricted or high-risk medications, such as balance checking, preparation, administration or discarding of unused amounts, must be undertaken by two authorised persons, with one being the witness (Northern Territory Government, 2017).

Second person checks prior to administration of a high-risk or restricted medication

An **independent check** by a second authorised person (e.g. an RN, NP or medical officer) should be carried out before certain high-risk medications or restricted medications are prepared and administered, and must include as a minimum:

- all intravenous medication
- high-risk medications such as insulin, heparin and warfarin
- medication administered to children aged under 16 years
- contrast dye
- radiopharmaceuticals for diagnostic or therapeutic purposes
- all restricted medications, irrespective of route (e.g. transdermal, intranasal), with the second person being the 'witness'.

The second person checking the collection, preparation and administration of a high-risk medication is responsible for:

- independently confirming the prescription, selection and amount of medication dispensed is correct
- for restricted medication, independently confirming the balance of medication in the **dangerous drug cupboard**, and that the amount removed is correct compared to what is recorded in the **dangerous drug register** (Figure 5.1)
- independently confirming that the dose, **diluent** and calculations are correct
- independently confirming that the automatic volume infuser (e.g. infusion pump, syringe driver) settings (e.g. rate, volume to be infused) have been correctly set
- independently confirming the identity of the patient
- for restricted medication, witnessing the transfer of medication to the patient
- for restricted medication, witnessing any unused medication being discarded

independent check This check should be made with no assistance from another party—the person responsible completes the entire check, including any calculations, from the original documentation and their own observations.

dangerous drug cupboard This is a separate locked cupboard securely attached to the wall or floor, purely dedicated for the storage of S4D and S8 medications or additional accountable medication as determined by local policy. All medication stored in the cupboard must accounted for in a dangerous drug register. **dangerous drug register** A dedicated register in which all transactions, administrations or discarding of restricted medications is recorded. **diluent** A substance used to reduce the concentration of (i.e. dilute) an injectable medication, such as normal saline (0.9% sodium chloride) or water, for injection.

Name, Form and Strength of Drug: Morphine (IV) 5mg/5mL Note: Each drug is to be entered on separate pages											
Date	Time	Patient's Name	Prescriber	IN	OUT	Balance	Amount given	Amount discarded	Name of person administering	Signature of person administering	Name of person witnessing	Signature of person witnessing
23/10/18	10:15	JOHNSON, Ann	Golding	0	1	15	3mg	2mg	A. Donovan	*A. Donovan*	R. Kelly	*R. Kelly*
23/10/18	16:00	From pharmacy		40	0	55			A. Donovan	*A. Donovan*	R. Kelly	*R. Kelly*
23/10/18	21:21	WRIGHT, Lee	Gallance	0	1	54	5mg		K. Kentwell	*K. Kentwell*	E. Ryan	*E. Ryan*

Figure 5.1 Example of entries in a dangerous drug register

- countersigning the administration on the medication chart against the signature of the administering person
- for restricted medication, countersigning the dangerous drug register against the signature of the administering person (Government of Western Australia, 2014; Tasmanian Government, 2014).

Additional important cognitive checks:

- Does the drug's indication correspond to the patient's diagnosis?
- Is the dosing formula (e.g. mg/kg, mg/hr, MIRCOg/min/kg) used to derive the final dose correct?
- Are the prescribed dose and frequency appropriate for this patient?
- Is the route of administration safe (e.g. impaired swallow) and proper for this patient?
- Is the infusion line attached to the correct port and labelled (if applicable)?
- Is the right monitoring in place (e.g. blood pressure monitoring in vasopressor administration)?

ETHICS IN NURSING

An understanding of ethics is essential for the delivery of safe, skilled professional care (NMBA, 2013b; Kangasniemi et al., 2015). Nursing, a profession focused on the quality of life and care of individuals, families and communities across the spectrum of health, is an ethical activity in itself. The primary aims of nurses are to do good, avoid or at least minimise harm, and to conduct themselves with integrity and dignity, including in the use of social media (AHPRA, 2014), to maintain public trust and confidence. Ethics is a branch of moral philosophy that is concerned with determining right and wrong in relation to people's decisions and actions. Bioethics, or healthcare ethics, is a specific domain of ethics used in healthcare that focuses on the moral issues that arise where ethics and life sciences meet (Avery, 2017). Bioethics has evolved into a unique discipline as a result of life-and-death moral issues encountered by healthcare professionals, patients and families. In recognition of the ever-expanding evidence base, increasing societal needs and changing socio-political values that shape nursing practice, a Code of Ethics for Nurses (NMBA, 2013b) was published as a guide for nurses to base their professional decision-making upon when faced with ethical issues. Ethical issues that nurses face in their daily practice range from providing quality care (Pavlish et al., 2011; Ulrich et al., 2010), to specific disease- and treatment-related decisions (Pavlish et al., 2012; Winterstein, 2012). The clinical activities in which nurses are involved on a daily basis regarding the care of their patients are based on respect for the patient's self-determination, best evidence and legislation (NMBA, 2013b), yet ethical dilemmas can still arise. An ethical dilemma is a complex situation where a difficult choice must be made between two or more alternate actions, which may result in a negative outcome for the patient. An action can be divided into three distinct facets: the motivation/intention of the action; the act itself; and the consequences of the act. Determining which action is right or wrong, good or bad, or the least harmful requires nurses to engage in a process of ethical analysis, which includes identifying which ethical concepts are involved.

Ethical concepts are often combined into frameworks, which provide support and guidance for ethical decision-making by enabling the important aspects of the situation to be highlighted and evaluated. Several ethical concepts and theories have been described within the nursing literature: principlism, utilitarianism, deontology and veracity. These are not intended to be used in isolation, but rather form part of an **iterative process**.

Principlism, a popular approach to ethics in healthcare, involves using a set of ethical principles drawn from a widely shared conception of morality. These include autonomy, beneficence, non-maleficence and justice (Beauchamp & Childress, 2012). The principle of autonomy states that an individual should have liberty from controlling influences and limitations to self-rule and make independent decisions. The principle of autonomy is sometimes described as respect. Respect for autonomy is a fundamental concept, both ethically and legally, that influences healthcare decisions. We can see it at work, for example, in the need to obtain informed consent from patients (Fry, 2008; Staunton & Chiarella, 2013).

iterative process
A process of reaching a decision by means of a repeated and converging cycle of operations.

Example

Mrs Green has been admitted to a ward with a suspected small bowel obstruction. During the admission, the treating physician informs you that Mrs Green will need a nasogastric tube to be inserted. During your nursing assessment, you discuss the initial management of small bowel obstruction and the use of a nasogastric tube to reduce nausea and vomiting. Mrs Green is quite hesitant about the use of a nasogastric tube and asks what is involved. You detail how the tube is inserted and checked to ensure it is placed correctly within the stomach. In discussing insertion of the nasogastric tube, you also describe common issues that can arise during and following the tube insertion, such as discomfort, gagging and sores at the nares. To ensure Mrs Green is informed, you ask her to repeat what she has understood regarding the rationale for inserting a nasogastric tube, common issues associated with their placement and how you will manage these.

Example

You are asked by a junior member of the nursing team to assist with re-siting a peripheral intravenous cannula. The patient, Mr Robinson, is 89 years of age and was admitted to the oncology ward for pain management due to bone metastases. During your nursing assessment, Mr Robinson states that his pain has been minimal since starting a new analgesia regimen. On reviewing Mr Robinson's medical chart, you notice that Mr Robinson has been charted regular oral analgesia and intravenous morphine for breakthrough pain. He has only required one dose of morphine since admission two days ago. There are no other intravenous medications charted. Mr Robinson describes two previous failed attempts at inserting a cannula, resulting in discomfort and restricted movement of his right hand. He would prefer that no further attempts were made. Reviewing the pain-management plan and Mr Robinson's response to oral analgesia so far, you outline how future breakthrough analgesia could be provided by other routes if needed, such as fentanyl lollipops, or how the current oral analgesia regimen could be revised to increase the degree of pain relief provided. Mr Robinson would like to pursue the use of oral analgesia and possibly fentanyl lollipops, and forego another cannula. You arrange for the pain team to visit Mr Robinson that afternoon to revise the use of intravenous morphine.

The principles of beneficence and non-maleficence state that the actions of nurses and the healthcare team are to provide appropriate and effective care (beneficence) while doing the least harm (non-maleficence) to the patient (Beauchamp & Childress, 2012). While these concepts are often paired, beneficence requires *taking* action to benefit others, whereas non-maleficence involves *refraining* from action that might harm others. The principles of beneficence and non-maleficence are often encountered during clinical decision-making.

Clinical decision-making is an integral part of nursing and vital to positive health outcomes for patients. In making clinical decisions, such as interventions or actions to restore, maintain or improve quality of life, nurses must weigh up the intended benefits to the patient against the possibility of or degree of harm. This process, in addition to respecting patient autonomy, must also consider the ethical principle of justice.

The principle of justice—the foundation of duty-based moral reasoning—is complex and difficult to define. However, within nursing discourse, justice is commonly used in two related senses: distributive justice and justice as fairness. Distributive justice pertains to the organisation and distribution of benefits and burdens equally among members of society. The only exception to this is where an unequal distribution is necessary to ensure that the least well-off can receive the basic benefits of society's productivity (Johnstone, 2011). Justice as fairness relates to a largely intuitive sense of justice—that is, based on personal opinions and preferences about how benefits and burdens are distributed and whether the resulting outcome is beneficial or harmful, and whether it is fair (Beauchamp & Childress, 2012). Nursing has a long and rich history of promoting justice in healthcare service provision and access, both locally and internationally. One famous example of a nurse promoting healthcare justice was Florence Nightingale (1820–1910) (Barritt, 1973).

Justice, whether denoting equality of opportunity, access to or distribution of benefits, is at the foundation of nursing's responsibilities to promote health, prevent disease, restore health and alleviate suffering. Further, justice is at the centre of nursing's responsibility to advocate for equity and fairness of health, social and economic resource allocation, especially for vulnerable populations (International Council of Nurses, 2012).

Utilitarianism theory judges the outcome of an action based on whether it provides the greatest benefit to the largest number, or the least possible balance of negative consequences. Utilitarianism theory reminds us that the consequences of our actions have moral significance, and must be taken into account (Kerridge et al., 2005). This ethical theory is observed through the economic evaluation used to prioritise provision of high-cost treatments for different medical conditions that receive financial subsidisation via the Pharmaceutical Benefits Scheme. This approach of economic evaluation is utilitarian, in that treatments and procedures shown to have the greatest health and economic outcome (i.e. efficacy) for the greatest number of patients are made more affordable through subsidisation, thus making treatment more affordable for all (Lu et al., 2008). The capacity to benefit the largest number of people is a necessary criterion from the perspective of distributive justice, as scarce resources (e.g. public funds) should be distributed to patients who have a reasonable chance of benefit (Beauchamp & Childress, 2012).

In contrast to utilitarianism theory, deontology places value on the intentions of the individual and focuses on following rules, obligations and duties. Deontology requires absolute adherence to these obligations, and acting from duty is viewed as acting ethically. One of the key criticisms in healthcare is that applying a strictly deontological approach to healthcare can lead to conflicts of interest between equally entitled individuals, which can be difficult or even seemingly impossible to resolve. However, deontology reminds us of the importance of rationality in moral judgement and of moral standards, independently of the consequences (Kerridge et al., 2005).

Example

Working as an agency nurse, you are allocated to the local day surgery unit, an area for which you are appropriately skilled given your background in working in general theatres. On arriving at the unit, the team leader assigns you to be a scrub nurse for today's gynaecological patient list. On reviewing the procedures being undertaken today, you notice that the last patient on the list is scheduled for a surgical termination of pregnancy. While abortion is legal within the state in which you are practising, and it is a personal right of individuals to request an abortion, it conflicts with your religious beliefs. The day surgery unit is very busy, and you are one of four agency nursing staff working this morning as several permanent staff have called in sick. You approach the nursing team leader to discuss the issue. The team leader suggests that if you can prepare the patient for the procedure and recover the patient after the procedure; another experienced nurse currently working in recovery can assist as scrub nurse for the surgical procedure.

Veracity is an ethical principle underlying the idea of trust and **fiduciary** relationships (Staunton & Chiarella, 2013), such as the nurse–patient relationship where the nurse is entrusted with the responsibility to act in the best interest of a patient or organisation. Veracity is a dual concept that refers to both the duty of being truthful and the obligation to respect confidentiality. Providing truthful information to patients about the risks involved in a proposed treatment and their healthcare needs facilitates autonomous choice and enhances patient decision-making. Conversely, using the patient's treatment outcomes in research without first obtaining permission would be a breach of confidentiality.

> **fiduciary** A person who holds a legal or ethical relationship of trust with one or more individuals, such as a nurse and a patient in their care.

To practise in an ethically sound professional manner, nurses need to balance ethical considerations with professional values and relevant legislation. The essence of ethical practice at all levels involves an individual or team identifying what the legal, ethical and professional standards required are and how these can be compassionately applied to the challenges of clinical practice. Making ethical decisions is not a solitary activity, particularly where decisions impact on others. Quality patient care relies on a team approach that supports the decision-making of the patient in a professional partnership where their views, wishes and values are respected and acknowledged.

Clinical situations that raise ethical questions, often with multiple complex factors, are challenging to navigate. In addition to considering the multiple clinical facts of the situation, patient values, preferences, privacy, and the concerns and values of the family must be considered. In some instances, a decision is needed quickly. Ethical frameworks provide a systematic approach to forming a balanced decision that incorporates the wants and wishes of the patient and family with the medical facts and achievable quality-of-life end-points. One such framework that commonly is used in clinical practice is the 'four-topics' method, or four-quadrant ethical framework, developed by Jonsen and colleagues (2006). The four-quadrant framework was developed to provide clinicians with a method for sorting through and focusing on specific aspects of ethical questions encountered in clinical practice, and for connecting context and circumstances to ethical principles (Figure 5.2). The four elements of the ethical framework are described below.

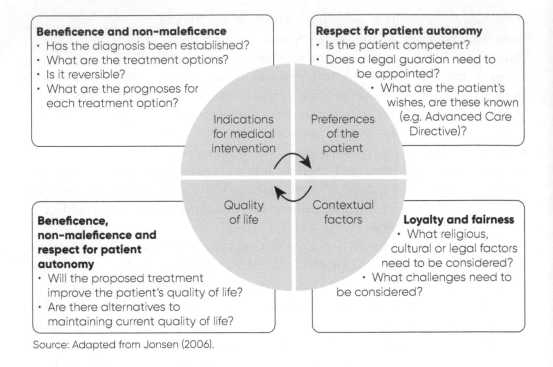

Source: Adapted from Jonsen (2006).

Figure 5.2 Four-quadrant ethical framework

Preferences of the patient

Factors to be considered include:

- respect for the patient's autonomy
- whether the patient is competent
- whether a legal guardian needs to be appointed
- the patient's wishes—are these known (e.g. Advanced Care Directive)?

Contextual factors

Issues to be considered include:

- loyalty and fairness
- religious, cultural or legal factors that need to be considered
- challenges that need to be considered.

Quality of life

Factors to be considered include:

- beneficence, non-maleficence and respect for patient autonomy
- whether the proposed treatment will improve the patient's quality of life
- whether there are alternative solutions to maintaining the patient's current quality of life.

Indications for medical intervention

Factors to be considered include:

- beneficence and non-maleficence
- whether the diagnosis has been established
- possible treatment options
- whether the condition is reversible
- the prognosis for each treatment option.

Summary

In this chapter, we looked at legal issues that may affect nurses, their practice and clinical decision-making. We defined the concepts of accountability and responsibility, and the legal responsibilities nurses have for particular patient groups, including those at risk of physical or emotional abuse. We examined in detail the importance of establishing a patient's consent to treatment and what is meant by 'duty of care'. We then looked at mental health and guardianship legislation, and how this relates to nursing. We also considered medication and poisons legislation.

Review questions

5.1 Which of the following are inappropriate grounds upon which to judge that a person is mentally ill or disordered?
a Religious beliefs
b Sexual orientation
c Immoral conduct
d Intellectual disability
e All of the above

5.2 Which of the following are WHO principles?
a Access
b Equity
c Effectiveness
d Efficiency
e All of the above

5.3 Capacity refers to an individual's ability to understand the information provided to them. What else does an individual have to be able to demonstrate?
a The ability to retain information
b An ability to fully converse in English
c The capacity to weigh up the benefits and informed risks

5.4 With regards to informed consent, the lead practitioner can request the patient's permission to allow a student to site an indwelling catheter. True or false?

5.5 An RN can carry out a non-urgent procedure without first seeking the patient's permission. True or false?

5.6 In what ways can consent be given?
a Verbal
b Written
c Implied
d All of the above

5.7 What is the most common form of consent in daily practice?
a Implied
b Verbal
c Written

5.8   Which ruling allows for practitioners to take action in urgent situations?
a   Doctrine of necessity
b   Samaritan's Law
c   Duty of care

5.9   Of the following 'rights of medication administration', which ones are incorrect?
a   Right patient
b   Right medication
c   Right standard precaution
d   Right dosage
e   Right route
f   Right time
g   Right protocol

5.10   Diazepam is an example of what class of drug?
a   S4
b   S4D
c   S8

5.11   Morphine is an example of what class of drug?
a   S4
b   S4D
c   S8

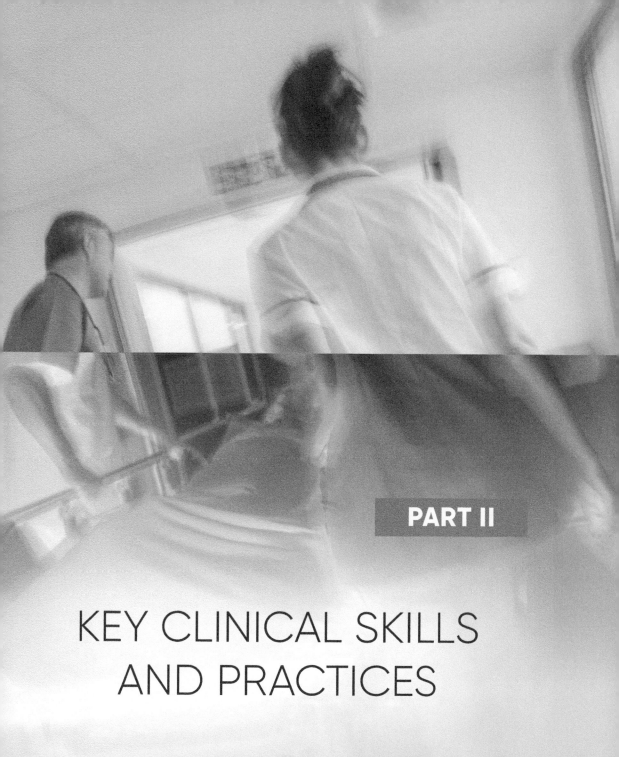

PART II

KEY CLINICAL SKILLS AND PRACTICES

6 HEALTH WORKFORCE CULTURE, TEAM DEVELOPMENT AND COMMUNICATION

Alister Hodge and Wayne Varndell

In this chapter, you will develop an understanding of:

- effective team communication
- working in teams
- conflict resolution
- workplace bullying
- multidisciplinary decision-making
- communication with patients and patient education
- managing complaints
- open disclosure
- violence and aggression in the workplace.

COMMUNICATION AND WORKING IN TEAMS

In today's health environment, being able to communicate effectively is of crucial importance for quality care delivery by the multidisciplinary team. Up to 89 per cent of a clinician's time involves communication, whether this is via face-to-face dialogue, telephone conversations or documentation (Kilner & Sheppard, 2010). During each admission, patients have contact with multiple care providers. One study found that a patient had over 50 different health professionals involved with their management over the course of only four days (O'Daniel & Rosenstein,

2008). This represents a multitude of instances where critical information must be transferred accurately.

The healthcare environment itself creates many impediments to effective communication. The clinical setting is often crowded, noisy and busy. Information transfer is often compromised through interruptions to conversations between health workers. An episode of poor communication can result in misinterpretation, a lack of critical information or unclear treatment plans, ultimately resulting in treatment error. Treatment errors may be **benign**; however, they can also lead to severe patient injury or even unexpected death (O'Daniel & Rosenstein, 2008). In episodes of accidental patient harm, the most frequent contributing factor reported is poor communication between clinicians (Altmiller, 2011; Kilner & Sheppard, 2010; Moroney & Knowles, 2006, O'Daniel & Rosenstein, 2008; O'Leary et al., 2010; Weller et al., 2014). Other impacts of poor communication include inefficient care delivery, clinician frustration and medication errors (Moroney & Knowles, 2006; Seago, 2008). Key areas where communication is critical for safety include patient handover, written documentation, interactions between health professions (e.g. nurse to doctor), transfer between treatment sites, escalation of care during patient deterioration and management of patients in high-acuity settings, such as the emergency department or operating theatre (Weller et al., 2014).

benign Not harmful in effect.

To improve the effectiveness of communication between yourself and other clinicians, consider three key themes: personal considerations, preparation and structure (Curtis et al., 2011).

Personal considerations

These prompt you to complete a brief self-appraisal. Question your own emotional state to identify whether you feel irritated, fatigued or time-pressured. Is this affecting your interactions with others? Also, consider the other clinician's perspective and individual pressures: are they also tired/stressed? Acknowledging these factors may help in controlling the tone of conversation.

Preparation

Taking time to collect your thoughts will improve the episode of communication. Consider what you want to achieve from the conversation, put together notes if required, and anticipate what the person you are contacting will need to know to make their decision—for example, the latest set of observations or pathology results.

Structure

The clinical environment is under constant time pressure, so communication must be clear, succinct and systematic. Effective delivery of information aims to minimise information to necessary details, prioritise the order of information by clinical urgency and deliver information in a systematic format that the receiver is likely to comprehend, and that facilitates decision-making. ISBAR is a commonly used framework to present information during clinical handover or **escalation** of the deteriorating patient (Jacques et al., 2009) (Table 6.1).

When escalating identified clinical deterioration, ensure that you notify the Nurse Unit Manager (NUM) as well as the treating doctor. Notification of the NUM enables allocation of appropriate nursing staff and equipment resources for the maintenance of patient safety. It also enables the NUM to further escalate the response if you do not acquire the necessary medical review.

Other patterns of communication can be used to help remove the chance of misunderstandings and are particularly useful during phone interactions. One such technique is *closed-loop communication*. This is a three-step strategy whereby the sender provides instruction, the receiver confirms what was communicated and seeks clarification as required, and the sender verifies that the message has been received and interpreted correctly (Weller et al., 2014).

escalation Refers to a situation where the clinician notes information that must be acted upon immediately. Escalation involves bringing this information to the notice of appropriate staff to enact needed change—for example, for a deteriorating patient, this would be the senior treating doctor, to make a decision regarding changes to the clinical management plan, and the Nurse Unit Manager, who may need to reprioritise nursing resources to assist in managing the patient.

Closed-loop communication example

Person 1: 'Mr Higgins in Room 4 has had a chemical splash to his eyes. Can you please irrigate his eyes with 1 litre of Hartmann's fluid, then re-check his pH?'

Person 2: 'Okay. Just to confirm, you want me to irrigate Mr Higgins' eyes with 1 litre of Hartmann's then re-check his pH afterwards?'

Person 1: 'That's correct—thanks.'

Table 6.1 ISBAR framework

Element	Action
Introduction	Identify yourself, your role and location, identify the patient.
Situation	State the patient's diagnosis/reason for admission and the current problem.
Background	What is the patient's clinical background?
Assessment	What is the current clinical condition of the patient (vital signs/physical assessment)?
Recommendation/ request	What do you recommend as a course of action, or what do you want the person you are contacting to do?

Source: Jacques et al. (2009).

Clinical example of ISBAR

Element	Action
Introduction	Hi, my name's Karen, I'm a nurse calling from 3 South surgical ward regarding a patient by the name of Gerald Smith, a 33-year-old male.
Situation	Mr Smith was admitted with appendicitis and has been awaiting theatre at the end of the day. However, he has had a deterioration in his clinical condition.
Background	Mr Smith's background includes: no known drug allergies, no regular medications or other significant medical history, and he has been fasted since 0700 hours.
Assessment	Clinically, he has deteriorated from his admission baseline. He is now pale and visibly distressed with abdominal guarding. Vital signs are GCS 15, blood pressure 100/50 mmHg, heart rate 20 beats per minute, respiratory rate 20 breaths per minute, and temperature 38.9°C.
Recommendation/ request	I would like to obtain an urgent medical review of the patient and a plan for response to Mr Smith's clinical deterioration.

Another technique is named 'step-back', and refers to stepping back from the clinical situation to gain an overview. The clinician responsible for the patient gains the attention of the team and summarises the situation and the plan, and seeks suggestions (Weller et al., 2014).

Step-back communication example

A new graduate nurse is talking to a Nurse Educator about their patient: 'Jenny, can I grab your time for a moment to run through my patient with you? This is Mrs Brown, a 28-year-old being admitted with severe tonsillitis. Her airway is patent and vital signs unremarkable at present, and she has IV access. The treatment plan includes Benzylpenicillin 2.4g IV, Metronidazole 500mg IV and Dexamethasone 8mg IV, and she has had a normal saline fluid bolus of 1 litre. Is there anything else I should think of before she goes to the ward?'

Nurse Educator: 'That sounds appropriate; however, ensure that adequate analgesia orders are provided on the medication chart as well.'

COLLABORATION AND WORKING IN TEAMS

Collaboration in healthcare is evident when different health professionals take **complementary roles**, and work together as a team to achieve an optimal patient outcome. Working in a collaborative team environment enables members to be more productive, and increases awareness and understanding of each other's knowledge and skills, leading to better informed decisions (O'Daniel & Rosenstein, 2008). Collaborative teams are associated with positive work cultures, and tend to be more successful in achieving organisational goals such as a reduction in error frequency, lower morbidity/mortality rates and shorter lengths of stay (Seago, 2008). Importantly, patients report greater satisfaction with their hospital experience when they believe they have been cared for by a functioning team, as collaboration between health professionals is thought to provide a more holistic approach to care (Mills et al., 2010).

complementary roles
When different health professions complete different aspects of management that together work towards the same over-arching goal of holistic patient care.

Multidisciplinary decision-making within teams

Multidisciplinary decision-making refers to making use of the broad knowledge and skill base across the health team to reach a decision about patient care. When the wider team has participated in the decision process, there is usually better adherence to clinical practice guidelines and evidence-based practice (Davies, 2009; Lamb et al., 2013). Multidisciplinary decision-making has also been linked to the development of a committed and productive team (Mickan & Rodger, 2000).

FACILITATORS AND BARRIERS TO EFFECTIVE TEAMS, AND STRATEGIES FOR ESTABLISHING AND SUSTAINING AN EFFECTIVE TEAM

Barriers to effective teams

To achieve a collaborative health team, numerous barriers must be overcome. Ideally, preparation should begin during undergraduate education. Communication patterns that support interactions between a nurse and patient are a common topic in undergraduate nurse education; however, until recently there has been little focus on improving information transfer between health professionals. On entry to the workforce, most graduates have yet to gain a solid grasp of their own role, let alone those of the numerous other disciplines with which they interact; however, a lack of understanding of other health professionals' roles, responsibilities and priorities can contribute to problems when interdisciplinary teamwork is required (Weller et al., 2014). To ensure you know what to expect from various members of the healthcare team, clarify with your educator the responsibilities of different levels of medical staff in the management of your patient, and the role that allied health professionals have to play in your patient's recovery. This will help you know who to approach for different aspects of your patient's care. The roles and responsibilities of various nursing and medical grades are explained in more detail in Chapter 3.

Psychological factors can also affect team interactions. For example, distinctions can be made between an 'in group' and an 'out group', where members of a professional group (e.g. doctors or nurses) view the attributes of their group as positive, and those of a different group in a more negative light. Another psychological barrier includes the hierarchical structures in healthcare that may result in a junior staff member being less willing to challenge a senior staff member despite patient treatment concerns (Weller et al., 2014).

Organisational factors can affect communication between teams. For example, an interdisciplinary meeting that various members are unable to attend can result in a lack of contribution by key stakeholders towards treatment decisions. Different forms of documentation across wards—for example, paper versus electronic—can also constitute an organisational barrier to communication (Weller et al., 2014).

Although all clinical environments and organisations are different, health teams may experience common barriers. These include:

- inter-professional rivalries
- different schedules and professional routines
- varying levels of qualification and status in the hierarchy
- differences in payment, reward and accountability
- personality differences
- differing personal values and expectations
- poor behaviour and disruption
- an emphasis on or a need for rapid decision-making
- people withholding their real views to maintain group harmony
- certain people vying for the spotlight
- members of the team failing to contribute
- a perceived loss of autonomy
- a lack of confidence in others' decisions (Davies, 2009; O'Daniel & Rosenstein, 2008).

Creating an effective team

Effective teams demonstrate positive attributes in three key areas:

1 team structure and organisational support
2 team processes and interactions
3 contribution by individual team members.

Being aware of these positive attributes will help you to model behaviours that support the functioning of the larger health team to deliver high-quality patient care. It may also help you to identify missing factors that need to be rectified for your team to function at its best.

- *Team structure and organisational support:* The team should have a shared purpose, suitable leadership and direction, with appropriate members and resources (Weller et al., 2014). The culture in an effective team is supportive

non-punitive environment
Healthcare is an extremely complicated environment with the potential for many things to go wrong. A non-punitive approach recognises that clinicians rarely make a mistake deliberately. Instead of punishing the person who made a mistake, the focus is directed towards understanding what contributed to the mistake in the first place (e.g. communication error, a lack of guidelines or education) so that this can be rectified and future occurrences prevented.

of interdisciplinary collaboration, with members functioning within a non-punitive and respectful atmosphere. Individuals have distinct roles and tasks, with clearly defined authority and accountability (O'Daniel & Rosenstein, 2008). Importantly, the aims and functioning of the team need to be supported by the larger organisation to enable sustainability.

- *Team processes and interactions:* A set of agreed processes must be in place to govern how the team members interact with each other and complete core business. Clear processes should be identified for team co-ordination, multidisciplinary decision-making, conflict management and performance feedback (Mickan & Rodger, 2000; O'Daniel & Rosenstein, 2008). A workable balance between member task participation is maintained to prevent individual burnout, and measurable processes and outcomes are used to identify achievement of the team's goals. Regular information sharing should occur via effective communication patterns, and shared responsibility for successes ensures that each member is recognised for their contribution towards the team's end goal. Increasingly efforts have been made to include the patient as an active member of the overall team, to ensure that decisions are made that reflect the patient's wishes (NSW Health, 2014; O'Daniel & Rosenstein, 2008).

- *Contribution by individual team members:* Team members actively participate in the creation of a clinical management plan and relevant aspects of care delivery, while demonstrating an appreciation for other specialties and what they contribute to the patient care episode (Davies, 2009; Doyle, 2008). Members of the team watch out for each other to identify when colleagues may require support during times of inappropriately high workload. High-functioning members demonstrate self-awareness and emotional maturity, whereby open discussion is utilised to resolve conflict and reach consensus on decisions (Davies, 2009). They are adaptable to alterations in the environment, and make relevant changes to patient management. Team members take into consideration other perspectives and ideas, and support a belief that the team's overall goal is more important than the individual (McComb & Hebdon, 2013; Weller et al., 2014).

Maintenance of positive team interaction requires a commitment to ongoing collaborative work structures from staff as well as leaders. This can further be supported via inter-professional education sessions in which team dynamics and desired patterns of interaction can be modelled and reinforced. Due to the high turnover of clinical staff in many locations, this requires inclusion of relevant teaching material during the orientation of new medical and nursing staff, along with modelling of desired behaviours by existing staff in the clinical environment (O'Daniel & Rosenstein, 2008).

CONFLICT RESOLUTION IN WORK RELATIONSHIPS

On entering the workforce, as in other areas of your life, you will eventually encounter people with challenging behaviours. Conflict in the work environment can come from numerous sources, including nurse–nurse, interdisciplinary and nurse–patient interaction. Conflict with colleagues is often the most distressing form to manage. Bullying, which is an ongoing pattern of behaviour that is intended to be offensive, intimidating, humiliating or threatening (NSW Health, 2013a), is discussed later in this chapter. Single instances of conflict are still challenging, and you should aim to acquire skills to resolve these situations in a way that encourages teamwork and patient safety (Altmiller, 2011).

Ideally, episodes of interpersonal conflict should be minimised through modelling of appropriate behaviour by senior staff, and be supported through the creation and implementation of an expected behaviour policy by senior management. This policy should outline the expected standards for appropriate communication and behaviour, while clearly noting the actions to be taken where an employee fails to comply (O'Daniel & Rosenstein, 2008).

Various strategies can be employed to manage conflict and resolve situations while maintaining professionalism and, most importantly, patient safety (Altmiller, 2011). One such strategy is cognitive rehearsal, which uses pre-formed statements to confront inappropriate behaviour or communication in a non-aggressive manner at the time it occurs. You avoid responding emotionally and consciously decide not to react. Instead, you step back and take the time to process what has been said before replying with a cognitively rehearsed 'shielding response'. Arming yourself with the ability to stop the situation makes it less likely that you will be targeted in a similar way in the future (Griffen, 2004) (Table 6.2).

In many situations, conflict is driven by an underlying concern about patient safety or disagreements regarding the appropriateness of a chosen clinical management strategy. It is crucial in these instances to keep the discussion focused upon

Table 6.2 Examples of shielding responses

Situation	Suggested response
Non-verbal innuendo—for example, raising eyebrows, making faces	'From your expression, I see there's something you wanted to say to me? It's okay to speak straight to me.'
Covert or snide remarks—for example, being mocked in an indirect fashion	'I tend to learn more quickly from clear directions and feedback. Is there some way we can talk in this fashion?'
Sabotage—for example, being deliberately set up to fail at a given task	'We know there's more to this situation than meets the eye. How about we talk about what happened?'
Arguing about trivial matters—for example, arguing about a non-work-related issue	'This isn't the time or place. Please stop.' (Move away or to a neutral location.)
Criticising a colleague while they are not present	'I wasn't there/don't know the situation, and don't feel comfortable talking about him/her. Have you spoken to him/her about it?'
Broken confidences—for example, 'Did you hear who just got a warning over excessive sick leave?'	'Wasn't that said in confidence? It sounds like information that should remain confidential/private.'

the patient to prevent extraneous personal factors from clouding the interaction. Two suggested strategies are reframing and graded assertiveness:

- *Reframing* helps you to redirect the line of communication or create an opportunity for re-evaluation of a potentially inappropriate treatment plan by focusing on patient safety. A simple technique is known as 'CUS', an acronym for 'concerned, uncomfortable and safe'. By using the words, 'I'm concerned, I feel uncomfortable with this, and I don't feel it's safe for the patient', you are able to highlight a potential safety threat (Altmiller, 2011).
- *Graded assertiveness* is another method you can employ to address concerns about a patient safety issue within a hierarchical clinical environment. The technique supports you to gradually escalate your concern with tact, while keeping the focus on the patient. Gentle cues may be all that is necessary to inform the other clinician that you have concerns regarding a management

plan or patient condition; however, this may be stepped up until you and your colleague are satisfied that individual concerns have been met (Curtis et al., 2011) (Table 6.3).

Table 6.3 Levels of graded assertiveness and examples of statements

Level	Example
Level 1: note initial concern with an 'I' statement	'I am concerned about ...'
Level 2: make an inquiry or offer a solution	'Would you like me to ...'
Level 3: ask for an explanation	'It would help me to understand ...'
Level 4: a definitive challenge demanding a response	'For patient safety, you must listen to me ...'

WORKPLACE BULLYING: WHAT CONSTITUTES BULLYING AND HOW SHOULD IT BE DEALT WITH?

Bullying is thought to be widespread in the nursing profession, with one study estimating over 80 per cent of nurses have experienced bullying at some time during their career or seen it happen to a colleague (Hutchinson et al., 2010). Bullying has far-reaching effects. For the victim, it can result in damage to psychological, psychosocial and physiological health. However, the damage caused by bullying does not stop with the victim, as the overall worksite suffers through decreased social cohesion and employee engagement, higher degrees of burnout and decreased staff retention (Allen et al., 2014; Douglas, 2014; Franklin & Chadwick, 2013, Hutchinson, 2009).

Single episodes of simple rudeness do not constitute bullying. Bullying is typified by an ongoing pattern of behaviour that is intended to be offensive, intimidating, humiliating or threatening (NSW Health, 2011b). Accepted definitions between the states see it as any repeated behaviour or treatment of a person or a group that is unreasonable, unfair, victimising, threatening, embarrassing or humiliating, or creates a risk to health and safety (Queensland Government, 2017; Victoria State Government, 2017; Tasmanian Government, 2016; Government of South Australia, 2014).

Bullying can come in a number of guises, from blatantly obvious verbal abuse through to subtle or covert acts (Douglas, 2014; Hutchinson, 2009).

Bullying takes three main forms: damaging reputation and professional competence; personal attack; and the use of work roles and tasks for attack. Examples of subtle forms of bullying include gossip, innuendo and exclusion. These are used by the bully to influence other staff members' opinions of the victim and affect their ability to work. During episodes of personal attack, bullying may include public humiliation, belittling or blaming. Examples of bullying through work tasks include withholding information needed to complete a role, frequent unnecessary interruptions and unfair allocation of work duties (Hutchinson, 2009).

Organisational factors are important in determining whether or not bullying becomes entrenched. If the unit culture accepts such behaviours without challenge, they will most likely increase in frequency. In work environments that are tolerant of bullying behaviours, nurses are more likely to report a fear of retribution if they complain, resulting in under-reporting and a lack of aid to the victim (Hutchinson, 2009; Hutchinson et al., 2010).

Not all behaviours that may seem unfair or that cause distress are bullying. For example, the employer can transfer, discipline, direct and counsel employees as long as they are acting reasonably. The following actions would not be considered bullying in isolation: allocating work, rostering, implementing policies, implementating change in work practices, and performance management (NSW Health, 2011b). Some of these necessary tasks of management can be used during subtle or covert forms of bullying; however, a single incident does not constitute bullying, and a reasonable person would need to consider the behaviour as offensive or intending to cause distress (Douglas, 2014).

The health organisation has a responsibility to combat and eradicate bullying cultures and behaviour from the workforce. In conjunction with zero-tolerance policies, harassment and discrimination legislation, and work health and safety policies and legislation, an important strategy to prevent and manage bullying in the workplace is education. It is critical that staff are educated about what constitutes bullying, what is acceptable/unacceptable behaviour in the workplace, how to identify bullying behaviour and how to respond to and report episodes of bullying. Unit culture has been identified as a major contributor towards acceptance of bullying behaviour, so the establishment of a workplace culture of respectful communication, empathy and compassion for fellow staff members is important to decrease the overall incidence (Franklin & Chadwick, 2013). In the event that an episode of bullying does occur, the organisation should have systems in place to support the victim through counselling and possibly mediation between the victim and perpetrator. Corrective measures towards the perpetrator of the bullying must also occur, including appropriate disciplinary action, and education regarding appropriate codes of behaviour (Hutchinson, 2009).

New graduate nurses historically have experienced higher rates of bullying than other staff members. By pursuing strategies to enhance structural empowerment in your workplace, you may be able to decrease episodes of bullying (Laschinger et al., 2010). Examples of these strategies are provided in Table 6.4. Identifying inappropriate behaviour as it happens, and calling the other staff member on it immediately, can also help to prevent the episode from becoming an ongoing pattern of behaviour. Refer to examples of 'shielding responses' in Table 6.2.

If you are experiencing bullying in the workplace identify your organisation's policies related to bullying and handling of grievances to discover what resources are available. Keep a diary of occurrences of bullying behaviour, documenting

Table 6.4 Strategies for enhancing components of structural empowerment

Component	Sample strategy
Opportunity	Pursue advanced education preparation. Identify available career and education pathways to guide your development.
Information	Become aware of over-arching departmental goals and key performance indicators.
Support	Pursue the development of a professional relationship with the educator or clinical mentor to support your development, and to provide feedback about and positive reinforcement of your achievements.
Resources	Make yourself available as a new graduate nurse stakeholder representative during the evaluation of new equipment or department projects.
Formal power	Avoid minimising your contribution to patient care, education and research during conversations with colleagues. Own your achievements.
Informal power	Honing your communication, collaboration and conflict management skills will support your development of informal networking skills at the unit level and presence within the worksite.

objectively and succinctly what happened and who was involved, and how it affected you at the time. If bullying is occurring digitally, keep a copy of all relevant emails, texts and posts.

Seek help early. Talking through what is happening with a trusted mentor or colleague can help to achieve a level of objectivity around what is happening, and how you may best respond to the situation. In many cases, your manager may be an appropriate person with whom to discuss the issue initially. If the bullying is from a direct manager, report it to an independent person such as a human resources representative, and also seek the early involvement of your union representative.

MANAGING COMPETING DEMANDS, RISKS AND DECISIONS

One of the key challenges you must overcome as a new graduate nurse is learning how to prioritise and complete necessary tasks in the management of your patient load. In the health setting, you will commonly have multiple activities and assessments to complete at any given time. As it is impossible to complete all simultaneously, you must be able to determine the highest priority for immediate attention, and decide what can be set aside for later management.

In many ward areas, nurses use *routines* to help them complete commonly required tasks. A routine is a customary way of managing tasks that usually occur each shift, and can reduce the cognitive demand of time management. Routines address what needs to be completed, as well as the order, timing and speed, and often synchronise with the routines of the wider health team (Waterworth, 2003). These routines usually cover tasks that apply to most patients, such as hygiene/showering, medication rounds and pressure care. When starting in a new clinical area, it is worth discussing with the educator what common tasks must be completed on a daily basis, and what structure/routine is recommended to achieve these in a succinct timeframe while fitting in with the needs of the multidisciplinary health team. Although useful in providing an initial structure to a shift, routines can potentially be dangerous if the nurse does not actively assess the individual clinical needs of the patient, and alter planned activities accordingly.

Completing a risk assessment is the first step towards ensuring patient safety. The risk assessment is a continuous process throughout your shift, seeking to identify issues that require alteration in treatment prior to them causing harm to the patient. The identification of risk to the patient is achieved via clinical assessment, and aims to find problems such as cardiovascular instability, falls hazard or medication side-effects (Groves et al., 2014). Once a risk has been identified, the nurse must make a *prioritisation* decision. Prioritisation is a critical skill for safe patient management, as you must be able to identify what is most important in a given set of tasks and sequence your work in response (Waterworth, 2003). In prioritising clinical risk to patients, employ the same assessment approach utilised in a resuscitation situation—that is, airway, breathing, circulation, disability to determine the hierarchy of which patient must be managed first. Simply put, consider what constitutes the primary threat to the patient's life. For example, the patient with respiratory compromise must take precedence over pressure care to prevent ulcer formation.

As a nurse, you are often expected to handle multiple tasks/interactions in rapid succession, such as documentation, monitoring technical equipment or preparing medications. In addition, many factors in the clinical setting will cause an interruption to general routine, ranging from a phone call to the clinical deterioration of your patient. Two main strategies are used to handle work demands and interruptions: *task-switching* and *multi-tasking*. As an example, if a nurse were asked a question while completing a task, they could stop what they were doing and reply (task-switching), or continue the activity while simultaneously providing an answer (multi-tasking) (Walter et al., 2014). Worryingly, for nurses, research into multi-tasking has shown that the quality of concentration and thought declines if a person tries to manage numerous tasks concurrently. Trying to complete related tasks at the same time or by alternating quickly between them has been associated with higher rates of error and increased time required to finish the task (Girard, 2007; Powell, 2005). This shouldn't come as a surprise, considering that it is common knowledge that driving while texting on a mobile phone increases the chance of a car accident.

Knowing the risks associated with multi-tasking and task-switching has practical use, as it allows you to decide when your full attention must be given to a task to ensure safety. Research has found that highly practised skills might be completed while you are thinking about something different; however, an activity that requires higher cognitive functioning, such as decision-making, requires the brain to switch to that particular task (Girard, 2007). Therefore, making a bed while talking to your colleague presents low risk, but taking handover while calculating a medication dosage presents an unreasonable chance of medication error and/or missed information.

COMMUNICATING WITH PATIENTS

A period of illness with resultant hospital admission is a time of high stress for patients and their families. Using effective communication strategies can affect how your patients perceive the clinical environment, health staff and the quality of the health service they receive. Basic needs of patients within the health setting may include:

- to feel safe
- to be treated with respect/courtesy
- to be involved in decision-making regarding treatment
- to know what is going to happen next during a course of treatment, and why
- to have confidence in the health system treating them
- to know what to do after hospital discharge.

Numerous factors affect communication between patients and health professionals. Paralinguistic features of communication refer to how we provide additional meaning to the words we use. They include both vocal and body language aspects.

Vocal paralinguistic features refer to how something is said, in terms of pitch, tone, pace, emphasis and volume. Each of these provide additional information to the patient about the situation. For example, a rapid pace of speech may indicate that the person is in a hurry, or a high tone may indicate nervousness or anger. During patient interactions, try to ensure that your speech remains slow and clear, and use a moderate to low tone to help provide a non-threatening demeanour and confident interaction. Body paralinguistic features refer to how we use our body to communicate.

Examples of body language include posture, touch, eye contact, proximity, facial expression and gestures. There is variability between cultures about the meaning of some behaviours; however, many are largely universal. Typical features that may help you communicate confidence during the clinical interaction include ensuring that your posture is not slouched, maintaining eye contact during speech, and ensuring that gestures made with hands and arms are purposeful and deliberate (Bigby & Ashley, 2008).

It is easy to forget that many of the terms and words we use to communicate ideas and treatment accurately between fellow health workers are likely to mean little or nothing to our patients, who may come from a different professional and educational background. Avoid the use of clinical jargon during patient interactions, as it will only create a barrier to the patient achieving an understanding about their own care. When conveying a clinical concept or information, endeavour to explain the concept in simple language and confirm the patient's understanding. Also, avoid the use of slang during communication to prevent potential offence or misinterpretation (Mullen, 2015). Psychological factors that affect interactions between the clinician and patient include attitudes and beliefs, prejudices, defence mechanisms, frame of mind/mood, stress and trust (Bigby & Ashley, 2008). As a nurse, be mindful of how each of these can affect your decision-making. Seek to understand your own core beliefs and prejudices to avoid incorrect cognitive leaps during the assessment process. An example of this would be deciding that an intravenous drug user presenting with abdominal pain is merely faking symptoms to access opioid medication, when in fact the patient may have acute appendicitis. As no person ever plans to become unwell, a key psychological factor for the patient during many health interactions is stress related to the illness or trauma event. Stress can negatively affect a patient's ability to process information and make a decision.

The environment in which the communication episode takes place will also affect the quality of information transfer. There are many environmental factors that are difficult to resolve in the clinical setting, where often only a curtain obstructs patients' vision of each other and does nothing to alter the transmission of sound or smell. However, every effort should be made to optimise a poor situation. Rooms or treatment spaces should be uncluttered and have adequate lighting. Ensure that invasive procedures and patient histories are conducted with privacy in mind. It is less likely that a patient will provide an honest answer to potentially sensitive questions, such as sexual health history, if they know someone else may overhear them. If a sensitive physical examination is in process—for example, a pelvic/vaginal exam—ensure adequate signage is on the outside of the door noting that the door is not to be opened.

Social factors such as age, gender, ethnicity and social status can affect communication (Bigby & Ashley, 2008). Factors associated with age, such as a decline in sight and hearing, must be considered. Cultural and gender factors should be considered: in some cases, the patient may be more comfortable if a procedure is completed by a clinician of the same sex.

Some general principles in communication that may help to facilitate a therapeutic relationship with patients include:

- addressing the patient by name
- introducing yourself and your role
- excusing yourself when you answer phones or other queries
- altering your communication style to suit the patient
- gaining consent of the patient and informing them of what you are about to do and why for each intervention and investigation
- keeping the patient and family up to date with the plan of care and also with any delays
- asking only one question at a time

- avoiding 'why' questions that may be interpreted as accusatory
- ensuring that any education is constructive, not condescending
- if the patient has difficulty giving you the information that you want, providing simple alternatives
- remaining aware of your own body language at times of stress.

PATIENT EDUCATION

Our aim in healthcare is to increase the patient's level of autonomy and ability to manage their own health. As such, patient education goals have altered from 'telling' them what to do to assisting development of skills and knowledge to manage and improve their own health (Comerford, 2010).

Two keys to successful patient education are reinforcement and keeping the message simple. Avoid intricate medical terminology or jargon, and explain the information in easily understandable language. During times of stress, information retention may be reduced. Aim for a strategy that supports retention of critical components for self-management. Always assess what the patient knows before starting, and choose three or four essential concepts on which to concentrate. When a concept is heard and explored multiple times throughout a session, it is more likely to be retained (Comerford, 2004).

When teaching adults, it is relevant to have a grasp of Knowles' adult learning principles:

- An adult will have greater interaction with learning when there is a perceived need.
- Do not re-teach something that is already understood. Move from the known to the unknown.
- Progress from simple concepts towards more complex ones.
- Active participation is more effective with adult learners compared with **didactic teaching** styles.
- If you are teaching a new skill, time is required to practise the skill and receive feedback.
- Adults also require reinforcement of learned skills through multiple opportunities to demonstrate the specific skill.
- Provision of timely feedback and early correction of misconceptions aid learning. This process can be targeted by asking a patient to paraphrase their understanding of taught content (Comerford, 2004).

didactic teaching
A situation where information is presented by a teacher to a student with little interaction—for example, a teacher presenting a topic from the front of the classroom.

Example of adult learning principles applied to a patient education session

A nurse, Roger, is undertaking a teaching session with a patient, Vera, regarding self-administration of Enoxaparin injections for Deep Vein Thrombosis (DVT). Roger starts by asking what Vera's understanding is of her diagnosis of DVT to clarify what she already knows so this is not re-taught. Roger then explains the role of the injection in the treatment, and what may happen if it is not administered; this ensures that Vera perceives a clear need to learn how to self-administer the medication. Roger encourages an interactive learning environment by inviting Vera to ask any questions as they go along, which also helps early identification of misconceptions requiring correction. Roger explains simple theory regarding administration of a subcutaneous injection, then invites Vera to paraphrase this information to check her understanding. Roger demonstrates how to administer the injection, then asks Vera to demonstrate the skill herself. Lastly, Roger follows up with feedback regarding needed changes in technique, or confirms that Vera is practising the skill correctly.

MANAGING COMPLAINTS

A complaint is an expression of dissatisfaction or concern regarding the health service that is made by a patient, family member or carer. Health consumer complaints frequently originate in communication issues, employee behaviour or perceptions of sub-standard clinical treatment. Patient complaints are an important source of evidence to ascertain why adverse events happen and, more importantly, how to prevent reoccurrence in the future. Competent management of complaints is required not only to improve health services, but also to rebuild community trust and decrease the chance of litigation (ACSQHC, 2005).

To ensure that high-quality care is delivered to patients, health services have instituted complaint management systems in each state. The Australian Commission on Safety and Quality in Healthcare (2005) recommends that a complaint-management system includes the following aspects:

- *It is committed to ongoing quality improvement:* a continuous quality improvement program exists that supports a consumer focus in relation to complaints.
- *It is accessible:* feedback from consumers is encouraged, with a dedicated system to support lodgement of complaints or concerns.

- *It is responsive:* all complaints are recognised and responded to in a timely manner.
- *It provides effective assessment of complaints:* all complaints are assessed by identifying risk factors, accountability and the request of the complainant to determine an appropriate response.
- *It achieves appropriate resolution:* complaints are managed in a fashion that is fair to all parties, is complete and achieves a just outcome.
- *It maintains privacy and open disclosure:* related facts and decisions are transparently discussed while ensuring confidentiality and privacy.
- *It has appropriate documentation and information-management systems:* all complaints are recorded to allow identification of trends and risks, and the review of individual cases, and to enable reporting upon how improvements in practice have been achieved in response.
- *It supports introduction of improvements:* complaints are used to improve the health service, and the complaint-management system is reviewed regularly to ensure it meets contemporary policy and practices.

In the event that a patient, carer or family member identifies a concern, you should be as helpful as possible, and aim to resolve the issue at the time. If this is not an option, help should be provided to assist the individual to make a formal complaint (Treanor, 2014). Make yourself familiar with the process of lodging a complaint within your particular institution. A clinical governance or clinical practice improvement department within the hospital or service commonly manages complaints. Other avenues may be via an incident information-management computer program where you can lodge the complaint on behalf of the patient, or direct phone lines and email addresses that the consumer can utilise.

Once a complaint is lodged, an acknowledgement letter is sent to the complainant. The complaint is then forwarded to the relevant manager to investigate and to provide a written response. Complaint investigations seek to identify system errors rather than apportioning blame to a particular staff member. The inquiring manager will then send their response to the department responsible for managing complaints, to be collated with any other responses from other investigating managers, before sign-off by the director of operations. Commonly, there are key performance indicators (KPI) to monitor responses to complaints. In NSW Health, for example, there is a KPI for a complaint to be acknowledged within five days, and to be investigated and a response created within 35 days (NSW Health, 2015a).

OPEN DISCLOSURE

Across Australia, thousands of patients receive health-related treatments each and every day. For the most part, optimal outcomes are achieved in challenging work environments. Despite best efforts, however, adverse events occur that result in patient harm. *Open disclosure* refers to the process employed by clinicians to communicate with the patient and family affected by the adverse event, and is considered a right of the patient, as well as a feature of good clinical and ethical health practice. The use of open disclosure is articulated in the Australian Open Disclosure Framework, and is mandated in the National Safety and Quality Health Service Standards for use in all Australian clinical settings (ACSQHC, 2013b).

The key elements of open disclosure include:

- an apology that includes the words 'I am sorry' or 'we are sorry'
- a clear explanation of what occurred
- provision of opportunity for the family and patient to convey their experience
- a conversation regarding the possible consequences of the adverse event
- an explanation of what is being done to manage the event, and how the organisation aims to prevent recurrence of a similar situation (ACSQHC, 2013b).

Open disclosure is a process of two-way communication between the healthcare team and the patient/family that may occur over several meetings. It does not, however, imply guilt or that a clinician or service has blameworthy facts to report, or constitute a legal process. Open disclosure seeks to address and balance the interests of clinicians, patients, managers and health organisations, as well as other stakeholder groups including professional organisations and medical indemnity insurers (ACSQHC, 2013b).

DE-ESCALATION OF AGGRESSION AND VIOLENCE IN THE WORKPLACE

Unfortunately, you are likely to be exposed to aggression and violence in the workplace at some time during your nursing career, and challenging communication encounters may occasionally deteriorate to the point of overt aggression or violence. Understanding some of the risk factors and precipitators for violence in the health setting is an important step towards helping you to decrease its occurrence. Mental health, geriatrics and emergency are three specialty areas that have been found to be high-risk areas for aggression and violence against health staff (Powley, 2013; Wharton & Ford, 2014). In the emergency department, the most common factors noted to increase the chance of violence include alcohol, drugs and waiting times for treatment (Hodge & Marshall, 2007). While patients are often the main aggressors, visitors and relatives are also common instigators of violence. Other common factors influencing or potentially triggering violence in any healthcare setting include:

- physical illness
- confusion
- delirium
- anxiety
- altered perceptions/paranoid ideas
- boredom
- heat
- excessive or constant noise
- lack of information
- having no right of appeal regarding decisions made
- lack of choice
- group/peer pressure
- staff shortages
- lack of understanding of how health staff prioritise workloads
- inadequate staff training
- perceived negative staff attitudes.

As a nurse, you should be aware that the way you approach a situation is important. If a situation is tackled in the wrong way, it may exacerbate the tension or create further aggression from the patient. The best way to control violence is through prevention; however, in the health setting it is impossible to eradicate all triggers for aggressive behaviour. If you notice signs of escalation towards a behavioural emergency, inform your manager so that the most appropriate personnel are allocated to deal with the situation, and call security if necessary. The most common behaviours preceding an episode of violence are confusion, irritability, boisterousness, physical and verbal threats and attacking objects, provocative behaviour, angry demeanour, pacing, loud speech, tense posture and frequent changes in body position (Hodge & Marshall, 2007).

The first strategy for stopping a developing incident from progressing to outright violence and aggression should be de-escalation. De-escalation requires defusing, negotiation and conflict resolution, with an aim of recognising signs of impending violence to prevent it in the first place (Hodge & Marshall, 2007). Remember that your first priority is to maintain safety for yourself and patients in your care (Table 6.5).

Table 6.5 Strategies for de-escalating violent behaviour

Promote safety	Communication strategies
Monitor for signs of violence (facial expression, posture).	Use calm respectful language (e.g. use appropriate titles, Mr/Mrs).
Approach the patient with caution.	Use open-ended sentences (e.g. How can I help you?).
Do not startle the patient (e.g. don't walk up behind the patient prior to announcing your presence).	Express your own feelings and let the patient know your concern (e.g. 'Our main aim is to keep you safe and provide treatment that will help you get better quickly, however, when you shout at staff, it makes it difficult for them to provide the care you need.').
Separate the patient from the group (e.g. invite the patient to move away from the group so you can discuss and help them resolve their problem).	
Avoid provocation (e.g. do not swear, shout, point, make accusations).	Tell the patient the effect they are having on those around them (e.g. 'Your behaviour and speech is frightening some of the patients around you.').
Avoid vulnerable positions (e.g. room with only one exit, or being backed up against a wall).	
Remove dangerous objects from the immediate vicinity (e.g. items that could be picked up and used as a weapon).	Model calm behaviour (e.g. open posture, relaxed expression, calm, slow speech in normal conversation volume).
Outline consequences of behaviours (e.g. if this behaviour continues, you will have to leave the department).	Establish rapport and dialogue with the patient (e.g. introduce yourself, reaffirm that you want to help the patient sort out their health complaint while maintaining safety for everyone present; try to find out what the patient wants).
Stay out of lunging distance from patient (e.g. maintain at least 1 metre distance between you and the patient).	

Source: Adapted from Hodge & Marshall (2007).

HEALTH INFORMATION SYSTEMS AND TECHNOLOGIES

Information technology and computers are a reality of our modern world, as is their incorporation into the health industry. The application of systems and technologies has increased sharply over recent years to assist clinicians in coping with the growing complexity and efficiency required in many areas of clinical practice. One such system has been the development of the electronic healthcare record, which has impacted greatly on the work of the clinician. The electronic medical record (EMR) is an electronic document detailing clinical data such as patient information, past medical history, vital signs, progress of treatment, diagnostic test orders and results, and medication orders. The introduction of EMR systems within hospitals has received mixed reviews by healthcare administrators, clinicians and nurses. While EMR has enhanced patient safety and provided a means of evaluating care quality and coordination, efficiency and staffing demand (Beck et al., 2013; Cipriano et al., 2013; Harper, 2012; Towsley et al., 2013), the design of the system and cumbersome data entry have been reported to slow or impede the delivery of care and nursing practice (Roman et al., 2016; Sockolow et al., 2012; Stevenson et al., 2010). For clinical documentation to be considered contemporaneous, the information being recorded must be accurate and entered in a timely fashion. The process of documenting patient care efficiently must be incorporated into the design and operation of health information systems and technologies if errors are to be avoided (ACSQHC, 2012; Bove & Jesse, 2010; Piscotty & Kalisch, 2014).

With increasing use of EMR and informational technology systems across all sectors of healthcare, including the provision of education, nurses need to develop computer literacy skills. The following is an outline of essential computer literacy skills.

- Nurses need to know how to retrieve, open and save files across common software programs such as Word and Excel, and have sufficiently developed keyboard and mouse control skills.
- Nurses should have sufficiently developed skills to be able to navigate a Windows desktop.
- Nurses need to be able to recognise when information is needed, and be able to locate, evaluate and use that information appropriately, such as searching for and retrieving basic information from research databases, use of email and finding patient education resources.
- Nurses must be able to read electronic charts and input patient data into the EMR system used within their area of employment, including electronic prescribing and automated dispensing systems if used.
- Use of EMR systems may vary within hospitals, and even between wards. The switch from paper records to electronic records, or a mix of the two, has raised new challenges for nurses—especially consistency of documentation.

A thorough understanding of the process of documentation and the systems used must form part of the orientation education period of new staff and nurses.

- Nurses need technical skills to navigate eLearning platforms or training software to access continuing education programs.
- Various human interaction devices, such as barcode scanners, are used to track patients and decrease human error—for example, confirming patient identity as part of medication administration or blood collection. Familiarity with these devices is essential, and again must form part of the orientation education period.
- Knowledge and use of nursing 'apps', while not major requirements, are useful for nurses working in a range of healthcare settings. Many apps have been designed to assist nurses in clinical decision-making, delivering care, providing appropriate information to patients, and accessing research and the latest clinical updates.

One of the challenges for nurses relating to health information systems is the goal of achieving seamless care. Patients access a range of care services, both within hospitals and in the community. Being able to share patient records in real time with other clinicians involved in the patient's care has been fraught with difficulty. Ensuring patient confidentiality and privacy when communicating with other healthcare services necessitates stringent security measures to be taken, including protection from unlawful wireless (e.g. wi-fi, bluetooth) or remote internet access. Using high-grade internet security, while necessary, presents an additional roadblock for community care providers in different healthcare districts, as the appropriate level of security is needed before access is granted. In addition, EMR systems may not be compatible across different sites, further limiting access to patient information. A common work-around is to use portable technology such as tablets or smartphones. However, the advent of health technologies and numerous mobile devices with the capacity to capture, monitor, store and transmit data wirelessly presents both opportunities and challenges.

Smartphones and other mobile computing devices are becoming an integral part of our daily lives, and have penetrated almost every industrial and professional field. Surveys suggest that over 70 per cent of nurses and physicians already use smartphones as part of their clinical practice (Dolan, 2012; Kiser, 2011). The use of such devices presents both opportunities and challenges for professional nursing practice, and while guidelines have been produced regarding mobile technology within the healthcare work setting, the effectiveness of their use ultimately lies with the individual clinician. The adoption of smartphone technology within today's healthcare industry has enhanced clinician and patient education, patient engagement (Doswell et al., 2013) and communication (Wu et al., 2011). Yet it has also led to the erosion of professional behaviours and attitudes, placing patient privacy, confidentiality and safety at risk (Westbrook et al., 2010). It is also a recognised infection-control hazard (Brady et al., 2007; Hassoun et al., 2004).

In 2015, there were over 165,000 medical applications available across all mobile device platforms (Constantino, 2015). While this may decrease the need of clinicians to commit and retrieve information from memory, there are growing concerns regarding the credibility of information provided by applications, due to the lack of robust regulation and peer-review processes (Haffey et al., 2013). Today, mobile devices can quickly combine high-resolution photography and messaging (e.g. text, voice) to allow more detailed information to be shared between clinicians (Hsieh et al., 2015). However, unless other methods are used, this information is sent using unsecure devices and networks. While higher quality information may greatly assist clinicians in managing patients, it may be prudent to make a conscientious effort to refrain from using smartphones in the clinical setting until data security and patient concerns regarding their use are addressed.

social media Refers to the online and mobile technologies that allow the creating and sharing (i.e. posting) of information, ideas, opinions, photos, videos and other forms of expression via virtual communities and networks, such as social networking sites, personal websites and blogs.

The use of **social media** is expanding rapidly. When used appropriately, it provides increasing opportunities for healthcare professionals and organisations to network, and to share knowledge and experiences. It can also be a vital tool for communicating essential information during a disaster event. Yet, while use of social media as a means of communication is widely accepted, it is not without risk. When posting information on social media, it is important to remember that the *Health Practitioner Regulation National Law Act 2009*, the Code of Conduct and the Guidelines for Advertising Regulated Health Services apply.

If posting on social media, you should ensure that what you publish:

- does not breach professional obligations (e.g. Code of Conduct or Ethics, contract of employment)
- does not breach confidentiality and privacy obligations (such as discussing patients or posting pictures of procedures, case studies, patients or sensitive material that may enable patients to be identified without prior consent)
- is not biased and does not make unsubstantiated claims, and
- does not use testimonials or purported testimonials in any capacity on any medium (AHPRA, 2014).

Summary

In this chapter, we have explored the vital issue of communication in the workplace. We have noted the importance of working effectively in teams in today's healthcare environment and how to develop collaborative approaches and achieve efficient decision-making. We have looked at conflict resolution, workplace bullying and managing competing demands. We then turned to communication with patients, including effective patient education strategies and managing complaints. We also looked at dealing with aggression and violence, and finally considered the use of health information systems in clinical practice.

Review questions

6.1 Problems in communication are one of the leading causes of adverse outcomes. True or false?

6.2 In relation to communication, what does ISBAR stand for?

6.3 When escalating identified deterioration in one of your patients, who should be made aware?
   a Treating doctor
   b Nurse Unit Manager
   c Both of the above

6.4 Common barriers to effective teams include:
   a Hierarchy: varying levels of qualification and status
   b Differences in payment, reward and accountability
   c Some members' failure to contribute
   d Different schedules and professional routines
   e Shiftwork

6.5 Effective teams demonstrate positive attributes in the areas of:
   a Team structure and organisational support
   b Clinical governance
   c Team process and interactions
   d Contribution by individual team members

6.6 Bullying refers to:
   a Occasional episodes of rudeness
   b An ongoing pattern of behaviour that is intended to be offensive, intimidating, humiliating or threatening

6.7 A risk assessment is a one-off activity completed at the start of your shift to see whether your patient requires a clinical review or change in therapy. True or false?

6.8 Routines can be dangerous if the nurse doesn't change their planned activities to match the individual clinical needs of the patient. True or false?

6.9 When conducting patient education, it is relevant to apply 'adult learning principles' to your teaching session. Some appropriate adult learning strategies are:
   a Not re-teaching something that is already understood
   b Using didactic teaching styles
   c When teaching a new skill, allowing time for practising the skill and providing feedback

6.10 Open disclosure is:
   a considered a feature of good clinical and ethical practice
   b mandated for use in all clinical settings
   c a process of two-way communication between the healthcare team and patient/family
   d a policy that seeks to decrease litigation costs for the health provider

6.11 Common factors that increase the chance of aggression and violence from patients and visitors include:
   a Lack of information
   b Confusion
   c Alcohol and drugs
   d Good communication
   e Perceived negative staff attitudes

7 ASSESSMENT, CARE DELIVERY AND DIAGNOSTIC REASONING

Alister Hodge and Wayne Varndell

In this chapter, you will develop an understanding of:

- patient assessment
- forming a management plan
- documentation
- common nursing models of care delivery
- how to delegate care and supervise practice
- how to develop a mentor relationship
- diagnostic reasoning in nursing
- identification of the deteriorating patient
- patient transfer and transportation
- basic life support
- medication administration
- nursing with a diverse culture
- illness, death and dying.

PATIENT ASSESSMENT

Competent physical assessment skills are fundamental to all nursing specialties. The ability to accurately assess the condition of your patient is vital in the creation of an appropriate plan of management. It can be very helpful to use a systematic approach when conducting a physical assessment.

In critical care areas such as emergency and the ICU, the primary/secondary survey and comprehensive physical assessment formats are utilised to guide time-critical and complete assessment of the patient. In some ward areas where the patient has a defined diagnosis, a focused physical assessment may be employed to examine affected body systems after completion of a general assessment.

Identifying immediate compromise on first interaction with the patient

The *primary survey* is a format used to systematically assess a patient for immediately life-threatening factors while simultaneously completing lifesaving treatment interventions (Cameron & O'Reilly, 2010). Although classically used in a trauma or medical emergency situation, the version of a primary survey provided in Table 7.1 is useful to structure a general assessment of baseline respiratory/ circulatory and neurological function. An informal primary survey should be completed on first contact with any patient. Much of the following information is gained from the foot of the bed through initial simple interaction with the patient—for example, the patient speaking in full sentences indicates a **patent airway** and absence of significant respiratory distress. During initial interaction with the patient, also consider the set-up of your clinical environment to ensure that items required during an emergency are present and working—for example, check oxygen/suction/presence of airway adjuncts (Table 7.1).

patent airway An airway that is open and clear of obstruction, allowing inhalation of oxygen and exhalation of carbon dioxide.

In a medical emergency, the ABCDEFG approach to assessment should be employed (Table 7.2). This structured assessment has been adopted by Between the Flags, a NSW Government program seeking to improve identification of deteriorating patients and their subsequent escalation of care (Jacques et al., 2009).

Table 7.1 Primary survey/general assessment for ward environment

System	Assessment activity
Airway	Check for evidence of airway obstruction/patency.
Breathing	Check respiratory rate, peripheral capillary oxygen saturation (SpO_2), skin colour, signs of respiratory distress, air entry, **adventitious airway noise**.
Circulation	Check peripheral pulse strength, heart rate, blood pressure, **skin colour/perfusion**, capillary refill.
Disability	Check level of consciousness: AVPU (Alert/responds to voice/responds to pain/unresponsive)

adventitious airway noise An abnormal sound heard from a patient's lungs or airways, e.g. wheeze.

skin colour/perfusion When assessing breathing, assessing skin colour can give an indication of oxygen saturation of haemoglobin. With adequate oxygen saturation of haemoglobin, the patient's skin will have colour. Poor oxygen saturation will be evidenced by pale skin, progressing to blue/cyanosed skin as oxygen saturation decreases. In relation to circulation assessment, a patient with normal blood pressure should be well perfused—that is, have colour to their skin. If they have low blood pressure, this will be evidenced by poor perfusion, pale skin and a capillary refill time of greater than 2 seconds.

Table 7.2 ABCDEFG assessment during a medical emergency

Stage	Activity
A: Airway	Look for: foreign bodies, **tracheal tug**.
	Listen for: snoring, gurgling, **stridor**, hoarseness, inability to talk in sentences.
	Feel for **tracheal deviation**, diminished air movement.
	Interventions: institute required airway adjuncts (e.g. jaw thrust), insert an oropharangeal/nasopharangeal airway, maintain spinal precautions if spinal injury suspected.

continues

Table 7.2 ABCDEFG assessment during a medical emergency *continued*

Stage	Activity
B: Breathing	Look for: paradoxical chest movement, **tachypnoea**, respiratory rate, accessory muscle use, skin colour. Check SpO_2.
	Listen for: absent or decreased breath sounds, unequal air entry, adventitious noises.
	Feel for: **subcutaneous emphysema**, **crepitus**, tracheal deviation.
	Interventions: apply oxygen, apply SpO_2 monitoring.
C: Circulation	Look for: pallor, peripheral perfusion, skin colour, obvious signs of external bleeding, distended neck veins.
	Listen for: muffled heart sounds.
	Feel for: palpate pulses for presence, quality, rate and rhythm, symmetry. Check blood pressure and heart rate.
	Interventions: institute haemorrhage control, ensure intravenous access is present in upper limbs.
D: Disability	Look for: level of consciousness by accurately using Glasgow Coma Scale. Check pupils for size, shape, reaction to light, **consensuality**. Check limb strength.
	Interventions: place in **left lateral position** if unconscious (if no evidence of spinal injury).
E: Expose	Expose patient to assess for injuries, haemorrhage, rash, bruising, wounds and preparation for secondary survey.
F: Fluids	Check fluid chart, calculate input vs. output balance. Check for losses from all drains and tubes.
G: Glucose	Look for: patient's glucose level. Check for signs of low glucose, which may include confusion, decreased conscious state, and sweaty or clammy skin. Interventions: give glucose if blood sugar level is <3 mmols/L or between 3 and 5 mmols/L with an accompanying decrease in consciousness level.

tracheal tug Caused by upper airway obstruction, it is an abnormal downward movement of the trachea during inspiration.

stridor An abnormal airway sound caused by turbulent airflow in the upper airway, high pitched in sound.

tracheal deviation The trachea should be midline as it descends past the supra-sternal notch. Movement of the trachea to left or right, i.e. deviation, is evidence of possible tension pneumothorax.

tachypnoea Describes abnormal fast respiratory rate.

subcutaneous emphysema Describes the presence of air trapped within the tissue below the skin, and has the sensation of rice paper under your fingers on palpation.

crepitus A grating sensation on palpation caused by the ends of fractured bone rubbing against each other.

consensuality Pupils should have a consensual response to light—for example, when light is shone into one eye, the opposite pupil should contract at the same time.

left lateral position Also known as recovery position. Decreases the chance that an unconscious person will aspirate in the event of vomiting.

CLINICAL ASSESSMENT

If no life-threatening factors are identified that require immediate action, a clinical examination incorporating history and physical assessment can be undertaken. A common format for this type of assessment used by medical, nursing and allied health professionals involves investigating the following:

- the presenting complaint
- history of the presenting complaint
- allergies
- medications
- past medical/surgical history
- when the patient last ate/drank, last menstrual period
- family/social history.

A comprehensive investigation such as this is used on first contact with a patient where there is no established diagnosis. The presenting complaint, history of presenting complaint and background history are evaluated in conjunction with the initial clinical impression of the patient. In light of the presenting clinical situation and background history of the patient, a relevant physical assessment that targets specific body systems is determined.

Further physical assessment may be approached in two different ways:

- In the critically ill patient, a comprehensive assessment should be completed. A head-to-toe or systems approach is often taken to guide this.
- For the patient with a readily identifiable complaint, it may be more appropriate to focus directly on systems relevant to the complaint—for example, for a patient with an isolated limb fracture, the relevant assessments may include musculoskeletal, neurovascular and pain assessment.

Findings from the physical assessment and history are used to guide further investigations and interventions.

FORMING A MANAGEMENT PLAN

Information gained from patient history and physical assessment determines an appropriate nursing management plan for your patient. Management plans will vary depending upon the patient's physical state or clinical condition under treatment. Areas that may often be considered in a nursing management plan include frequency and type of observations required, eating/drinking status, type of monitoring required—for example, cardiac/SpO_2—pressure care required, fluid balance monitoring, wound-management plan, pain-management plan, mobility aids needed and medical/allied health reviews required.

Clarify with your educator or Nurse Unit Manager whether there is a pre-existing management template that you are expected to use. Many organisations have clinical pathways that provide an evidence-based standard to guide patient management. Clinical pathways commonly guide post-operative management for numerous surgical interventions—for example, total hip replacement; however, the appropriateness of a generic plan must be assessed against the clinical status of the patient.

DOCUMENTATION

Accurate, readable and relevant documentation is critical to optimal care delivery in the clinical environment. Poor documentation has multiple ramifications for the patient as well as the provider. Information missing from a patient's record impacts upon subsequent clinical decisions of the wider health team. An over-arching clinical management plan can only be formed after consideration of patient clinical progress, investigations, previous interventions and subsequent response. However, if this information has not been documented, the proposed management plan may prove inadequate for the actual clinical situation.

Accessibility of your documentation is affected by legibility and formatting.

Another clinician may be deterred from reading your documentation if they have to decipher poor handwriting, non-standard abbreviations (see the list at the end of the book) or read through a large block of text to find a specific detail. You will also be dependent upon the accuracy of your own documentation if called to defend your patient management in court (Townsend, 2007). As time moves on and the number of patients with whom you come in contact steadily increases, you will not be able to recall specifics of all care episodes; therefore, you will be relying on the accuracy of your documentation to remember the event. Lastly, unless there is documented evidence of the care provided, your verbal recall of the event will not be given the same degree of consideration in court (Townsend, 2007).

The healthcare record should be an integrated multidisciplinary document, with sequential entries sufficiently detailed to:

- provide effective communication to the healthcare team
- provide continuity of a patient's care across service boundaries (subject to confidentiality)
- clearly describe the patient's progress (including clinical incidents, should they occur) and health outcomes, including assessment, implementation and evaluation of patient care (Strategic Relations and Communications, 2012).

Documentation must be written in close time proximity to the events described. Avoid writing notes in retrospect—for example, at the end of the shift or the next day. All entries in the patient's record should be your accurate and complete statement of fact, or of clinical judgement relating to care, treatment and/or professional advice given (Strategic Relations and Communications, 2012). Entries must not contain prejudicial, derogatory or irrelevant statements about the patient or others involved in the patient's care. Figure 7.1 is an example of the documentation of a comprehensive assessment.

The strengths of this form of documentation include the following:

- Writing under headings enables the reader to locate a specific area of interest without reading the whole document.
- It allows the writer to use minimal sentence structure and text, therefore decreasing recording/writing time; the use of accepted abbreviations can further reduce the amount of text written.
- The history and physical assessment record pertinent information required to determine a plan of care.
- The plan of care has evidence of appropriateness through documented history and physical assessment.

The example shown in Figure 7.2 below details the review of an admitted ward patient using a focused assessment format.

Nursing notes

12.03.09. **Time:** 1840.

Patient: 24-year-old female

Presenting complaint: Inversion injury right ankle

History of presenting complaint: While running this morning, inversion injury occurred to right ankle on uneven ground. Unable to weight bear after injury.

Allergies: No known drug allergies

Regular medications: Nil

Past medical history: Nil

Physical assessment: Alert, orientated, well perfused, nil respiratory distress

Vitals: Blood pressure 110/60 mmHg, Heart rate 65 bpm, respiratory rate 14 bpm, temperature 36.5°C, Glasgow Coma Scale 15. Pain: rates pain 4/10.

Right knee: No abnormality detected

Right ankle/foot:

Inspection: Swelling at lateral malleolus.

Palpation: Bony tenderness lateral malleolus and base of 5th metatarsal.
Tender over the lateral ligaments of ankle.

Movement: Decreased range of movement of ankle.

Weight bearing: Unable to weight bear on right foot.

Neurovascular assessment: Dorsalis Pedis and Posterior Tibial pulses present. Normal sensation. Foot pink, Capillary refill <2 seconds.

Impression: ?fracture ?sprain

Investigations: Right ankle and foot X-ray.

Interventions: Rest/ice/compression/elevation of ankle.

Analgesia: paracetamol 1 g, ibuprofen 400 mg.

Plan: Review pain post analgesia, await X-ray.

Signed: Bob Dole RN

The main reason the patient has sought medical care stated in a few words.

How the presenting complaint occurred, e.g. how, what, why, when, and subsequent signs and symptoms experienced.

Regular medications are identified. A medication history is another source of information that may guide investigations or assessments.

Physical assessment of a limb injury generally includes as a minimum:
- inspection—what does it look like?
- palpation—what does it feel like, does it cause the patient pain when touched?
- movement—is there an alteration to the range of movement of the joint?
- neurovascular assessment—what is the state of nerve and blood supply like?

Dorsalis pedis and posterior tibial pulse are two key pulses assessed during a neurovascular exam of the lower limb. Normal sensation—indicates sensory function of nerves in the foot is intact. Capillary refill < 2 seconds—on pressing on a nail bed or skin, the skin will blanch, then go pink as blood returns to the capillary bed. The time taken to re-perfuse is referred to as capillary refill time; a time of < 2 seconds is an indication of adequate limb perfusion with blood.

Plan articulates what the next stages of clinical management will entail.

In an inversion injury the ankle is turned inward with force, typically causing injury to the ligaments on the lateral aspect of the ankle.

Known drug allergies or reactions are sought and documented to avoid administration during treatment.

Past medical history is a key source of additional information that may guide additional investigations, physical assessments conducted and possible differential diagnoses (range of diseases/injuries) that could create the signs and symptoms observed during the initial assessment.

Physical assessment begins with a general clinical picture of the patient to demonstrate that airway/breathing/circulation/disability is adequate and not requiring immediate intervention. In this case, it is provided by the statement 'Alert, orientated, well perfused, nil respiratory distress'.

Possible diagnoses are listed simply as the 'impression' drawn by the clinician, another term commonly used for this is 'differential diagnoses'.

Investigations are the tests that will be completed to confirm or discard the initial impression and form a concrete diagnosis.

Interventions are what you do as a clinician to treat the problems identified during your assessment.

Figure 7.1 Nursing notes: comprehensive assessment

Figure 7.2 Nursing notes: focused assessment

Nursing notes

12.04.11. 1730hrs.

Admission reason: 26-year-old male, appendicitis. Admitted from emergency department, awaiting theatre.

Physical assessment: Alert, orientated, pale, radial pulse present, nil respiratory distress.

Vitals: Blood pressure 100/60 mmHg, Heart rate 105 bpm, temperature 38.5°C, respiratory rate 18 bpm, SaO2 96% on room air. Glasgow Coma Scale 15.

Respiratory system: Talking in full sentences.

Cardiovascular system: Strong radial pulse. IVC right wrist. IVT N/saline 1L 4/24 infusion running.

Abdomen: Involuntary guarding present, rigid abdomen.

Pain: Rates pain 8/10. Appears distressed.

Renal: Urine output >30 mL/hr.

Plan: Notify doctor/nurse manager of worsening acute abdomen needing urgent review and escalation. Request second IVC to be sited. Nil by mouth. Continue intravenous fluids. Give pain relief: morphine. Reassess pain and observations in 15 minutes.

Signed: Bob Dole RN

Annotations:

The reason why the patient is in hospital, stated in a few words.

Physical assessment begins with a general clinical picture of the patient to demonstrate that airway/breathing/circulation/disability is adequate and not requiring immediate intervention. In this case, it is provided by the statement 'Alert, orientated, pale, radial pulse present, nil respiratory distress', and a full set of vital signs. It then continues into specific body systems relevant to the diagnosis and clinical picture of the patient.

Urine output is a key indicator of whether there is adequate blood pressure to achieve end organ perfusion. An expectation of urine production is 0.5 mL/kg in a young adult. This would mean that, for an average adult of at least 60 kg, the patient should be producing 30 mL/hour or more.

Talking in full sentences is a key feature to document overall respiratory stability. For a patient to be talking in full sentences, they must have a patent airway, and breathing slowly enough that they can communicate normally.

Strong radial pulse—this is key evidence demonstrating that the blood pressure of the patient is adequate to perfuse brain/organs and limbs. IVC is abbreviation for intravenous catheter; it is documented to demonstrate the current level of venous access. IVT is an abbreviation for intravenous therapy, and notes the current type and speed of intravenous fluid resuscitation in place.

Involuntary guarding and a rigid abdomen are features of an acute abdomen where there is irritation of the lining of the abdominal cavity, the peritoneum, causing the abdominal muscles to spasm. In the situation of appendicitis, this may be an indication of rupture.

The strengths of this form of documentation include the following:

- Writing under headings enables the reader to locate a specific area of interest without reading the whole document and allows the writer to use minimal sentence structure and text, therefore decreasing recording/writing time.
- The recorded physical assessment presents a clear clinical picture of an acute abdomen requiring escalation.
- The plan of care has evidence of appropriateness through documented history and physical assessment.

For ongoing notes after your initial assessment, document by exception—that is, note any changes in clinical condition and your response, or changes in management plan.

NURSING MODELS FOR CARE DELIVERY

The two most common structures for care delivery in Australia are currently *primary nursing* and *team nursing*. In primary nursing, decision-making regarding an ongoing nursing plan is completed by the nurse delivering bedside care (Manthey, 2009). The primary nurse is responsible for conducting clinical assessments and ongoing patient-management activities, and for interacting with the medical/allied health teams regarding patient treatment. The nurse is also expected to competently identify the deteriorating patient, implement appropriate interventions and notify relevant health personnel. Primary nursing can provide several benefits, such as facilitating continuity of care for the patient, with the primary nurse being assigned to the same patient's care during the duration of their admission. In team nursing, two or more nurses work in a team to provide care to a group of patients. Ideally, the team incorporates a senior nurse working in a constructive relationship with a junior nurse to complete patient care activities. In a functioning team, the structure provides professional development opportunities by creating a learning environment for discussion of patient care issues while providing a support structure for new nurses. It may also contribute to earlier detection of deteriorating patients through increased supervision by a senior clinical staff member.

Following is an example of how team nursing can be implemented during a shift.

- The two nurses work as a team over their assigned beds to ensure support for each nurse is available throughout the shift and that heavy workloads are shared.

- New admissions are completed together: one nurse acquires and writes the history while the other nurse conducts interventions/investigations such as an ECG, measuring vital signs, attaching a monitor.
- Ongoing documentation is completed by each nurse for half of the patients managed together.

At shift change the following occurs:

- Both nurses attend a bedside handover for their patients.
- After completing an informal primary survey during handover to identify any patients requiring immediate intervention, both nurses start a systematic examination of each patient: one nurse checks bedside documentation not assessed during handover, while the other nurse checks drains, wounds, monitoring, fluids attached. The nurses assist each other in any repositioning of patients required. Each nurse clearly communicates their findings to their teammate as the review takes place. The Nurse Unit Manager and treating doctor are notified of any patient identified as having signs of deterioration. Medications requiring administration are noted and charts put aside for later.
- After patients have been assessed, the team has a brief discussion to clarify the tasks requiring completion for each of their patients and agrees upon what must take priority. Items that will be easier to complete with the help of two are noted so that they can be done together.
- The two nurses share the load of medications over the team's allocated patients.
- The two nurses in the team are to verbally touch base with each other at least every 30 minutes to ensure that they are aware of any developments/changes/need for help.
- At the change of shift, each nurse within the team is responsible for handing over half of the patients.

DELEGATION OF CARE AND SUPERVISION BY THE NEW GRADUATE NURSE

Although new to the clinical environment, as a new graduate nurse you may have to delegate a work task to another clinician during a shift. Graduates often feel uncomfortable doing this; however, the ability to delegate tasks appropriately is an important skill for you to master. Most commonly for the graduate, delegation of workload will be to Assistants in Nursing (AINs) or nursing students. Nursing tasks that may be appropriate for delegation to an AIN include feeding, turning, assisting the patient to walk, performing hygiene duties and checking vital signs.

If you decide to delegate a task to an AIN or student, be aware that you are still accountable for the safe completion of that particular task. This means you must provide an adequate degree of supervision to ensure that the task is completed satisfactorily, and that any relevant data obtained are interpreted and acted upon where needed (Bittner & Gravlin, 2009).

Before delegating work to another clinician, check the appropriateness of your request by considering the patient's condition and its complexity, and the scope of practice, competence and workload of the AIN (Bittner & Gravlin, 2009; Hudspeth, 2007; Kendall-Raynor, 2012; Saccomano & Pinto-Zipp, 2011). This is important, as inappropriate delegation may increase the chance of harm or compromise management of your patient. A task should only be delegated to a healthcare worker who has the knowledge, skill and opportunity to complete it. A 'five rights' rule has been proposed to simplify the process. To apply the five rights of delegation, ensure you are delegating the right job, in the right situation, to the right clinician, with the right instructions, under the right degree of supervision and subsequent evaluation (Hudspeth, 2007).

Effective communication is essential to successful delegation. As in any interaction regarding clinical care, your communication with the AIN should be clear and concise. You should identify what type of information is required post completion of the task, and any findings about which you must be immediately informed (Kendall-Raynor, 2012). Confirm that the AIN understands the task that you have asked them to do, and that they accept responsibility for its completion. Ensure you provide an opportunity for the AIN to ask any questions, and use your professional judgement to determine whether the other clinician requires direct supervision during completion of the task (Hudspeth, 2007).

Your ability to successfully delegate a task will be influenced by your professional relationship with the other worker involved. A positive relationship evidenced by trusting, respectful interactions will likely aid delegation and subsequent task completion. The style of communication used is important to achieve engagement from your colleague. Ensure you are polite and respectful, and provide a rationale for the delegation (Bittner & Gravlin, 2009; Potter et al., 2010).

Keep in mind that delegation is not merely a tool by which to decrease your personal workload. It is a method to achieve efficient completion of overall patient care by the health team. Attempting to delegate tasks to another clinician that you could have completed more efficiently yourself is unlikely to be received well, and will ultimately place strain upon team relationships if it becomes a pattern of behaviour.

MENTORING

Supportive relationships are key to developing supportive work environments, and growing dynamic and confident staff. Nurses commonly transition between roles, specialties, workplace cultures and environments many times throughout their careers (Creasia & Parker, 2001). Nurses transitioning into a new workplace or assuming a new role, such as Nurse-in-Charge, need support to provide safe and competent care to patients while adapting and filling in the gaps in their clinical and organisational knowledge (Health Education and Training Institute, 2012). To ensure patient care is safely and competently delivered, mentorship from a senior experienced staff member is essential. Defining mentoring is challenging due to the use of interchanging terms such as coaching, preceptoring, supervision and teaching (Butterworth et al., 1998; Milton, 2004), and how such interventions are operationalised within the work environment. Broadly speaking, mentoring can be defined as a voluntary, collaborative and professional relationship between an experienced individual (the mentor), who contributes to the personal and professional growth and career development of, and serves as a role model to, a less experienced, aspiring individual (the mentee) (Atkins & Williams, 1995; Stewart & Krueger, 1996). Mentoring has three key differences from other development interventions:

1 Mentoring does not involve assessment.
2 While a mentor may be more experienced, there is an equality in the relationship as the mentor is not in a managerial position.
3 The mentor is not necessarily at a higher academic level.

Advantages and disadvantages

A mentoring relationship can occur at any time in an individual's career, and continues for more than just a few days or during a probationary period. Mentors have a critical role in transitioning staff new to the workplace or experienced staff assuming a new role, as well as the development of the mentee's professional career. Mentors can greatly help mentees to gain confidence, as well as experience and knowledge that is not easily gained through formal education, such as workplace culture and politics, formal and informal norms, beliefs, values and expectations. Mentoring can have a positive impact on novice nurses' ability to perceive and actively cope with stress, leading to a more resilient and responsive workforce (Demir et al., 2014). Through mutual goals and shared accountability, mentors influence and shape the professional standards and practice of their mentee, ultimately enhancing quality of patient care and safety (Committee on Quality of Health Care in America, 2001; Institute of Medicine, 2011). It is therefore critical that the mentor has consummate standards of practice and ethics, and that the mentor and mentee recognise their responsibilities and communicate effectively. Poor mentorship, or a mentor–mentee relationship filled with conflict, can risk jeopardising patient care and potentially could compromise the careers of both mentor and mentee (Health Education and Training Institute, 2012).

Choosing a mentor

Mentors should be good, active listeners. Further, effective mentors should be altruistic by not projecting their preconceptions or prejudices onto the mentee's issues or goals. Instead, effective mentors demonstrate sensitivity, empathy and enthusiasm, prioritising the mentee's needs and interests over their own. A good mentor should serve as a role model in terms of integrity, honesty, high professional standards and ethics (Strauss et al., 2013). Accomplishments in teaching, practice development and research are also important, and will greatly assist in examining and consolidating expert knowledge and skills. Other characteristics of a good mentor are:

- enthusiasm for teaching students and peers
- experience and knowledge of postgraduate courses and their content
- good time-management skills
- being flexible and approachable
- being well respected within the workplace for setting and maintaining high standards of care and practice
- possessing a strong history of mentoring and assisting staff in their academic and professional career planning.

A single mentor may be able to adequately deal with most of the clinical and professional issues that arise as a part of a mentee's development. However, people have different strengths. A mentee interested in undertaking clinical research or pursuing endorsement as a Nurse Practitioner may require a second mentor who has experience, knowledge and skills in that field for guidance and support. Your mentor may be able to point you in the direction of other mentors to assist in areas of development outside his or her own experience. This second mentor may exist within the workplace, but is more likely to be based within a university if you are pursuing higher degree qualifications (e.g. Master of Research or

Nurse Practitioner). You would identify them based upon the area of specialty (e.g. chronic care, critical care).

Getting the most out of your mentor

Getting the most out of your mentor is about building a reciprocal and professional relationship, which requires spending time with your mentor. Setting time aside to meet may seem obvious, but not meeting at all or with any regularity will waste key development opportunities for both the mentor and mentee, such as setting goals and providing feedback (Blass & Ferris, 2007; Tracey & Nicholl, 2006). Mentors are better able to assist in identifying and shaping the necessary steps needed if your career goals and aspirations—both short and long term—are known to them. When arranging to meet with your mentor, be on time and be prepared. If you need to cancel a meeting, make sure your mentor is informed. Don't rely on email. You should also expect this of your mentor.

Mentees should also ask about their mentor's career goals, clinical and professional interests and experiences within the department and organisation to gain insight into future directions, trends and opportunities that may not previously have been considered. Maintaining a running agenda or professional development plan that details a summary of each meeting and goals, objectives and actions will also keep the mentor–mentee relationship focused, timely and on track. In addition to setting aside time to meet with your mentor, arranging to work alongside the mentor can greatly increase the quality and depth of support and feedback provided. Being able to observe your mentor in action can better demonstrate the standard of practice to be developed, including skills and professional behaviours required to be mastered. It also provides the mentor with the opportunity to observe your clinical practice and conduct, and to provide more meaningful feedback (Milton, 2004; Strauss et al., 2013).

One of the strengths of an effective mentor–mentee relationship is the ability to give and receive critical feedback. While friendship between mentor and mentee may develop, it is not necessary for a successful mentor–mentee relationship to exist—indeed, some mentors feel that friendship may interfere with their ability to honestly and critically appraise without personal conflict (Milton, 2004).

As with any relationship, conflicts can and will occur. Everyone makes mistakes, and no one is perfect. Addressing and resolving conflict as soon as possible is essential to maintaining a strong mentor–mentee relationship. An appropriate space for the discussion needs to be identified, preferably away from the clinical area. Resolving conflict will rely on communicating openly and directly with each other (avoid emailing, instant messaging and social media), maintaining professionalism, honesty, trust and respect. Identifying a mediator may be necessary; they should be a senior individual who is both objective and neutral, and whose judgement is respected and trusted by both the mentor and mentee. Summarise the issue and your viewpoint before meeting. Remain objective, and allow plenty of time to listen and clarify each other's perspectives and feelings on the issue. Be flexible about ways to handle the problem, to ensure a solution can be developed that works for both of you. Be mindful that the issue may only be a symptom of a larger and sometimes different problem (family–work balance issues, depression, bullying in the workplace) (Foster-Turner, 2006). However, if a solution is unable to be found, it may be necessary to end the mentoring relationship.

DIAGNOSTIC REASONING IN NURSING

Before an effective patient-management plan can be created, the nurse must first obtain appropriate clinical information, and subsequently interpret this information correctly to identify a clinical problem or diagnosis that requires an intervention. Having an understanding of how you reached a decision is important to prevent avoidable diagnostic errors. With this in mind, two common theories of diagnostic reasoning will be discussed in detail: hermeneutical theory and information processing theory.

Ritter (2003) and Benner and Tanner (1987) provide a useful explanation of these two models. In hermeneutical theory, intuition is seen as fundamental to the decision-making process, allowing the nurse to absorb cues from the patient, environment and situation to form an understanding of the clinical scene as a whole. Previous experience and exposure to many similar events are seen as prerequisites to intuitive thought and understanding of a given situation. Intuitive thought is said to be enabled through:

- pattern and similarity recognition, where a nurse identifies similarities between past experiences and the current one
- understanding the illness experience of the patient, achieved through empathy for the patient's situation
- skilled know-how, where the nurse can complete an activity competently, but may be unable to explain the specifics of how the skill is completed
- understanding when an event is more important than it was on a previous similar occasion, and having the ability to alter the interpretation of events after considering alternatives.

In information processing theory, the clinician is viewed as a problem-solver, where understanding is required to achieve a goal, solve a problem or complete a task. It is marked by sequential stages of:

- cue/information gathering
- creation of a hypothesis
- interpretation of the initial information gathered, leading to further focused information gathering and subsequent hypothesis evaluation.

The accuracy of the generated hypothesis is dependent upon the knowledge of the clinician, as a superior knowledge base will likely enable better interpretation of identified cues (Paans et al., 2010; Ritter, 2003). Interestingly, advanced practitioners tend to collect less, but more accurate, data to generate an accurate diagnosis when compared with less experienced clinicians (Zunkel et al., 2004).

Figure 7.3 shows an example of diagnostic reasoning in practice, recorded in the patient's medical record.

The clinical assessment shown in Figure 7.3 was documented in the following sequence:

1   presenting complaint or main reason for seeking healthcare
2   history of the presenting complaint
3   past medical history
4   physical assessment
5   identification of relevant investigations and interventions
6   impression or list of possible diagnoses
7   plan.

Although the ordering of the documentation closely reflects the actual sequence of events, nurses frequently make additional assessments and clinical judgements during the consultation period that often do not appear in the documentation.

A more realistic description of the process follows below:

- General survey of patient via 'eye-balling'. This brief inspection provides much information, as groups of symptoms displayed are fitted into a clinical impression of the patient. From this impression, a decision will be made about whether the patient is displaying compromise to airway, breathing, circulation or disability that requires immediate intervention, prioritised assessment or immediate referral and escalation. This information also forms a basis for comparison against the patient's presenting complaint to see whether the

---

Nursing notes

12.03.09.   1840hrs.

Presenting complaint: 26-year-old male, foot injury right ankle.

History of the presenting complaint: Inversion injury to right ankle while walking. Pain and swelling to lateral aspect foot, unable to bear weight since.

Background history:

Allergies: No known drug allergies.

Medications: No regular medications taken.

Past medical and surgical history: Nil.

Physical assessment:

Alert, orientated, well perfused, nil respiratory distress.

Vitals: Blood pressure 120/60 mmHg, heart rate 85 bpm, respiratory rate 16 bpm, temperature 36.5°C.

Pain: Rates pain 7/10.

Right knee: No abnormality detected.

Right ankle/foot:

  Inspection: Swelling at base of fifth metatarsal and lateral ankle.

  Palpation: Bony tenderness base of fifth metatarsal. Tender over lateral ligaments.

  Movement: Decreased range of movement.

  Weight bearing: Unable to bear weight on right foot.

Neurovascular: Dorsalis Pedis and Posterior Tibial pulses present. Normal sensation. Foot pink, Cap refill <2 sec.

Impression: Possible fracture base of fifth metatarsal bone.

Investigations: Right foot X-ray.

Interventions: Rest, ice, compression, elevation. Give analgesia: paracetamol 1 g, Endone 5 mg.

Plan: Review pain post analgesia, neurovascular observations, await X-ray.

Signed: Bob Dole RN

Figure 7.3 Nursing notes: example of diagnostic reasoning in practice

picture 'fits'. Possible **differential diagnoses** for the cluster of symptoms seen are already being formed by the assessor at this time.

differential diagnosis
A list of possible diagnoses that could account for the patient presentation.

- A description of the presenting complaint (PC) is acquired from the patient.
- A history of the presenting complaint (HPC) and associated signs and symptoms is acquired from the patient.
- Background history is acquired: the PC, HPC and background history are evaluated in conjunction with the

initial clinical impression of the patient. A list of differential diagnoses that could cause the clinical presentation is formed. With these differential diagnoses in mind, a relevant physical assessment that targets specific body systems is determined.

- Physical assessment of relevant body systems is then completed: information gathered here is used to support, exclude or add further differential diagnoses.
- A formal list of differential diagnoses is documented, with the clinicians' main concerns for management and treatment listed first.
- Investigations: post consideration of history and physical assessment findings, a list of further investigations that will contribute to confirming or excluding the listed differential diagnoses, or that may contribute to a decision regarding appropriate treatment or referral, is made.

Aspects of this assessment process fit both within an intuitive/heuristic and analytical model of reasoning. Upon initial contact with the patient (general survey, PC and HPC), the clinician forms an impression of the situation—or, to put it another way, matches what they see against known 'patterns' of presentation for particular clinical complaints. This situation is also checked for similarities to/ differences from previous experiences of a disease process. This pattern/similarity recognition fits within the hermeneutical model of diagnostic reasoning.

This mode of cognitive evaluation is useful during a rapid assessment of a patient where time-critical intervention may be needed, and where multiple clinical cues may be available from inspection alone to diagnose a major event, such as **haemodynamic compromise** or threatened airway.

haemodynamic compromise
Haemodynamics is the study of blood movement. Compromise of blood flow is manifested in a drop of blood pressure and tissue perfusion.

Through the lens of the hermeneutical model, diagnosis is made without being able to rationalise the particulars of the situation that lead to the diagnosis. Benner and Tanner (1987) describe this as understanding without a rationale. At this point, however, the reasoning model crosses to the analytical path, as the initial clinical impression must be deconstructed within the clinician's mind to identify what cues have actually led them to their initial impression. This initial impression also marks the site at which description of the information processing model in the literature begins. The information processing model commences with acquisition of a set of facts or cues, acquired via the PC, HPC and general survey. Upon reflection of findings during this initial phase, a hypothesis of what may have caused this set of symptoms is formed. Without this analysis, relevant cue/fact gathering cannot subsequently take place.

The acquisition of the patient's background history, coupled with a rationalised physical assessment and list of investigations, fits with the information processing model, where specific cue gathering occurs to evaluate a set of hypotheses. Ritter (2003) argued that the completion and recording of a physical assessment is an example of skilled know-how, where the nurse completes an activity competently, but is unable to explain the specifics of how the skill is completed. It could be argued that a clinician should be able to explain technically how a skill is completed, as well as why it is done. Otherwise, you could not be sure that the skill has been completed in a way that will provide valid information for consideration. In the case study above, if a rationale had been provided as to why each element of the physical assessment had been performed, this would accord with the targeted gathering of information to support or rule out a hypothesis under the information processing model. The evaluation of the gathered information from history, physical assessment and investigations to test differential diagnoses also falls within the information processing model.

Both the hermeneutical and information processing models have some strengths and weaknesses. Pattern and similarity recognition within hermeneutic diagnostic reasoning enables a clinician to rapidly attain an impression of the situation with which they are dealing, and therefore start appropriate treatment earlier. However, relying on intuition, as described by Benner (2001), presents the patient, clinician and fellow health professionals with multiple problems. Merely understanding that something is wrong without being able to articulate the specific problem means that communication of a clinical situation to another clinician or the patient will be compromised. This was evidenced in a clinical account recorded by Benner (2001), in which a nurse recognised that the patient was deteriorating, but was unable to articulate any clinical signs or symptoms to prove that the concern was legitimate, and as a result was unsuccessful in gaining a review of the patient. Relying on intuition to guide management may have consequences from a legal viewpoint if something goes wrong in the patient's treatment. Being unable to provide a rationale or evidence for a particular diagnosis would be indefensible, as it would preclude another person from seeing how or why the clinician came to a particular conclusion (Lamond & Thompson, 2000).

In contrast, the information processing model could be argued to hold more benefits than negatives in the clinical setting. The early development of a hypothesis enables the clinician to focus upon a problem and then pursue questions, physical assessment and investigations to prove or disprove the differential diagnoses (Zunkel et al., 2004). The use of an analytical approach in decision-making also means that a clinician can explain how and why they have come to a conclusion, and therefore can also justify their clinical decision to others. This approach does ignore the fact that humans tend to respond to recognised patterns. If the clinician does not recognise the effect of pattern recognition upon diagnostic reasoning, it may result in the clinician jumping immediately to an incorrect treatment path without testing their diagnosis against clinical assessment findings.

It is argued that there is still a place and time for both models, with Lamond and Thompson (2000) stating that in a messy environment with many cues and little time, intuitive thought is potentially the best cognitive strategy. However, in a situation presenting few cues and ample time for investigation, an analytical model such as information processing would be the favoured cognitive model.

It has recently been argued that human problem-solving is likely to involve a mix of both intuitive thought in the form of pattern and similarity recognition and analytical processes. One study of Nurse Practitioners suggested that they used the hermeneutical model approximately 45 per cent of the time, and the information processing model the other 55 per cent of the time (Ritter, 2003). Croskerry (2009) noted that medical doctors also used a blend of intuitive and analytical reasoning during the diagnostic process. In the review of the patient assessment process performed in the study, it was found that pattern recognition on initial meeting of the patient likely influenced identifying target areas for further clinical assessment and cue gathering to support analytical cognitive processes.

As a clinician, you should be aware of what has influenced you in achieving a diagnosis and deciding on a line of treatment, and whether it is based purely upon intuition or conscious analysis of the presented evidence. If a hypothesis attained via intuition is not tested via analysis of obtained cues and investigations, it is possible that you may arrive at an incorrect diagnosis through an error in not recognising an atypical disease presentation.

THE DETERIORATING PATIENT

Many hospitals have Rapid Response Systems (RRS) that can be enacted by clinical staff to gain an escalated response to patient deterioration. The response is commonly in the form of patient review by a Medical Emergency Team (MET), sometimes also known as a Rapid Response Team (RRT). METs are composed of doctors and nurses, usually from critical care areas such as the Intensive Care Unit (ICU) or emergency department (Jones, 2010). The MET response aims to commence rapid treatment of an acutely unwell patient identified by trigger criteria, in an attempt to reduce the occurrence of cardiac arrests and other serious adverse events (SAEs) (Jones, 2010).

Multiple studies have demonstrated a deterioration within recorded vital signs in up to 84 per cent of cases prior to an SAE (Jones, 2010). As a result, the most common triggers for MET activation are based on vital sign derangement. In the hospital environment, the clinical deterioration of a patient is most commonly gradual—allowing time for intervention and prevention if identified sufficiently early (Jones, 2010). Criteria used by METs as triggers are typically 'late signs' of a deteriorating patient.

There has been debate surrounding the utilisation of earlier signs of clinical deterioration to prompt medical review and improve outcomes. The Signs of Critical Conditions and Emergency Responses (SOCCER) study developed a list of early and late signs of deterioration associated with cardiac arrest (Table 7.3) that can help prompt clinical concern and escalation of patient care (Jones, 2010). Many signs of deterioration, such as modest hypotension (80–100 mmHg), are common. If identified early, targeted interventions can usually rectify the situation and prevent subsequent harm to the patient.

If a risk of deterioration is identified, physically assess the patient via the ABCDEFG framework (see Table 7.2 earlier in the chapter). If early or late signs of deterioration are located through this physical assessment, escalate patient review according to your facility's RRS policy.

Common factors that contribute to a failure to identify a deteriorating patient include:

- observations not being completed for extended periods of time, leading to vital sign changes being missed
- a failure to identify the importance of documented deterioration
- not recording the observations
- inappropriate delay to medical review and change in management (Beaumont, 2008).

The factors listed above should prompt you to ensure that:

- completed observations are relevant to the patient condition and repeated at an appropriate time interval
- documented information should be compared against previous recordings to note any deterioration
- escalation of care must be systematic. If the required response is not provided, the situation must be escalated to the next level, and your Nurse Unit Manager notified of the situation.

Table 7.3 Early- and late-warning signs of patient deterioration

Early-warning signs

Poor peripheral circulation	$PaCO_2$ 51–60 mmHg
Systolic blood pressure 80–100 mmHg	pH 7.2–7.3
Heart rate 40–49 or 121–140/min	Base deficit –5 to –8 mmol/L
Systolic blood pressure 181–240 mmHg	Any seizure
Note decreased urine output	Complaint of chest pain
Urine output <200 mL/8 hours	Uncontrolled pain
Alteration in consciousness level	New pain
Glasgow Coma Scale (GCS) 9–11	Pain changed location
A fall in GCS of >2	> expected blood loss
Partial airway obstruction	New bleeding at any site
Respiratory rate 5–9 or 31–40/min	> expected drain fluid loss
SpO_2 90–95%	Blood sugar level 1–2.9 mmol/L
PaO_2 50–60 mmHg	Blood sugar level 16–25 mmol/L

Late-warning signs

Cardiac arrest	PaO_2 <50 mmHg
*Systolic blood pressure <80 mmHg	$PaCO_2$ >60 mmHg
*Heart rate <40 or >140/min	pH <7.2
Systolic blood pressure >240 mmHg	Base deficit < –8 mmol/L
Urine output <200 mL/24 hours	*2 or more seizures with no return to baseline
*unresponsive to verbal command	*Failure to reverse variable within 1 hour
*GCS ≤8 *Airway obstruction/stridor complete	Excess blood loss unable to be controlled by local staff
*RR <5 or >40 breaths/min	Blood sugar level <1 mmol/L
SpO_2 <90%	Blood sugar level >25 mmol/L

* = common MET call criteria

PATIENT TRANSFER AND TRANSPORTATION

Patient transport/transfer refers to the movement of a patient outside of the treatment area, whether this is to imaging, transfer to a different ward, or transport to a different hospital. Moving any patient outside of a treatment area comes with added risk if there has not been adequate preparation to manage possible alterations in clinical condition. Critically ill patients are prone to instability on movement, due to altered physiology; therefore, the decision to transport or transfer must be justified, with the perceived benefit outweighing the risk (Warren et al., 2004).

Consider who should be on the transfer team. Is the patient sufficiently stable and is their condition sufficiently low risk to allow transfer with only a porter, or will the patient require additional healthcare staff to supervise and possibly intervene in the event of clinical deterioration? The transferring team should be able to provide an equivalent standard of care during transport to that available in the ward of origin or target destination (ACEM et al., 2003). If you are uncertain about the level of supervision necessary for your patient, check with the Nurse Unit Manager and/or treating doctor, as an unstable patient may require a porter, nurse and physician to accompany the transfer. Staff must have the appropriate knowledge and skill to deal with possible clinical events while en route, and must also be able to use the transport equipment correctly. Ensure that at least one member of the transfer team is familiar with the layout of the facility to which the patient is being moved. This will reduce the time needed for the transit.

What equipment will be required to allow you to quickly identify changes in clinical condition or response to interventions during the transfer? Equipment should be determined by the patient's clinical condition, diagnosis and degree of therapeutic interventions required (ACEM et al., 2003). If unsure, always confirm with your Nurse Unit Manager. All equipment taken should be secured to the bed to prevent injury to the patient and staff, or damage to the equipment itself.

Monitoring for the unstable patient may include:

capnography Measures the amount of CO_2 in an exhaled breath, known as 'end-tidal CO_2', or 'ETCO$_2$' with a normal range of 35–45 mmHg. Capnography is used to help assess the adequacy of ventilation, i.e. the movement of air in and out of the lung.

- ECG displaying heart rate and rhythm
- blood pressure (non-invasive blood pressure/arterial line)
- pulse oximetry
- **capnography** (for ventilated patient).

Necessary equipment may include:

- portable oxygen
- suction
- ventilator
- defibrillator
- bag/valve mask
- resuscitation pack containing all necessary drugs and equipment for airway management and resuscitation.

Prior to leaving, ensure that the patient is stabilised and safe for transport (Warren et al., 2004). If the need for intravenous medication or fluid resuscitation en route is a possibility, ensure adequate intravenous access has been inserted and is patent. Airway, breathing, circulation and disability should be managed, monitored and controlled prior to departure. Potential issues must be identified early and corrected. There are no agreed criteria for what blood pressure and heart rate is deemed sufficiently stable for safe transfer. The final decision should be made by the most experienced physician involved in the patient's management, and take into consideration a risk versus benefit analysis of what will be achieved by the transfer. Wilkes (2010) suggests that a systolic blood pressure of at least 90 mmHg without requirement for additional fluids after correction of estimated losses would be a minimum requirement of haemodynamic stability prior to transfer. Conversely, stability is relative in some conditions—for example, ruptured Abdominal Aortic Aneurysm (AAA), penetrating trauma or severe head injury. These conditions cannot be cured or resolved in the ward or emergency environment, so the aim of the transfer or retrieval team in these situations is rapid assessment, minimal intervention and rapid movement to an area where definitive management can occur—for example, the operating theatre. In these emergency situations, transport is considered a treatment in itself (Holliday & Pearce, 2007).

In preparation for transport, you will be required to assist with assessment of your patient. The simplest method of completing a rapid assessment is the primary survey, as noted earlier in the chapter. If alterations in clinical condition are noted, escalate these findings to the treating doctor and Nurse Unit Manager so that appropriate interventions can be made to combat further deterioration. In cases of clinical deterioration, the transfer destination may no longer be appropriate—will a nurse responsible for six other patients on a general surgical ward be able to safely manage the patient with limited resources, or will your patient now require a high dependency unit to deliver the level of care and supervision required? If there is a risk of deterioration requiring invasive interventions during transit, it may be safer to complete the same interventions in a controlled environment prior to leaving. For example, if a patient's airway is at risk of becoming compromised due to decrease in consciousness level, elective insertion of an endotracheal tube may be indicated.

Lastly, if you will be handing over care of the patient to a different team, make sure they know you are coming. Talk to the clinician responsible at your patient's destination on the phone, and provide a structured handover of your patient's diagnosis, clinical condition and ongoing management plan using an ISBAR framework (explained in Chapter 6). This will ensure that the receiving department is aware, and has the staff and equipment resources available to manage the patient on arrival (Warren et al., 2004).

BASIC LIFE SUPPORT

Cardiopulmonary resuscitation (CPR) refers to the delivery of chest compressions in combination with rescue breathing. CPR aims to maintain sufficient circulation to preserve brain function in the short term until specialised treatment is available.

The current Basic Life Support (BLS) algorithm is:

D Danger?
R Responsive?
S Send for help
A Open Airway
B Normal Breathing?
C Start CPR (30 chest compressions: 2 breaths)
D Attach Defibrillator (AED) and follow prompts
Continue CPR until responsiveness or normal breathing returns (ANZCOR, 2016).

A reference to 'not breathing' has been replaced with the prompt question 'normal breathing?' The clinician is now to commence CPR if there is a combination of 'victim unresponsive and not breathing normally'. This is due to a high incidence of agonal breaths (gasping) post cardiac arrest being mistaken for adequate evidence of breathing. There is decreased focus on checking for a pulse by health professionals as it is an unreliable indicator of the need for resuscitation. If the patient is noted to be 'not breathing normally', CPR commences first with chest compressions, then breaths. CPR ratio remains 30 compressions to two breaths. The target rate of compressions is 100–120/minute. There is now a recommendation to change the rescuer delivering compressions every 2 minutes to decrease fatigue and to maintain correct compression depth and rate (ANZCOR, 2016).

MEDICATION ADMINISTRATION

Registered nurses predominantly administer medication to patients. As such, the responsibility to ensure that medication is administered safely lies predominantly with nursing. There are approximately 230,000 medication-related hospital admissions per year, 30 per cent of which are patients aged over 75 years, with an estimated cost of A$1.2 billion. Medication errors account for under 10 per cent of medication administrations in hospital, with additional errors in documentation of medication in discharge summaries occurring at a rate of two per patient, of which three-quarters are preventable (Roughead, 2016; Sharp, 2010). Common antecedents of medication administration errors include wrong patient, wrong dose, wrong calculation and wrong situation.

Most registered nurses would be familiar with the five rights of safe medication administration:

- RIGHT drug
- RIGHT patient (with two ID bands on)
- RIGHT dose
- RIGHT time
- RIGHT route.

However, with growing patient complexity, increasing workloads and nurse accountability, nurses must ensure that medication is administered for the right reasons, not simply dispensing medication blindly by following a drug chart. To improve safety, an additional five 'rights' have been generated:

- RIGHT reason—medication is used for the correct prescribed reason, such as 'for patient agitation'
- RIGHT documentation (includes clarity of prescription)
- RIGHT patient education—ensuring that the patient is fully familiar with the medication they are about to receive
- RIGHT assessment—assessing the patient's condition to ensure it is still appropriate for them to receive the prescribed medication
- RIGHT evaluation—reassessing the patient's pain levels or verifying serum drug levels (e.g. **warfarin**) are within safe limits.

> **warfarin** An anticoagulant that limits the blood's ability to form clots.

Listed below are the administration, recording, witnessing and checking procedures for controlled medications.

- *Schedule 8 drugs:* Substances that are addictive or have potential to be addictive require two Registered Nurses to check, sign out and witness the drug's administration.
- *Schedule 4D drugs:* Substances that may be abused and likely to cause dependency require two staff members, one of whom must be a Registered Nurse, to check and sign out.

NATIONAL INPATIENT MEDICATION CHART

A critical component in the delivery of safe healthcare is the written communication allowing dispensing and administration of medications. A major initiative was launched by the Australian Commission on Safety and Quality in Healthcare to improve the safe use of medicines, and decrease harm from medication errors through the nationwide implementation of a standardised medication chart. A common medication chart called the National Inpatient Medication Chart (NIMC) was developed and subsequently endorsed by the federal Health Minister in 2004 for mandatory implementation in all Australian public hospitals by 2006 (ACSQHC, 2004). The benefits of standardising the charting of medication means that the same chart will be used at any site where a doctor or nurse works, or wherever a patient is managed in a hospital (ACSQHC, 2004). In some states and territories, electronic medication charts have been introduced.

Summary

In this chapter, we have looked at the principles involved in undertaking patient assessment, including the primary survey, to determine any life-threatening issues. We covered the clinical assessment and the formation of a management plan, including the importance of documentation. We examined nursing models of care delivery, the delegation of care and supervision, mentoring and the principles of diagnostic reasoning. We noted how to identify signs of a deteriorating patient, issues involved in patient transfer, basic life support and medication administration.

Review questions

7.1   What are some of the common factors contributing to a failure to identify the deteriorating patient?
a   A lack of observations completed for a lengthy time period leading to vital sign changes not being detected
b   The failure to recognise the importance of documented deterioration, or no action being taken outside recording the observation
c   A delay in receiving medical attention, even when the deterioration was identified
d   All of the above

7.2   Although a definition of haemodynamic stability is not agreed upon for the purpose of safe transportation of patients, a systolic blood pressure of 90 mmHg and no requirements for additional fluids post correction of estimated losses would be a minimum requirement. True or false?

7.3   In adult BLS, what is the compression to ventilation ratio?
a   15:2
b   30:2

7.4   In the adult BLS algorithm, if the patient is unresponsive and is found to be not breathing, what should the rescuer continue straight to?
a   Check for a pulse
b   Give two rescue breaths
c   Commence compressions

7.5   There is a decreased focus on checking for a pulse in the health setting, as it is an unreliable indicator of the need for resuscitation. True or false?

7.6   What is the target compression rate in CPR?
a   100 per minute
b   80 per minute
c   120 per minute
d   60 per minute

7.7   How often should the person giving compressions be changed?
a   Every 2 minutes
b   Every 4 minutes

7.8   S8 drugs require the following procedure:
a   Two RNs must check, sign out and witness the administration
b   Two staff members, one of whom is an RN, must check and sign out the drug; however, only one RN is required for administration

7.9   S4D drugs require the following procedure:
a   Two RNs must check, sign out and witness the administration
b   Two staff members must check and sign out the drug; however, only one RN is required for administration

7.10   A basic survey of airway, breathing, circulation and consciousness level should be completed on contact with every patient. True or false?

7.11   Areas that are commonly considered in a nursing management plan include:
a   Cardiac or SpO_2 monitoring
b   Fluid balance
c   Wound management
d   Pressure care
e   Changes in medication dosage
f   Medical or allied health review required

7.12   Documentation should ideally be completed:
a   Contemporaneously
b   At the end of a shift

7.13   If delegating care to a student nurse or AIN, you are not accountable for what they do. True or false?

7.14   The five rights of delegation include:
a   The right job
b   In the right situation
c   To the right clinician
d   The right medications
e   The right instructions
f   The right supervision and subsequent evaluation

8 NURSING WITHIN A DIVERSE CULTURAL ENVIRONMENT, AND DEATH AND DYING

Alister Hodge and Wayne Varndell

In this chapter, you will develop an understanding of:

- nursing within a diverse culture
- illness, death and dying.

The Australian population comprises a rich blend of peoples from diverse cultures and backgrounds. As such, the provision of healthcare to diverse populations is a challenge faced by all nurses within the Australian workforce. Race, ethnicity, religion, language and economic status all have significant influence on a person's physical and mental health; therefore, the provision of patient-centred holistic care requires the nurse to also consider cultural aspects that may affect management of the health episode. The term 'culture' reflects the belief systems, values, attitudes, thoughts and actions of a societal group (Omeri & Raymond, 2009).

A considerable proportion of the Australian population consists of immigrants, with 6.9 million Australians having been born overseas. This represents around 28.5 per cent of the total population (ABS, 2017a). Australia also has a rich Aboriginal and Torres Strait Islander heritage reaching back between 50,000 and 60,000 years prior to British settlement in 1788 that has made a unique contribution to Australian society. While Australia's national language is English, in 2016 there were more than 300 separately identified languages spoken in Australian homes, with 21 per cent of Australians speaking a language other than English at home (ABS, 2017b).

The benefits of our diverse community have been embraced at all levels of Australian government and enshrined in policy. The government uses the term 'multicultural' to describe the diversity of culture and language within Australian society, and the benefits that an inclusive model bestows upon all citizens. Over the past 60 years, Australia's immigration policy has matured and evolved into the current model that strives toward unity in diversity. Multiculturalism values diversity and aims to utilise the knowledge and skills of people from all cultural backgrounds to enable equal contribution to society, while simultaneously celebrating Australian traditions and acknowledging the multifaceted nature of our continually evolving culture (Department of Social Services, 2003; Omeri & Raymond, 2009).

The four core principles of the Multicultural Australia United in Diversity Policy

1 **Responsibilities of all:** All Australians have a civic duty to support those basic structures and principles of Australian society, which guarantee us our freedom and equality and enable diversity in our society to flourish.

2 **Respect for each person:** Subject to the law, all Australians have the right to express their own culture and beliefs, and have a reciprocal obligation to respect the right of others to do the same.

3 **Fairness for each person:** All Australians are entitled to equality of treatment and opportunity. Social equity allows us all to contribute to the social, political and economic life of Australia, free from discrimination, including on the grounds of race, culture, religion, language, location, gender or place of birth.

4 **Benefits for all:** All Australians benefit from productive diversity—that is, the significant cultural, social and economic dividends arising from the diversity of our population. Diversity works for all Australians (Department of Social Services, 2003, p. 9).

Diversity is not limited to cultural differences. Other characteristics of diversity in the patient population may include economic status, language, level of education, religion, age, disability, refugee and asylum seeker status, and a rural or remote versus a metropolitan home. Each of these characteristics has an impact on a potential management plan, and on the approach taken to ensure that the patient maintains an active role in determining their path back to optimal health.

For example, patient education resources need to consider the culture/age and education background of the target population to improve the effectiveness of the program (Omeri & Raymond, 2009).

An expectation of all Australian health staff is to achieve 'cultural competence' in delivering healthcare. This refers to the care provider having sufficient knowledge and sensibility regarding culture to meet the needs of individual patients and their families, and reflects a set of behaviours, practices and attitudes that embrace and respect cultural differences. To achieve this, nurses should consider completing a cultural self-assessment. What are your own cultural attitudes, beliefs, values and practices? Improved self-awareness will help to prevent you from perpetuating discrimination and prejudice through inappropriate cultural stereotyping. On commencing work, identify resources available within your health network to assist in care provision to the population accessing your service. These services will include various services such as phone translation and religious visitors (Omeri & Raymond, 2009).

ILLNESS, DEATH AND DYING

Caring for the patient who is dying or who has died is an inevitable part of nursing, and one that will have a profound impact upon the family and those closest to the patient—including you. The impact of death in our society is easily underestimated. While evidence-based guidelines now exist to help with the care of patients who are dying, which include symptom control, psychosocial support and bereavement care, too many patients die an undignified death with uncontrolled symptoms (e.g. pain, distress) and with too little support provided to relatives (Ellershaw & Ward, 2003). Caring for patients who are nearing death or who have died, and their families, is an essential part of nursing practice, and is one of the greatest privileges of being a nurse.

In order to care for dying patients, it is essential to examine the concept of 'dying'. Dying is a complex process, and in a hospital setting where the culture is often focused on 'cure', the pursuit of treating illness when recovery is uncertain may come at the expense of the comfort and dignity of the dying patient. Recognising the key signs and symptoms of dying is an important clinical skill. During the journey to death, the signs and symptoms of approaching death are unique to each person and their condition (Ellershaw & Ward, 2003).

If death is gradual, generally at one to three months prior to death the patient may reach a stage where they sleep or doze for increasing amounts of time, eat and drink less, become withdrawn and are less communicative. At one to two weeks prior to death, the patient may become increasingly bed-bound, will be very fatigued and may experience increasing pain. Patients may also experience congested breathing due to retained secretions at the back of the throat, disorientation and/or hallucinations. Changes in the patient's vital signs also occur during this stage of dying, including loss of appetite and thirst, which may make taking oral medications difficult (Kennedy et al., 2014). When death is imminent, the patient—if not already unconscious—may drift in and out of consciousness; eventually all bodily systems will cease to function and the patient will die.

Caring for a person after death is enormously important and a privilege; it is the final act that you, the nurse, will carry out for a patient in your care. Traditionally steeped in ritual, and often referred to as 'last offices', this act can achieve closure for the nurse and the family (Andrews, 2013). Caring for a patient who has died and providing after-care for the family are a significant process, which encompasses highly developed sensitive communication skills, spiritual care, familiarity with health and safety guidelines, religious and cultural practices, and bereavement care (Pattinson, 2008).

Care of the deceased is often a ritualistic process, which may simply involve washing and dressing the deceased in a particular manner. Essential elements to consider when providing care after death include honouring the spiritual or cultural wishes of the deceased and their family while ensuring legal obligations are met; preparing the deceased for transfer to the mortuary or collection by an authorised funeral services provider; affording family members and/or significant others (e.g. religious leader, celebrant, family elder) the opportunity to participate in the process of preparing the deceased and supporting them to do so; maintaining the privacy and dignity of the deceased person and their relatives at all times; ensuring that appropriate personal protective equipment is worn and used correctly at all times; respecting the wishes of the deceased and/or their legal guardian concerning organ and tissue donation; and returning the deceased person's personal possessions to their relatives (Quested & Rudge, 2003).

Nurses remain the first and continuing point of contact for families even after the patient has died; you will often be the first person to contact the patient's family and to meet them when they arrive at the ward. It is essential to remember that the care given at this time is extremely important. How family members react to the news of their relative dying or when viewing the deceased's body will vary, even if they have experienced the death of a relative or significant other before. They may also be unable to process information or instructions. Memories of the events surrounding the death and what occurs immediately afterwards may be intense and vivid, often remaining with the family and you for a long time. The impact of the loss of their relative may be acute or delayed. Essential family after-care includes preparing the family for what they might see; inviting the family into the bed space or room; being available to accompany family members but respecting their need for privacy should they require it; anticipating questions; offering the family members the opportunity to discuss care at that time or in the future; offering to contact relatives or a chaplain on behalf of the family; and advising the family about bereavement support services that can be accessed and how to access them, such as the social worker.

Legal issues

Nurses' responsibility to a deceased patient continues until the body leaves the clinical environment. This requires the continuing need for excellent documentation standards until the body is removed. Death must be verified by a medical officer before last offices commence. This is to ensure that any legal circumstances requiring referral to the Coroner or police have been considered prior to preparing the body for viewing or transport to the mortuary. Deaths reported to the Coroner for investigation are largely unsuspicious, and are typically the direct or indirect result of accidents. Reportable deaths are outlined within the relevant state or territory coronial legislation (e.g. *Queensland Coroners Act 2003*) and include, but are not limited to:

- violent or unnatural deaths
- sudden deaths where the cause is unknown
- where there are suspicious or unusual circumstances
- where the person has not been attended by a doctor in the six months preceding the death
- where death was not the reasonably expected outcome of a health-related procedure
- where the person was in or temporarily absent from a mental health facility where they were receiving involuntary treatment.

As part of a coronial investigation, a post-mortem (or autopsy) may be required to discern the cause of death (Coroner's Court (New South Wales), 2015a). The larger role of the Coroner is to protect lives and the wellbeing of others by bringing to the notice of relevant authorities any practices, policies or laws which could be changed to prevent similar deaths in the future (Coroner's Court (New South Wales), 2015b).

General principles in preparing the deceased patient (Coroner's case)

In general, nothing should be done to a body after death if it is a Coroner's case. All intravascular devices including peripheral cannulas, needles, intragastric tubes, all drains and airway devices (e.g. nasopharyngeal, oropharyngeal, endotracheal, tracheostomy tubes) should be left in situ. All intravenous fluid bags and feed lines attached to the body must accompany the body (Hills & Albarran, 2010a). All sharps or items of equipment left in situ should be firmly secured to the body in such a way that the risk of sharps injury or leakage is minimised. Any sharps or equipment not required to remain in situ should be removed for disposal or reprocessing and documented in the healthcare record.

The body should not be washed even if the surface is soiled so that all surface contamination can be observed by the forensic pathologist and duly assessed. For instance, when death occurs shortly after a motor vehicle accident or by violent assault, washing may remove vital trace evidence such as paint flakes or glass chips or an offender's blood and hairs, which may be relied upon to determine what happened, or the identity of the offender (Hills and Albarran, 2010b). The body should be placed only in a plastic body bag in accordance with local policy. Documentation should reflect how the body was managed, with items (e.g. clinical or personal property such as rings) left in situ.

Limbs and jaws must not be tied and orifices should not be plugged as these activities can leave marks that may make forensic examination difficult. Any material sucked from the stomach and/or any vomitus from suspected poisoning cases should be retained, appropriately labelled and forwarded with the body for chemical analysis.

General principles in preparing the deceased patient (non-Coroner's case)

Unless contraindicated, preparing the deceased for transfer includes washing the patient, performing oral hygiene, brushing hair and ensuring the bed space is neat and tidy. Family members should be given the option of seeing their loved one before or after last offices. If relatives want to be involved with cleaning and dressing the deceased, depending upon the condition of the deceased's body (soiling, blood and trauma) and the immediate area, you may want to perform the initial wash to remove most of the detritus and to tidy the immediate area prior to inviting the relative in to assist with the final wash.

Collect clean linen, towels, wash items such as soap and water, toothbrush and toothpaste, a shroud or patient gown, body bag, equipment to remove catheters and intravenous devices including temporary dressings (Hills & Albarran, 2010a). Make sure you are wearing the appropriate personal protection equipment (mask, visor, apron, gloves, etc.) in accordance with local policy. Ensure that the patient's dignity and privacy are maintained throughout. Ensure that you have assistance throughout the procedure, as you will need to reposition the deceased several times. Raise the bed to a suitable working level.

The following guide is intended to help you with preparing the deceased.

1 If there are no religious objections, place the patient supine and straighten their limbs. **Rigor mortis** can begin as soon as 10 minutes after death, beginning with the face. Remove catheters and other invasive devices (e.g. cannulas, airway devices).

> **rigor mortis** The progressive stiffening of muscles after death.

2 Remove any clothing and pack personal possessions into a bag labelled with the patient's details (e.g. full name, healthcare record number, date of birth) in accordance with local policy. Clothing and any items removed from or remaining on the body must be documented in the patient's healthcare record. Relatives may wish for the patient's possessions to be returned to them. Any items collected and by whom must be documented in the patient's healthcare record. If identification bracelets were removed or grossly defaced, these must be replaced.

3 Wash the body gently, paying attention to the hands and face. Clean the patient's mouth—a toothbrush and toothpaste are fine. Use moistened swab sticks to wipe excess toothpaste free from the mouth, and suction as required. If the patient has dentures, clean and replace them, again using a toothbrush, but with lukewarm water instead (Hills & Albarran, 2010a). Occasionally the patient's mouth can sag open, and this may be distressing for the family to see. Place a rolled-up towel under the patient's chin; remembering to remove it once last offices have been completed.

4 Brush the patient's hair into their preferred style. If this is not known, ask the family for advice.

5 To preserve the patient's corneas in case of possible corneal donation, irrigate the patient's eyes with normal saline (0.9 per cent sodium chloride) and close the patient's eyes. Occasionally, the patient's eyes may be partly or fully open, which can be unsettling for the family and staff. If this occurs, repeatedly massage the eyelids down and to the side. Alternatively, placing saline-soaked

gauze over the closed eyelids may help (Hills & Albarran, 2010a). The gauze should be removed when the body is being viewed, and then replaced to keep the corneas moistened. If possible, apply moisturiser to the patient's lips.

6 Change the bottom sheet if possible, and place an absorbent sheet under the patient to capture any soiling. Dress the patient in a clean gown or shroud. Cover the body with a clean sheet, and place a fresh pillow under their head. Position the body so that at least one arm is outside the top sheet palm down.

> **livor mortis** A deep reddish-purple colour that forms on the sides of the face, earlobes, neck and posterior surfaces of the body because of blood pooling in the dependent regions of the body; usually starts 30 minutes after death.

Elevate the head of the bed to at least 30 degrees to lessen **livor mortis**. If possible, move the bed away from any walls so that family members have more space to approach the bed and/or sit around the deceased.

7 Before leaving the room, ensure the space immediately around the bed is clear of equipment and cords. Lower the bed, and provide chairs so that the family can sit. There is a temptation to lower the lights in the room; however, this can make it difficult for visitors to navigate around the room safely. Provide boxes of tissues and access to water.

8 Before bringing family to the deceased, explain what they might see. For many, it will be the first time they will have seen a dead person. Afterwards, spend time with them, orientate them to the room and tell them how to call you if needed.

9 Everybody's reaction to the death of a loved one is unique and different. Responses can range from silence to quiet sobbing, loud chanting or prayer, anger, yelling, fainting, flailing and/or throwing themselves over the body or onto the ground. Remain calm and be supportive (Hills & Albarran, 2010b). While it is highly unlikely that any shouting, anger or violence will be directed towards you, you should remain conscious of your own personal safety.

10 If there are large numbers of visitors, it may be necessary to identify a senior family member to coordinate the flow of visitors to prevent overcrowding of the immediate area and the ward.

11 Prior to transporting the deceased to the mortuary, ensure that identification band details are correct, and that any mortuary tags are well secured to the deceased and body bag in accordance with local policy. Summon extra assistance to help place the deceased into the body bag. Review and update any documentation.

12 Escort the deceased to the mortuary. Double-check the patient's identification band, and complete the required mortuary documentation, such as the mortuary register in accordance with local policy.

OVERVIEW OF RELIGIOUS AND CULTURAL BELIEFS AT THE TIME OF DEATH

It is important that nurses have a basic understanding of the impact of culture and religious beliefs regarding caring for the patient who is sick, dying or has died and their family. The intensity, duration and frequency of the grief process may vary based on the manner of death, duration of illness, the individual family and cultural beliefs. Customs concerning death, dying, grieving and illness vary across cultures and are often heavily influenced by religion. Religions span national, geographical, cultural and ethnic boundaries, and may be the focus of individual or family identification. Religions and spiritual observances play an important role in caring for an individual's and their family's social, psychological and cultural needs.

Australia has a rich social make-up that includes a diverse Aboriginal and Torres Strait Islander population, a British colonial past and extensive immigration from many different countries and cultures, and has one of the most culturally and linguistically diverse populations in the world.

How cultural and religious customs are practised varies depending on the country of origin, the level of acceptance within wider society and the degree of observance of the individual or family members themselves. As such, it can be challenging to predict how any one patient or family member may understand or apply them in the context of illness and dying. Therefore, nurses should encourage patients and family members to interpret how religious/cultural values may be pertinent to their care while in hospital regarding personal needs, interaction with staff (e.g. same-gender requirements) and decisions about treatment (e.g. end of life).

According to the 2016 Census, the predominant religion in Australia was Christianity with about 52 per cent of the population (around 12.2 million people) identifying as Christian (ABS, 2017c). This group comprises over 70 different Christian denominations, with the major denominations being Catholic (22.6%); Anglican (13.3%); Uniting Church (3.7%); Presbyterian and Reformed (2.3%); and Eastern Orthodox (2.6%). Other major religions represented in the Census included Buddhism (2.4%), Islam (2.6%), Hinduism (1.9%) and Judaism (<1%). Some 30.1 per cent of Australians (over 7 million people) reported having no religion (ABS, 2017c).

Aotearoa New Zealand

Aotearoa New Zealand is a former British colony. The population of Aotearoa New Zealand is smaller (4.7 million) than that of Australia, and is largely bicultural with an indigenous Māori population comprising 14.9 per cent and 67.7 per cent being descendants of British settlers known as Pākehā (Statistics New Zealand, 2013). The Māori culture embraces the importance of the family (*whanāu*) and being in harmony with the physical, natural and spiritual world. Maintaining a balance in life through practising culture and adhering to the laws of *tapu* is of great significance.

Tapu (restricted or sacred) and *noa* (unrestricted or blessed) are key concepts that underpin many Māori practices, many of which align with good health and safety practices. *Tapu* is the strongest force in Māori life, and breaching it (*hara*, meaning violation) could incur the wrath of the Gods. *Noa*, on the other hand, lifts the *tapu* from a person or object (Herbert, 2001). While *tapu* and *noa* remain part of the Māori culture today, their application and adherence to can vary between each tribal group (known as *iwi*). Engaging with the patient and family is essential to optimise cultural respect and avoid distress. Hospitals should have clear guidelines to assist you in your care and practice, such as:

- not passing food over the patient's head
- not using pillowcases for any other purpose
- using different flannels for washing the head and body
- when washing, starting from the neck, then moving down to the genital and then anal areas
- keeping food separate from anything that comes into contact with the body or body fluids—for example:
  - A separate designated lift is to be used at all times for transporting food, as lifts used to move waste bins, cleaning trolleys, the deceased or patients to and from the wards or theatre, can become contaminated with body fluid.
  - Combs and brushes are not to be placed on the surface where food is placed.
  - Tables or workbenches used for food or medication are not to be used as a place to sit.
  - Separate designated fridges and freezers are used for food or medication and not for any other purpose.
  - Drinking water containers are not used for any other purpose.
  - Bedpans/urinals and food are not present at the same time or placed on surfaces used for food.
  - Bedpans/urinals are stored in their own designated area (Mercy Hospital, 2016).

Depending on *iwi*, customs and beliefs (*tikanga*) may vary; therefore, it is important to actively engage with the patient and their family to find out how individuals may wish to be treated during or after their death (Higgins, 2011).

Where a person has been unwell for a period of time and their death is anticipated, there will generally have been a gathering of *whanāu* and friends to their home or hospital bedside. This is a special time when the person dying has access and is accessible to both the spiritual and the physical world. Any words spoken by the dying person are of great importance and significance, with those present privileged to hear them (Herbert, 2001). For many Māori, *karakia*, meaning blessings or prayers, are essential for protecting and maintaining their spiritual, mental, emotional and physical health, whether prior to a routine operation or during illness or death. *Karakia* should be encouraged. Time should be made available for *karakia* to occur, with interruptions kept to an absolute minimum.

Once death has occurred, the body (*tapupaku*), is considered *tapu* (sacred) and is subject to more sensitive and restrictive practices. This includes placing a bowl of water in the room with which family members can sprinkle themselves prior to entry and on exit, which is a symbolic way of keeping the world of the living and the dead separate. The deceased should not be left alone at any time until they are buried, which may mean you are required to watch over the deceased until a family member arrives. A *whanāu*, *hapu* or Māori organisation (*iwi*, Runanga Māori Authority) has the option to carry out the appropriate *tikanga* pertaining to their own deceased person's rituals, practices and philosophies relating to their *whanāu*, *hapu* or *iwi* (Herbert, 2001). The family of the deceased may also perform their own blessing and rituals according to the deceased person's culture, religious beliefs or philosophies.

Maori believe that the spirit (*wairua*) of the deceased continues to exist after death, visiting places familiar to the deceased before heading to Te Rerenga Wairua (the top of the North Island) to depart this earth. If no autopsy is required, the deceased is washed and dressed by the family prior to transferring the deceased into the care of a funeral director. If an autopsy is required, the deceased is transferred to the mortuary (Hope, 2011).

The room in which the person has died is *tapu*. Once the deceased has been moved from the room, it must be blessed by an approved celebrant, including any linen, equipment and the healthcare record of the deceased, returning it back to its ordinary, normal use, from *tapu* to *noa*, before another patient uses the room (Mercy Hospital, 2016). The door of the room or cubicle curtains must remain closed until the blessing is complete. A sign can be placed on the outside of the room/cubicle to alert staff that blessing of the room is required. The body is usually buried rather than cremated so it can be returned to Papatuanuku (mother earth).

Australian Aboriginal and Torres Strait Islander people

For some Aboriginal and Torres Strait Islander people, the time before and following death is subject to a number of customary practices. While death is inevitable, understanding its meaning and significance is essential for providing the best care for all patients and their family members at their final stages of life. For Aboriginal and Torres Strait Islander people, the term 'passing' is the preferred and accepted terminology to use when discussing death or dying, due to the spiritual belief around the life cycle (Queensland Health, 2015).

Aboriginal and Torres Strait Islander people are two distinct and diverse cultures. While customary practices may vary between and within some Aboriginal and some Torres Strait Islander tribal groups, they are deeply sacred. Where possible, definitive guidance should be sought from the patient, the family and/or the Aboriginal and/or Torres Strait Islander Health Worker or Hospital Liaison Officer—particularly in grief and loss circumstances it is paramount to ensure not only local but also family-specific cultural protocols are adhered to and respected the best that they can be, to ensure care is delivered with the utmost respect. Further, being aware of the resources available, such as the hospital Aboriginal or Torres Strait Islander Advocate, can greatly assist in providing meaningful care.

Providing comfort and pain relief is important regardless of ethnicity or race. While we are all susceptible to pain, how we experience and express it varies. Some Aboriginal and Torres Strait Islander people may not openly complain about pain or discomfort, being reserved and reluctant to be of any trouble to healthcare staff. Further, Aboriginal and Torres Strait Islander people may wish to keep men's and women's business separate and may not disclose pain or suffering to someone not of their gender in fear of breaching this cultural protocol. Ask if the patient would like to consult with someone of their gender. Some Aboriginal and Torres Strait Islander patients are accompanied by a close family member, to support and, if necessary, act as an interpreter. A hospital-approved interpreter should be sought with consent from the patient; however, there may be distrust between Aboriginal and Torres Strait Islander tribal groups.

Patients and family members are vulnerable during the final stages of life. It is therefore critical to actively engage and build a rapport with any patient and their family to build trust, enhance communication and to deliver meaningful care. Where a person has been unwell for a period of time and death is anticipated, there may be a gathering of immediate and extended family and friends as a mark of respect for the patient. A family member may request to stay overnight with the patient, and this should be accommodated and where necessary negotiated in line with hospital policy and cultural protocol. Access to a chaplain should be made available if requested. To avoid infringing upon cultural protocols, ask the patient or one of the senior members of the family in private about who would be the most appropriate contact person in case of health deterioration or passing. Engaging with the local Aboriginal and Torres Strait Islander Advocate can assist in this process.

Death is very traumatic for family and friends of the deceased, which can extend to involve the whole community. At the time of passing certain cultural protocols will be set in motion. Extended family and relatives provide support to the immediate bereaved family, as well as feeding, transporting and housing mourners, and communicating about the death of their relative to the wider family members (Queensland Health, 2015). In some Aboriginal cultures, it is taboo to mention the name of the deceased person, which may include writing the name of the deceased person. It some Aboriginal cultures, it is also culturally inappropriate for non-Indigenous healthcare workers to contact and inform the next of kin of a person's passing. Cultural protocol of the Western Island group of the Torres Strait requires certain in-laws to undertake the role of 'Marigeth' or Spirit Hand, who is given the primary role of caring for the grieving family, informing family members of the person's passing and acting as the main communication point between the family, relatives and services such as funeral services. The Marigeth is also the person you would contact if open disclosure interviews were required.

It is natural to want to console family members following the death of their relative; however, customary practices following death differ between Aboriginal and Torres Strait Islander people. In some communities, respect is conveyed by avoiding eye contact with family members, or a silent handshake without eye contact can suffice. Listening to the family will greatly assist in identifying how you can help and maintain cultural respect.

Buddhism

Buddhists follow a list of religious principles with very strong emphasis on mindfulness and meditation and do not worship any gods or a single God. Most Buddhists believe a person has countless rebirths, which inevitably include suffering. Buddhists seek to end these rebirths by purifying the heart and letting go of all yearnings toward sensual desires and attachments (Boyett, 2016).

The importance of mindfulness and the awareness of all of life's experience may affect patients' or family members' decisions about pain relief, out of worry that analgesics may unduly cloud awareness. Nurses are encouraged to be very specific about any effect the analgesic may have on the individual's level of awareness (Andrews, 2013). Conversely, relief from pain by using analgesia may enable greater concentration and mindfulness. Non-pharmacological pain-management options may be more acceptable and should be explored with the patient and their family. In some instances, however, while Buddhism focuses on the relief of suffering, Buddhists may refuse analgesics in preference to maintaining clarity of consciousness and mental alertness. Clarification of the patient's wishes about the use of analgesics in the days and hours before death is very important for developing an ethical pain-management plan.

Patients or families may pray or chant out loud. Patients may use a string of beads during prayer. Families sometimes wish to place a picture of the Buddha in the patient's room. Requests to burn incense or candles can be handled by suggesting alternatives, such as placing flowers or scented cushions in the room or setting up a small electric light (Parkes et al., 2015).

As a patient approaches death, medical and nursing staff should minimise actions that might disturb the patient's concentration or meditation in preparation for dying. Similarly, family members may keep their physical distance from the patient's bed, becoming quiet so as not to disturb the patient's concentration. In Buddhist tradition, death is conceived as a crucial time of transition in the cycles of birth and rebirth, a process that has karmic implications in the next life (Boyett, 2016).

After a person dies, Buddhists believe that the body of the deceased is not immediately devoid of the person's spirit, so there is continued concern about disturbing the body. Such a belief may also be an impediment to discussing organ donation. Staff should try to keep the body as still as possible and avoid jostling during transport. Families may request that, after a patient has died, the patient's body be kept available to them for a number of hours for the purpose of religious rites. All such requests should be negotiated carefully, maximising the opportunity for accommodation in recognition of the religious significance (Andrews, 2013).

Christianity

A Christian refers to a follower of Jesus Christ, who may be Catholic, Protestant, Anglican, Baptist, Pentecostal, Mormon, Gnostic or a follower of another branch of the religion. There are differences between the branches, but generally a Christian follows the teachings of Jesus Christ. Jesus Christ's virgin birth, death and resurrection are held to be central to a belief in eternal life after earthly death. This belief is held with varying intensities, so it is important to ask a patient or family if they would like a Protestant chaplain or their own minister or Pastor to visit to offer support. This support could include comforting, prayer and reading of the Bible (Boyett, 2016).

There are no prescribed protocols for handling a deceased person (Andrews & Boyle, 2012). However, the Christian belief that all people are made in God's image and bear his likeness requires that bodies must be treated with utmost respect. Autopsy, organ donation and cremation are generally considered acceptable; however, you should inquire about the family's views.

Catholicism

Catholicism is a Christian **denomination**. The Catholic Church has its origin in the life and mission of Jesus Christ (Andrews & Boyle, 2012); however, special honour is given to the Virgin Mary because of her role as the mother of Jesus. A Catholic refers to a Christian who follows the Catholic religion as transmitted through the succession of Popes of Rome and the Vatican Empire across history (Boyett, 2016).

> **denomination**
> A distinct religious body that is defined by its doctrine, a set of beliefs/teachings, and church authority (for example, the Bible).

Catholics worship within the local community parish, and continuing contact with the parish is an important aspect of the spiritual care of a Catholic patient, which health emergencies and illness can interrupt. Access to the patient's local priest is important; however, during emergencies the hospital chaplain should be contacted.

Catholics believe that while God does not cause pain and suffering, these exist to further human growth. The Catholic Church subscribes to the principle of totality, which means that medical treatments, such as analgesia, are allowed as long as they are used for the good of the whole person (Carroll & Shiraishi, 1995). While fasting is advocated for healthy individuals between the ages of 18 and 62 years on certain significant religious days such as Ash Wednesday, Good Friday and the Fridays of Lent, individuals who are sick or infirm are not bound to this practice (Toropov & Buckles, 2011).

Sacraments and blessings are highly important, especially before surgery or whenever there is a perceived risk of death. The sacramental requests most commonly made by patients are the Sacrament of the Sick, Confession and Holy Communion (Andrews, 2013). During illness, Catholics may request the Sacrament of the Sick (formally known as the Last Rites), which includes anointing of the individual, holy communion (receiving a wafer and wine, normally grape juice) if able and a blessing from a priest. It can also include prayers for the sick and members of the family. A private, quiet environment should be provided if possible. Confession (how God forgives sins, cleanses the body of unrighteousness and reconciles that person with God) involves disclosing wrong actions and thoughts to God through either private prayer or private disclosure to a priest. The priest will then propose an act of penance, which might include prayer, a work of mercy or an act of charity, and provide counsel on how to live a better Christian life.

Individuals may request baptism. Baptism is the first and chief sacrament of forgiveness of sins because it unites the individual with Christ, and is a serious matter for Catholics. In non-emergency situations, the hospital chaplain or local priest can be contacted to perform the baptism. However, in an emergency and in the absence of a priest, any baptised Christian can perform the baptism by 'sprinkling water onto the head of the person three times, while saying, "<Person's name>, I baptise you in the name of the Father, and of the Son, and of the Holy Spirit", notifying the local priest or hospital chaplain immediately after the emergency baptism' (Andrews, 2013).

After a person dies, leave any items of religious significance in place, which may include religious statues and pictures of the Virgin Mary or Jesus Christ. While removal of these items is permitted if it is unavoidable, such as when needing to perform a chest X-ray or MRI scan, removing them in other situations, such as following death of the person, may cause distress to family and community members (Parkes et al., 2015).

The body of the deceased person is washed, taking care to leave religious objects such as chain and cross in place on the body (this should be documented in the deceased patient's notes), then legs and arms are laid straight, before a shroud is placed on the body. The body should then be wrapped in a sheet prior to placing the deceased person's body into the mortuary bag. Family members may wish to assist in preparing their relative's body and should be encouraged to do so. A priest can sometimes be requested to pray for the family and the soul of the deceased. Access to chaplaincy support should be provided.

Hinduism

Hinduism is the world's oldest living faith and third largest religion. Hinduism has no central doctrinal authority, so how individuals practise their religion will vary. Generally, Hindus believe that the soul is eternal and that it passes through successive cycles of birth and rebirth; reincarnation is accepted as fact.

Hinduism encourages the acceptance of pain and suffering as part of the consequences of karma. It is not seen as a punishment, but as a natural consequence of past negative behaviour, and is often seen as an opportunity to progress spiritually. This may affect triaging or the monitoring of pain levels as Hindu patients may not be forthcoming about pain and may prefer to accept it as a means of progressing spiritually (Parkes et al., 2015). However, this behaviour may be less prevalent in Australia, especially among young people. A Hindu patient may wish for a Pandit (priest) to be present to perform certain rituals, including tying a sacred thread around the neck or wrist, placing a few drops of water from the River Ganges into the patient's mouth or placing a sacred tulsi leaf (holy basil) in the patient's mouth.

A Hindu patient—especially a Hare Krishna follower—may wear sacred tulsi beads (a string of small wooden prayer beads) around their neck. It is important that these be on the body at the time of death. If it is necessary to remove these beads, they should be retied around the wrist (preferably the right). Patients may wish to read or recite religious chants and prayers. However, some patients may prefer to listen on a personal media player or small radio. Disregard for modesty can cause considerable distress to Hindus, and in particular to Hindu women. Even in a healthcare context, women are generally reluctant to undress for examination. A same-sex health provider may be preferred, and should be inquired about with the patient.

Hindus believe that the time of death is determined by one's destiny, and they accept death and illness as part of the crucial transition in the cycles of birth and rebirth. As such, the patient and their family may prefer no medical treatment in end-of-life situations if it merely prolongs the final stages of a terminal illness. Under these circumstances, it is permitted to disconnect life-supporting systems. However, suicide and euthanasia are forbidden in Hinduism. Hinduism supports the donation and transplantation of organs; however, the decision to donate or receive organs is left to the individual (Andrews, 2013).

A deceased Hindu's body is usually washed by close family members, normally led by the eldest son. If removal is not necessary, all jewellery, sacred threads and religious objects should be left in place. Family members may want to carry out a number of pre-death rituals such as tying a thread around the person's neck or wrist, and after death, they may request to wash the patient's body (Parkes et al., 2015). The deceased patient's family may prefer to reposition the body after death. There may be a strong desire for death to occur in the home rather than in the hospital. Family may request that there be constant attendance of the deceased's body, and a family member or representative may wish to accompany the body constantly, even to the morgue (Andrews, 2013).

Hindus are usually cremated as soon as possible after death (Queensland Health, 2011). Hindus generally regard autopsies as unacceptable; however, autopsy is permitted if required by law. Healthcare providers should consult with the family of a deceased Hindu patient before proceeding with an autopsy.

Islam

Followers of Islam are called Muslims. There are two types of Muslims—Shi'ite and Sunni—so beliefs and customs may differ. Muslims believe there is the one almighty God, named Allah, who is infinitely superior to and transcendent from humankind. Allah is viewed as the creator of the universe and the source of all good and all evil. Everything that happens is Allah's will (Andrews & Boyle, 2012). He is a powerful and strict judge, who will be merciful towards followers, depending on the sufficiency of their life's good works and religious devotion.

Islam has strict rules regarding what foods are permissible and which are forbidden. The main prohibited foods are pork and its by-products, alcohol, animal fats and meat that has not been slaughtered in accordance with Islamic rites. While most foods prohibited by Islam may be easy to identify, some—such as vanilla essence that contains alcohol, and ice-cream that may contain the pork derivative gelatine—may not be so obvious (Parkes et al., 2015). Spend time with your patient and their family to find suitable meal options.

In addition to strict dietary requirements, fasting is an integral part of Islam, especially during the month of Ramadan. For all healthy, adult Muslims fasting during Ramadan is compulsory; during this time, Muslims are not permitted to eat or drink anything—including water—from dawn until dusk. Muslims will consume a pre-dawn meal before fasting during the day until sunset. Muslims may also fast on other days prescribed by Islam, but this is voluntary. Muslims who are pregnant, breastfeeding, menstruating, experiencing temporary illness or travelling are exempted from fasting, but are required to make up for the fast at a later date (Parkes et al., 2015). Individuals with ongoing illness are exempted from fasting and may offer a *fidyah*, a donation such as food or money to those in need, as an alternative. While Muslims are fasting, they may take some medications and treatments without breaking their fast, which include injections, blood tests, transdermal medications (e.g. fentanyl patch) and gargling. However, ear or nose drops, suppositories, pessaries or inhaled medications will break the fast. Muslims diagnosed as having intellectual or cognitive disability or severe mental illness are absolved from all obligatory requirements of Islam, which includes praying, fasting and pilgrimage (Andrews & Boyle, 2012).

Muslim patients may express strong religious and cultural concerns regarding modesty, especially treatment by someone of the opposite sex. A Muslim woman may need to cover her body completely before anybody enters the room. Time must be provided to allow Muslim women to dress appropriately. Physical assessment of a Muslim woman should only occur when a family member is present, unless agreed to by the patient. Further, the clinician performing the examination of a Muslim patient should be of the same sex as the patient to minimise distress. Casual physical contact by non-family members of the opposite sex, such as shaking hands or passing a medication cup may not be permitted—not out of rudeness or disrespect, but for reasons of modesty. Similarly, some Muslims may even avoid eye contact. However, Islam allows exceptions to its rules in emergency situations (Andrews & Boyle, 2012).

Pain-control measures and blood transfusions are permissible; however, euthanasia is forbidden. The permissibility of organ and tissue transplant or donation is a personal choice. Visiting the sick and dying is strongly encouraged; therefore, there may be large numbers of visitors. At death—in hospital or elsewhere—the body must not be left naked or uncovered, and the body should be wrapped in a plain sheet while still unwashed. The body of the deceased should face Mecca or the East. If possible, staff of the same gender as the patient should handle the body, preferably with disposable gloves. If possible, the body is commonly buried within 24 hours of death; embalming and cremation are not permitted. Autopsy is permitted for legal or medical reasons only. In Islam, public grief is allowed for only three days, which allows non-family members to visit. After three days, the family is left to grieve privately.

Judaism

The term 'Jewish' reflects both a people and a religion. Worldwide, there are approximately 13 million Jewish people. Jewish people may be grouped into one of four ethnic groups: Ashkenazim, Sephardim, Mizrahi (or Oriental Jews) and Yemenite Jews. There are an increasing number of divisions within Judaism, each varying in its interpretation of Jewish law (known as *halakhah*) and practice of Jewish religious traditions (Andrews, 2013). The larger divisions include: orthodox, conservative, reformed, reconstructionist, humanistic and renewal. In traditional Judaism, there is one indivisible God (Bonura et al., 2001). Most Jewish men will cover their heads during worship and follow kosher dietary laws.

Family and community members will provide food for the patient unless kosher food can be provided. Kosher food should not be re-heated using a microwave or oven that has been used for non-kosher food unless double-wrapped. Prayer and ritual hand-washing varies across the divisions of Judaism. Where possible, care should be provided by healthcare workers of the same gender as the patient, or if this is not possible a chaperone must be present—although this requirement again varies across the divisions of Judaism. Engaging with patient and family members can greatly assist in optimising patient care while avoiding breaching cultural and religious practices.

Where matters of health are involved, particularly where there is danger to life, most of Judaism's rituals are set aside in the interests of sustaining life. Judaism teaches that all actions that may protect or prolong life should be taken, so organ transplants, blood transfusions, life support and pain control are all acceptable. Judaism teaches that the body is a gift from God, so all attempts at maintaining the health of the body and the soul are extremely important (Andrews & Boyle, 2012).

When a Jewish person becomes ill, family and friends are obligated to visit, so you can anticipate many visitors. These visits will be highly valued and comforting to the patient and the immediate family. Further, when a person is critically ill or dying, a family member will stay with the patient until death. If possible, the dying patient is encouraged to recite the confessional or affirmation of faith known as the *shema* before death, otherwise family members will recite the *shema* for the patient. In instances where there are no family members or friends to support the patient, contact the nearest synagogue or hospital rabbi (Andrews & Boyle, 2012).

Jewish people believe that the spirit leaves the body at the time of death. To allow the soul to depart, the body is to be left alone and untouched for half an hour after death. Following this, Judaic law requires that the body is not to be left alone. In some orthodox divisions of Judaism, the eldest son or relative may want to close the eyes and mouth of the deceased. Individuals of the opposite gender of the deceased are not permitted to touch the body of an orthodox Jew (Parkes et al., 2015).

Do not wash the deceased person's body. The body should be laid flat with legs extended and arms and hands (palm up) placed at the sides of the body. Incisions should be covered, and the body—including the head—covered with a sheet. Any dressings with the deceased patient's blood on them must be left in place. In some instances, the family may want to align the body of the deceased with the feet pointing towards the door. The family may contact the Chevra

Kadisha (Burial Society), which will prepare the body for burial. The body should be buried within 24 hours. Orthodox Jews do not permit cremation; autopsy is permitted if required by law (Parkes et al., 2015).

Sikhism

Sikhism was established in northern India by Guru Nanak Dev Ji. The Guru Granth Sahib, sometimes called the Adi Granth, is the spiritual text and is regarded as the eternal living Guru. Sikh beliefs include universal acceptance of all humanity; belief in one God; equality of all persons; and equality of the sexes. The Sikh way of life is based on remembering God with every breath; honest work and family life; sharing and living as an inspiration and support to the community; and control of desire, anger, greed, attachment and pride (Andrews & Boyle, 2012). Sikhs believe in reincarnation and that all humans suffer. Suffering stems from two sources: failure to control the mind and failure to appreciate God's creation. There are several sects within Sikhism, with some practices differing from those of orthodox Sikhs.

Many Sikhs are vegetarians. Animal-based medications and thickeners should be avoided, as they may contain gelatin. Alcohol is also not permitted. During the patient's stay in hospital, family members may bring *karah parshad*, a sacred pudding made from butter, sugar, flour and water. Family members' participation in caring for the patient, including provision of sacred or general food items, should be encouraged if appropriate (Parkes et al., 2015).

A devout Sikh may want to follow the daily ritual of private prayer, a bath in running water and meditation. Sikhs known as Amritdhari Sikh wear the five signs of their faith, sometimes referred to as the Five Ks: *Kesh* (hair), a Sikh must not cut hair from their body (males wear turbans); *Kachera*, special underwear similar to boxer shorts; *Kirpan*, a small sword often worn in a shoulder belt; *Kara*, an iron wrist bangle; and *Kanga*, a small wooden comb. If any of the five Ks need to be removed, discuss this with the patient and their family. For example, it may be possible to cover the hair with a cloth, or keep one leg in the *Kachera* instead of completely removing it.

Sikhs may have a large extended family, which can include members of the wider Sikh community. When a person is ill, many people may visit. Family members may request to stay with their relative, and want to participate in caring for the relative. This should be supported wherever possible. After the person dies, the family may wish to prepare the relative's body and this should also be encouraged wherever possible. The body is first washed and then wrapped in a white shroud, being careful to leave the five Ks in place. The head will be wrapped in a turban. If no family is available, the head of the deceased should be kept covered (Henley & Clayton, 1982). Relatives may prefer traditional washing and preparation of the body for cremation. Cremation should occur as soon as possible after death.

Summary

In this chapter, we have considered the challenges of nursing within a diverse culture, the definition of multiculturalism in Australia and the principle of cultural competence. We also explored the nurse's role to care for terminally ill patients and supporting a patient's family through death and dying, as well as examining a variety of faith-based practices for dealing with a dying patient or someone who has died.

Review questions

8.1   Cultural capability is defined as:
   a   The demonstrated capacity to act on cultural knowledge and awareness through a set of core attributes that are acquired through a lifelong learning process
   b   Being aware of different religious practices between cultural groups
   c   Knowing how to say hello, please and thank you in the languages of your most commonly treated patient groups

8.2   Characteristics of cultural capabilities include:
   a   Components are static and unchanging
   b   Language and religion
   c   Holistic, transferable and responsive, and can be adapted to new and changing contexts
   d   Understanding practices around death and dying

8.3   Cultural safety education focuses on:
   a   The knowledge and understanding of the individual nurse, rather than learning about cultural groups other than their own
   b   Religions of other cultural groups

    c Health practices of other cultural groups
    d How to communicate effectively

8.4   The three stages of cultural safety are:
    a Language, health, communication
    b Introspection, creativity, language
    c Awareness, sensitivity and safety

8.5   How many different languages are known to be spoken in different Australian homes?
    a 10–20
    b 50–100
    c 200
    d >300

8.6   What percentage of Australians speak a language other than English at home?
    a 5 per cent
    b 10 per cent
    c 21 per cent

8.7   What is the predominant religion in Australia?
    a Christianity
    b Catholicism
    c Islam
    d Judaism

8.8   If the deceased is subject to a coronial investigation (i.e. Coroner's case), can you remove the indwelling catheter?
    a Yes
    b No

9 NURSING AND ABORIGINAL AND TORRES STRAIT ISLANDER HEALTH

Roianne West and Alister Hodge

In this chapter, you will develop an understanding of:

- the Aboriginal and Torres Strait Islander Health Curriculum Framework
- the diversity of first peoples
- contemporary challenges in Aboriginal and Torres Strait Islander health
- the history of Australia's first peoples and the post-colonial experience
- racism and anti-racism in healthcare
- social determinants of health
- the Commonwealth Department of Health's 'Closing the Gap' commitment
- partnerships with first peoples, health professionals, organisations and communities
- Aboriginal and Torres Strait Islander nursing knowledge
- the Congress of Aboriginal and Torres Strait Islander Nurses and Midwives (CATSINaM)
- leadership, advocacy and effecting change
- cultural safety in healthcare
- reflection
- culturally safe communication.

It is well known that nurses are considered the backbone of Australia's healthcare system. For this reason, the nursing profession has great potential and strategic placement to lead improvements in health outcomes for Australia's Aboriginal and Torres Strait Islander people (West, 2014).

ABORIGINAL AND TORRES STRAIT ISLANDER HEALTH CURRICULUM FRAMEWORK

In order for the nursing profession to lead change in Aboriginal and Torres Strait Islander health education, cultural safety and anti-racism training need to become an integral aspect of nursing education, extending nursing's already comprehensive repertoire of skills (West, 2014). Good healthcare outcomes for Aboriginal and Torres Strait Islander people require nurses to be both clinically and culturally capable.

To this end, the Australian Nursing & Midwifery Accreditation Council (ANMAC) has introduced accreditation standards relating to the mandatory inclusion of Aboriginal and Torres Strait Islander health education, including cultural safety, in nursing curricula (ANMAC, 2014). Since its introduction, there have been a number of approaches by schools of nursing to address this standard. Mostly led by nursing academics who do not have an Aboriginal or Torres Strait Islander background, with little more education and experience in the area than the students they are attempting to teach, content has been inconsistent. In the academics' defence, most did not have access to the Aboriginal and Torres Strait Islander education on offer today.

More recently, the Commonwealth Government endorsed an Aboriginal and Torres Strait Islander Health Curriculum Framework (the Framework) for universities. The Framework has been developed to address this inconsistency among all health professions and higher education providers regarding how the Aboriginal and Torres Strait Islander curriculum is implemented.

The Framework responds to, and builds on, widespread evidence and recommendations from numerous reports, studies and consultations to actively develop greater cultural safety in health service delivery. The aim of the Framework is to provide a model for higher education providers to successfully implement Aboriginal and Torres Strait Islander health curricula, with clear learning outcomes and associated cultural capabilities (Department of Health, 2014). Ensuring that all nurses develop cultural capabilities before graduating from higher education is one way of enhancing the profession's health service delivery to Aboriginal and Torres Strait Islander people.

The National Aboriginal and Torres Strait Islander Health Plan 2013–2023 (NATSIHP) mandates 'the centrality of culture in the health of Aboriginal and Torres Strait Islander peoples and the rights of individuals to a safe, healthy and empowered life' (Department of Health, 2013b). The development of cultural capabilities for the nursing profession is paramount for the successful implementation of the Plan. Table 9.1 shows the Aboriginal and Torres Strait Islander Health Curriculum Framework, including cultural capabilities and key descriptors. This chapter will expand only on the key descriptors identified in **bold** in Table 9.1.

Graduate Cultural Capability Model

The Graduate Cultural Capability Model from the Framework (Figure 9.1) identifies the capabilities that new graduate nurses should have developed after undertaking studies in a tertiary setting where the Framework has been implemented (Department of Health, 2014):

- respect
- communication
- safety and quality
- reflection
- advocacy.

Cultural capability

The Framework uses the notion of 'cultural capability' as its foundation. Cultural capability entails the demonstrated capacity to act on cultural knowledge and awareness through a set of core attributes that are acquired through a vigorous process of lifelong learning. Importantly, capabilities are holistic, transferable and responsive, and can be adapted to new and changing contexts (Duignan, 2007; Stephenson, 1999). This agility is necessary, given the diversity of Aboriginal and Torres Strait Islander patients and health contexts.

DIVERSITY IN ABORIGINAL AND TORRES STRAIT ISLANDER CULTURES

Australia has been inhabited continually for between 50,000 and 60,000 years by the country's first nations peoples, known as Aboriginal and Torres Strait Islander peoples (Health Education and Training Institute, 2014; Horton, 2015; Mooney, 2013). Many different Aboriginal and Torres Strait Islander communities existed

Table 9.1 Aboriginal and Torres Strait Islander Health Curriculum Framework Cultural Capabilities and Key Descriptors

Each capability has a number of key descriptors that articulate required attitudes, values, skills and knowledge that students need to demonstrate to develop the associated capability.

Respect
Recognise Aboriginal and Torres Strait Islander peoples' ways of knowing, being and doing in the context of history, culture and diversity, and affirm and protect these factors through ongoing learning in healthcare practice.
Key descriptors:
  Topic 1.1 History of Australia's First Peoples and The Post-Colonial Experience
  Topic 1.2 First Peoples Culture, Beliefs and Practices
  Topic 1.3 Diversity of First Peoples Cultures
  Topic 1.4 Humility & Lifelong Learning

Communication
Key descriptors:
  Topic 2.1 Cultural Safety in Healthcare: Terminology and Definition
  Topic 2.2 Culturally Safe Communication
  Topic 2.3 Strengths Based Knowledge and Communication
  Topic 2.4 Partnerships with First Peoples Health Professionals, Organisations and Communities

Safety and Quality
Apply evidence- and strengths-based best-practice approaches in Aboriginal and Torres Strait Islander healthcare.
Key descriptors:
  Topic 3.1 Population Health
  Topic 3.2 Social Determinants
  Topic 3.3 Clinical Presentation

Reflection
Examine and reflect on how one's own culture and dominant cultural paradigms influence perceptions of and interactions with Aboriginal and Torres Strait Islander peoples.
Key descriptors:
  Topic 4.1 Self-reflexivity
  Topic 4.2 Cultural Self and Healthcare
  Topic 4.3 Culture of Australia's Healthcare System
  Topic 4.4 Racism and Anti-racism in Healthcare
  Topic 4.5 White Privilege

Advocacy
Recognise that the whole health system is responsible for improving Aboriginal and Torres Strait Islander health. Advocate for equitable outcomes and social justice for Aboriginal and Torres Strait Islander peoples and actively contribute to social change.
Key descriptors:
  Topic 5.1 Equity and Human Rights in Healthcare
  Topic 5.2 Leadership, Advocacy and Affecting Change

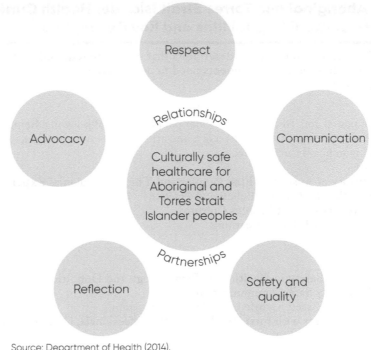

Source: Department of Health (2014).

Figure 9.1 Cultural capability model

across Australia, speaking different languages and with various local beliefs and practices (Mooney, 2013). In 1788, there was an estimated Aboriginal and Torres Strait Islander population of 750,000 people, with approximately 700 languages spoken throughout Australia, and over 400 Aboriginal nations (Watts, 2015). In 2013, the estimated Aboriginal and Torres Strait Islander population was 698,000 people (Australian Indigenous HealthInfoNet, 2013). Table 9.2 shows the distribution of Aboriginal and Torres Strait Islander peoples across Australia.

Figure 9.2 shows the geographical distribution of Aboriginal and Torres Strait Islander people, demonstrating that urban and large regional centres have the highest numbers of Aboriginal and Torres Strait Islander people. Some 79 per cent of Aboriginal and Torres Strait Islander people lived in non-remote areas and 21 per cent lived in remote areas in 2015. Queensland and New South Wales hold more than half of all Aboriginal and Torres Strait Islander people in Australia (ABS, 2015), with the majority of Aboriginal and Torres Strait Islander people residing in an urban setting (ABS, 2011) and the minority (approximately 25%) living in remote and very remote settings (ABS, 2015).

Table 9.2 Aboriginal and Torres Strait Islander population by Australian state and territory

State or territory	Aboriginal and Torres Strait Islander people (no.)	Proportion of total Aboriginal and Torres Strait Islander population (%)
New South Wales	220,902	31.0
Queensland	203,045	28.5
Western Australia	93,778	13.1
Northern Territory	72,251	10.1
Victoria	50,983	7.1
South Australia	39,800	5.6
Tasmania	25,845	3.6
Australian Capital Territory	6707	0.9
Australia total	713,311	100.0

Source: Adapted from AIHW (2015c).

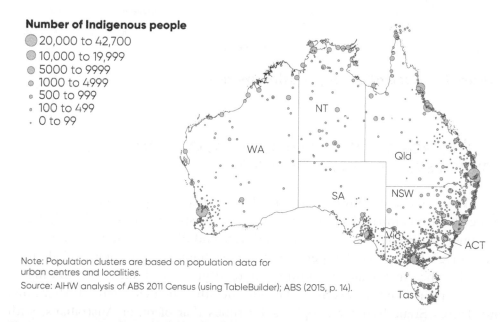

Number of Indigenous people
- 20,000 to 42,700
- 10,000 to 19,999
- 5000 to 9999
- 1000 to 4999
- 500 to 999
- 100 to 499
- 0 to 99

NT

WA

Qld

SA

NSW

Vic

ACT

Tas

Note: Population clusters are based on population data for urban centres and localities.

Source: AIHW analysis of ABS 2011 Census (using TableBuilder); ABS (2015, p. 14).

Figure 9.2 Geographical distributions of Aboriginal and Torres Strait Islander people

Figure 9.3 shows the age structure of the Australian population, by Aboriginal and Torres Strait Islander and non-Indigenous status. It shows a growing and very young population.

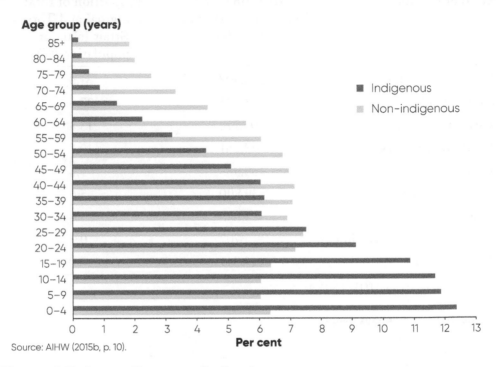

Source: AIHW (2015b, p. 10).

Figure 9.3 Australian population by age

CONTEMPORARY CHALLENGES IN ABORIGINAL AND TORRES STRAIT ISLANDER HEALTH

The Aboriginal and Torres Strait Islander population experiences significantly poorer health compared with the rest of the Australian community. Probably the most disturbing statistic is the death rate and life expectancy of Aboriginal and Torres Strait Islander people; it brings home the immense challenges faced by the Australian community in rectifying the issues contributing to poor Aboriginal and Torres Strait Islander health. The death rate of Aboriginal and Torres Strait Islander people is 1.9 times that of other Australians, with life expectancy ten to 11 years less than for non-Indigenous males and females (HETI, 2014).

The rates of morbidity within Aboriginal and Torres Strait Islander communities outstrip those of other Australians in many areas. The following are some examples.

- *Chronic kidney disease (CKD)*. In 2012–13, the rate was 3.7 times higher for Aboriginal and Torres Strait Islander people compared with other Australians, and accounted for 45 per cent of all hospitalisations for Aboriginal and Torres Strait Islander people (ABS, 2015).
- *Cardiovascular disease (CVD)*. In 2012–13, Aboriginal and Torres Strait Islander people were 1.2 times as likely to report having CVD as other Australians, and one in eight Aboriginal and Torres Strait Islander people over the age of two was reported as suffering from CVD (ABS, 2015).
- *Social and emotional wellbeing (SEWB)*. In 2012–13, Aboriginal and Torres Strait Islander people were hospitalised at twice the rate of other Australians, and the suicide rate was almost twice the rate as that for other Australians. For 15–19-year-olds, the suicide rate was five times as high as the rate for other Australians in this age group (ABS, 2015).
- *Diabetes*. In 2012–13, 11 per cent of Aboriginal and Torres Strait Islander adults had diabetes and 4.7 per cent were at risk of developing the disease. Indigenous people were 3.3 times as likely to have diabetes as other Australians. In 2008–12, diabetes was the underlying or associated cause of death in 20 per cent of Aboriginal and Torres Strait Islander deaths (ABS, 2015).

HISTORY OF AUSTRALIA'S FIRST PEOPLES AND THE POST-COLONIAL EXPERIENCE

The health of the country's Aboriginal and Torres Strait Islander peoples prior to 1788 was generally better than that of most people in Europe at the time (Watts, 2015). Many diseases endemic to Western and Asian cultures did not exist within Aboriginal and Torres Strait Islander communities. The arrival of Europeans in Australia devastated the health landscape for the Aboriginal and Torres Strait Islander population, with the introduction of previously unknown diseases. The introduction of these diseases—especially smallpox—decimated the Aboriginal population, resulting in significant loss of life with secondary damage to the fabric of existing societies through depopulation and social disruption (Australian Indigenous HealthInfoNet, 2013).

Although the introduction of new diseases was the main cause of Aboriginal deaths, direct conflict, dispossession and occupation of Aboriginal homelands by non-Indigenous people also led to increases in mortality, as colonists sought similar resources that were prized by the original inhabitants (Horton, 2015).

The ongoing movement of settlers across Australia, in conjunction with the impacts of disease and conflict, seriously challenged the ability of the Aboriginal and Torres Strait Islander population to achieve healthy lives by ruining traditional food sources, devaluing their culture, splitting families and dispossessing entire communities (Australian Indigenous HealthInfoNet, 2013). Aboriginal and Torres Strait Islander people who had been dispossessed of their land for farms and settlements became dependent on European food and clothing. They were also exposed to alcohol, which was used as a means of trade by the British, contributing to further damage to traditional social and family structures (Watts, 2015). The resulting loss of autonomy contributed to the establishment of a cycle of dispossession, demoralisation and poor health (Australian Indigenous HealthInfoNet, 2013).

RACISM IN HEALTHCARE

Larson et al. (2007) proposes racism as a root cause of the extreme socio-economic and health disadvantage suffered by Aboriginal and Torres Strait Islander people. Racism is experienced on three levels: institutional, interpersonal and internalised. *Institutional* racism relates to policies and practices employed by government and institutions that result in Aboriginal citizens receiving less benefit than other Australians from the same policy. *Interpersonal* racism describes discriminatory interactions between people, such as demeaning comments or behaviours. *Internalised* racism, also referred to as oppression, alludes to the effect of racism on the individual that may result in decreased self-esteem, and more depression and hostility (Larson et al., 2007). The appalling health of Australia's Aboriginal and Torres Strait Islander people is undeniably related to the impact of colonisation (Sinclair, 2004), racism and oppression (Paradies et al., 2008).

SOCIAL DETERMINANTS OF HEALTH

Although many of the disadvantages faced by the Aboriginal and Torres Strait Islander community have their origins in historical impositions, the ongoing perpetuation of disadvantage is founded in contemporary social determinants of health, including education, employment, housing, income, access to services, racism and incarceration (Australian Indigenous HealthInfoNet, 2013). Many Aboriginal and Torres Strait Islander people have a broader understanding of health, inclusive of the physical, social, emotional and cultural wellbeing of an individual and the whole community, and aim to create an environment in which each individual is able to achieve their full potential as a human being, thereby bringing about the total wellbeing of their community (National Aboriginal Health Strategy Working Party, 1989).

Dudgeon and colleagues (2014) describe elements commencing with *social wellbeing* as being important social determinants of health. They go on to say that these social determinants do not occur in isolation, but rather impact 'health' both at the same time and cumulatively. *Emotional wellbeing* relates to mental wellbeing (or mental ill-health), and to cognitive, emotional and psychological human experience, including fundamental human needs such as the experience of safety and security, a sense of belonging, self-esteem, values and motivations, and the need for secure relationships. Dudgeon and colleagues (2014) state that *cultural wellbeing* relates to Aboriginal and Torres Strait Islander people's capacity and opportunity to sustain and (re)create a healthy, strong relationship with their Aboriginal or Torres Strait Islander heritage. Finally, *community wellbeing* relates to the fundamental right to identity and understanding of self within Aboriginal and Torres Strait Islander cultures. This broader understanding is paramount for improvements in Aboriginal and Torres Strait Islander health outcomes.

THE COMMITMENT OF THE COMMONWEALTH DEPARTMENT OF HEALTH

Closing the Gap

The Australian government, Australia's health workforce and Aboriginal and Torres Strait Islander communities have a shared challenge to confront the social determinants of health that are perpetuating the cycle of lower-quality health experienced by Aboriginal and Torres Strait Islander people. In 2008, the Council of Australian Governments (COAG) committed to six targets to rectify the disadvantage experienced by Aboriginal and Torres Strait Islander people in education, life expectancy, child mortality and employment (COAG, 2009). The policy framework to achieve these ambitious targets is called Closing the Gap (CTG). The policy is a long-term framework acknowledging that improving opportunities for Indigenous Australians requires intensive and ongoing effort from all levels of government as well as communities, individuals, charity and 'for-profit' organisations. The CTG policy aims to build on the 2008 National Apology to Aboriginal and Torres Strait Islander Peoples (COAG, 2014). The agreement aims to:

- close the gap in life expectancy within one generation (by the year 2031)
- halve the gap in child mortality of Aboriginal and Torres Strait Islander children by 2018
- guarantee access for all Aboriginal and Torres Strait Islander four-year-olds to early childhood education
- halve the gap in reading, writing and numeracy achievement for Aboriginal and Torres Strait Islander children by 2018
- halve the gap in Year 12 achievement rates by Aboriginal and Torres Strait Islander students by 2018
- halve the gap in employment outcomes between Aboriginal and Torres Strait Islander people and other Australians by 2018 (COAG, 2009).

To achieve the CTG aims, and for the nursing workforce to provide services to Aboriginal and Torres Strait Islander people commensurate with those provided to other sectors of the wider community, health workers must understand the differences and barriers that can inhibit the patient–carer relationship.

PARTNERSHIPS WITH ABORIGINAL AND TORRES STRAIT ISLANDER HEALTH PROFESSIONALS, ORGANISATIONS AND COMMUNITIES: INDIGENOUS NURSING KNOWLEDGE

Colonisation aimed to denigrate and eradicate Aboriginal and Torres Strait Islander culture, ways of knowing, ways of being and ways of doing (Martin, 2003). Despite this approach, Aboriginal and Torres Strait Islander ways of knowing, ways of being and ways of doing remain today, and it is this knowledge that the nursing profession has to capitalise on to close the gap in health outcomes between Aboriginal and Torres Strait Islander people and other Australians. Aboriginal and Torres Strait Islander knowledge is not possible without the people from whom it originates, and Aboriginal and Torres Strait Islander nursing knowledge is not possible without Aboriginal and Torres Strait Islander nurses (West, 2014). Only Aboriginal and Torres Strait Islander nurses can speak with cultural authority in nursing.

Unfortunately, Aboriginal and Torres Strait Islander nurses currently make up only 0.8 per cent of the nation's nursing and midwifery workforce, and only 1414 of these are registered nurses. Based on 2011 census data (ABS, 2011) and population parity of 3 per cent, we require 5400 Aboriginal and Torres Strait Islander Registered Nurses in Australia; this is four times the number we currently have. However, this is more than just an equity issue, so when we factor in burden of disease, conservatively allowing for only twice the burden of disease, we require at least 10,800 Aboriginal and Torres Strait Islander Registered Nurses, which is 8.5 times the number we have currently (CATSINaM, 2015a, 2015b).

In order to achieve an increase in the participation of Aboriginal and Torres Strait Islander people in the nursing workforce, we have to increase the number of Aboriginal and Torres Strait Islander people completing university nursing programs (West et al., 2010). If we are committed to improving the health outcomes for Indigenous Australians, an Indigenous nursing workforce is essential (West, 2014).

CONGRESS OF ABORIGINAL AND TORRES STRAIT ISLANDER NURSES AND MIDWIVES (CATSINaM)

CATSINaM is the peak representative body for Aboriginal and Torres Strait Islander nurses and midwives in Australia. CATSINaM's purpose is the recruitment and retention of Aboriginal and Torres Strait Islander people into nursing and midwifery, with the aim of closing the gap in health for Aboriginal and Torres Strait Islander peoples. One of the ways by which CATSINaM aims to achieve this is through collaborating with nursing and midwifery education providers to increase awareness and understanding of the issues that impact on Aboriginal and Torres Strait Islander health (CATSINaM, 2015a, 2015b).

LEADERSHIP, ADVOCACY AND EFFECTING CHANGE

Given the disproportionate representation of Aboriginal and Torres Strait Islander peoples in all sectors of Australia's healthcare system, and the strategic position in which nurses are placed, all nurses need to obtain the necessary leadership skills to advocate for equitable health outcomes and culturally safe services for Aboriginal and Torres Strait Islander clients, and need to develop resilience to manage resistance to change from others (Department of Health, 2014). When working with Aboriginal and Torres Strait Islander patients, leadership is most effective when it respects culture and is deliberately and consciously committed to learning about and building solutions from the best of all cultures, inclusive of Aboriginal and Torres Strait Islander cultures, non-Indigenous cultures, nursing and midwifery cultures and the culture of the healthcare system (West, 2014). The health of Aboriginal and Torres Strait Islander people is a concern and responsibility of all clinicians, and as a new graduate nurse you can show leadership by modelling appropriate behaviour through the delivery of culturally safe care. As nurses comprise over half of the Australian health workforce, nurse leaders from health services policy and academia need to collaborate to strategically build the cultural capability of the nursing workforce (West, 2014).

CULTURAL SAFETY IN HEALTHCARE: TERMINOLOGY AND DEFINITION

Cultural safety education focuses on the knowledge and understanding of the individual nurse, rather than learning about cultural groups other than their own. A nurse who can understand their own culture and the theory of power relations can be culturally safe in any context, irrespective of the patient's cultural background. However, given the effects of historical relations between Aboriginal and Torres Strait Islander people and other Australians on the contemporary health status of Aboriginal and Torres Strait Islander Australians, this process is of critical importance. According to Ramsden (1992), *cultural awareness* is the first step in the process of learning cultural safety. Cultural awareness involves acknowledging and understanding difference, while *cultural sensitivity* is an intermediate step where critical self-reflection by the student begins. Cultural safety is an outcome of this learning that enables a safe, appropriate and acceptable service, as defined by those who receive it (Figure 9.4).

Practical examples of culturally respectful strategies a nurse could undertake include:

- engagement in the Aboriginal and Torres Strait Islander health curriculum at university
- engagement of Aboriginal Hospital Liaison Officers during care episodes

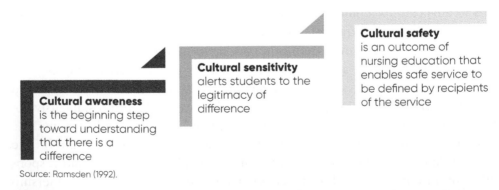

Cultural safety
is an outcome of nursing education that enables safe service to be defined by recipients of the service

Cultural sensitivity
alerts students to the legitimacy of difference

Cultural awareness
is the beginning step toward understanding that there is a difference

Source: Ramsden (1992).

Figure 9.4 The process of achieving cultural safety in nursing practice

- undertaking additional professional development in Aboriginal and Torres Strait Islander health education, including but not limited to health service-provided training
- acknowledgement of Traditional Owners as appropriate with guidance from health service Aboriginal and Torres Strait Islander leadership
- with the patient's permission, physically co-locating Aboriginal and Torres Strait Islander inpatients together with other individuals who speak the same traditional language or are from the same community if it is culturally appropriate
- becoming aware of and adhering to the health service's Aboriginal and Torres Strait Islander health strategies, including Aboriginal and Torres Strait Islander health workforce developments (Australian Health Ministers' Advisory Council, 2004).

REFLECTION

Reflection is one of the five capabilities identified in the Aboriginal and Torres Strait Islander Health Curriculum Framework, with the learning outcome of recognising the influence of your own culture and identity, your professional (nursing) culture and identity, and the culture of the Australian healthcare system on your perceptions of Aboriginal and Torres Strait Islander people. Key elements include self-reflexivity, cultural self and healthcare, culture of Australia's healthcare system, racism and anti-racism in healthcare, and white privilege (Department of Health, 2014).

The Framework (Department of Health, 2014) uses the work of Walker and colleagues (2015) in developing its arguments for the importance of critical reflection. Walker and colleagues state that critical reflection of an experience, situation or performance facilitates a deeper level of learning, understanding and conscious decision-making to potentially improve and transform professional (nursing) practice. Walker and colleagues (2015) describe the stages of critical reflective practice (adapted for nursing) as:

(i) *Defining* and discussing the issue and its key themes;
(ii) *Reflecting* on how your own culture (life experiences and worldview) and your nursing culture, influences your understanding of the issue. Further reflect on how this influences your perceptions of and interactions with Australia's First Peoples in healthcare;
(iii) *Analysing* the viewpoints and assumptions of others and the dominant cultural paradigm relating to the issue and how this influences your perceptions of and interactions with Australia's First Peoples in healthcare;

(iv) *Discussing* what you have learnt from this reflective process and how this might contribute to your lifelong learning within your nursing;

(v) *Reflecting* on what you have learnt from undertaking this critical reflection process including the potential this process has to transform your nursing practice.

See Figure 9.5 for the critical reflective practice model.

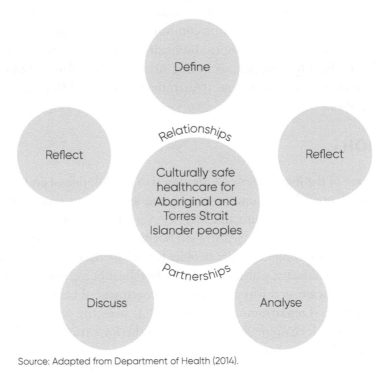

Source: Adapted from Department of Health (2014).

Figure 9.5 Critical reflective practice model

DEFINING 'CRITICAL' IN THE CONTEXT OF ABORIGINAL AND TORRES STRAIT ISLANDER HEALTH EDUCATION

Aboriginal and Torres Strait Islander knowledge

Numerous Aboriginal and Torres Strait Islander authors have demonstrated how mainstream services, including universities and healthcare services, unconsciously work to exclude, harm and disadvantage Aboriginal and Torres Strait Islander populations (Walker et al., 2015). Aboriginal authors Martin (2003) and Rigney (1997) highlight the importance of embedding and applying Aboriginal terms of reference—that is, ways of knowing, ways of being and ways of doing—into policy and program development that impacts Aboriginal people. The work of Martin and Rigney provides strategies for how universities and healthcare systems can be culturally responsive and sensitive to the needs of Indigenous Australians.

Central to engaging in transformative education and service delivery in the 'intercultural space' (Nakata, 2007; Nakata et al., 2012) is understanding the history of Australia's first peoples and the post-colonial experience, and the impact that racism and its associated stereotypes and assumptions have had, and continue to have, on the contemporary health status of Aboriginal and Torres Strait Islander people. Being critically reflective here requires all healthcare workers to be prepared to challenge racism and its associated assumptions and stereotypes. This process can be emotionally confronting and expose vulnerabilities, powerlessness and feelings of being out of place. However, having the ability to work outside your own comfort zone is crucial to the development of the growth of cultural capabilities (Walker et al., 2015).

The following examples show where *critical* reflective practice can be valuable:

- in developing partnerships and relationships with Aboriginal and Torres Strait Islander health professionals and organisations to challenge current beliefs and practices regarding Aboriginal and Torres Strait Islander health
- when analysing the enablers and disablers within the healthcare system to deliver high-quality, comprehensive, equitable, culturally safe healthcare to Aboriginal and Torres Strait Islander people
- in developing resilience to manage resistance to change
- in providing a framework to examine your own responses to applying a strengths-based approach in Aboriginal and Torres Strait Islander health
- in providing a framework *and* a vehicle to move from reflection to action in challenging racist and colonial discourses
- in transforming experiences into knowledge and deeper wisdom and application in personal and professional lives (Department of Health, 2014).

Culturally safe communication

Depending upon the community in which you are working, alterations to clinical interaction may be required to achieve an optimal health experience for patients, ensuring patients understand their illness and have the opportunity for input regarding any proposed treatment.

A key aspect of any clinical interaction is communication. Studies into

Aboriginal and Torres Strait Islander patient–health worker interactions have identified critical miscommunications that often went unrecognised by both patient and clinician on issues such as diagnosis, treatment and prevention, but that are important for a successful outcome. One study by Cass and colleagues (2002) identified six main areas that impeded effective communication between the patient and treating clinician:

1 *Lack of control:* for example, staff commonly have control over the decision as to whether an interpreter is required and the clinician controlled the topic of discussion and style of verbal discourse.
2 *Modes of discourse:* for example, in some Aboriginal cultures the 'question–answer' interview style of Western health interactions is considered rude. This may result in a patient feeling it is impolite to give what they view as a negative answer, so instead they say whatever they believe the interviewer wants to hear.
3 *Cultural and linguistic distance:* English is a second language for many Aboriginal people living in rural and remote communities; conversely, most treating health professionals have no ability to communicate in the patient's first language. Culturally specific terminology can also present problems during health discussions—for example, discussion of quantitative measures while explaining medicine or diagnostics might have little or no meaning for certain linguistic/cultural groups.
4 *Lack of shared knowledge:* an understanding of the pathophysiology of the disease being treated is needed to enable meaningful discussion around treatment with a patient. If a shared understanding of the topic is not present, effective communication is compromised. This is a common challenge for health interactions throughout the wider community as well.
5 *Lack of staff training in cross-cultural communication:* in many cases, clinicians delivering care to Aboriginal and Torres Strait Islander patients have had minimal formal training in relevant communication issues.
6 *Limited use of interpreters* (Cass et al., 2002).

Consider your own and the patient's body language and non-verbal communication. Non-verbal communication patterns vary widely between cultural groups, and it is important to understand key local practices that may affect the maintenance of a therapeutic relationship (Omeri & Raymond, 2009).

Poor communication often severely impacts the uptake and appropriate usage of medications by Aboriginal patients. Aboriginal health workers have identified that inappropriate use of medications is related to issues including literacy level, medication information often being confusing and difficult to understand, and

Aboriginal patients feeling uncomfortable about requesting advice from clinicians regarding use of the medication (Hamrosi et al., 2006).

Some strategies have been suggested to improve communication with Aboriginal and Torres Strait Islander patients:

- Ensure you have had appropriate education in cross-cultural communication issues to enable Aboriginal and Torres Strait Islander patients to arrive at informed choices.
- Provide your patient with the option for, and access to, interpreter services for clinical discussions.
- Engage with educational resources that promote a shared understanding of the relevant health complaint and related treatment options.
- Display humility and compassion, and maintain a friendly demeanour during your interactions. Being officious or overly assertive may not be well received.
- Engage in reflection to monitor the effectiveness of your staff–patient communication, to ensure that episodes of miscommunication are minimised.

In any health interaction with an Aboriginal or Torres Strait Islander patient, the health professional should consider the belief system of the patient and the impact this may have on communication and management. A clear explanation should be provided of the disease and cause. The biomedical explanation must be respectful of any traditional explanation that the family or patient may voice, as differences in beliefs to the origin or cause of the illness or disability may affect the management and subsequent compliance with any suggested management plan. The discussion of treatment options must respect the wishes of the patient and family, including the use of traditional medicine if this is requested or suggested (Maher, 1999). The clinician must also maintain awareness of body language and verbal communication strategies to enable clear understanding and patient interaction with the health episode.

Summary

In this chapter, we have considered the importance of the Aboriginal and Torres Strait Islander Health Curriculum Framework in providing a model for higher education providers to successfully implement Aboriginal and Torres Strait Islander health curricula. We have looked at the contemporary health challenges faced by Aboriginal and Torres Strait Islander people and the contribution of colonisation, racism and ongoing social determinants such as education and employment to poor health outcomes. The Australian government's Closing the Gap strategy has been considered together with initiatives to improve cultural awareness, culturally safe practice and communication.

Review questions

9.1   The Australian Nursing & Midwifery Accreditation Council (ANMAC) introduced accreditation standards relating to the mandatory inclusion of Aboriginal and Torres Strait Islander health education into nursing and midwifery courses:

a   Because good healthcare outcomes for Aboriginal and Torres Strait Islander people require nurses to be both clinically, and as importantly, culturally capable

b   To meet new 'Closing the Gap' targets

c   As a response to changes in mandatory training requirements in public hospitals

9.2   In what year did the Commonwealth Government endorse the Aboriginal and Torres Strait Islander Health Curriculum Framework for universities?

a   2000   c   1788

b   2016   d   2008

9.3   The National Aboriginal and Torres Strait Islander Health Plan 2013–2023 (NATSIHP) mandates what as being central to healthcare?

a   Patient advocacy   c   Culture

b   Clinical knowledge   d   Clear communication

9.4   Which of the following cultural capabilities are identified in the Aboriginal and Torres Strait Islander Health Curriculum Framework?

a   Respect, communication   c   Reflection and advocacy

b   Safety and quality   d   All of the above

9.5   Prior to 1788, approximately how many different people, how many different Aboriginal and Torres Strait Islander languages and how many nations existed on the Australian continent?

a   100,000 people; 50 languages; 200 nations

b   750,000 people; 700 languages; 400 nations

    c   50,000 people; 20 languages; 5 nations

    d   1,000,000 people; 500 languages; 400 nations

9.6   The majority of Aboriginal and Torres Strait Islander Australians live in:

    a   Non-remote areas (urban and large regional centres)

    b   Remote areas

9.7   Which of the following statements is true of the age of the Australian Aboriginal and Torres Strait Islander population?

    a   It is static

    b   It is an ageing population

    c   It is a growing and very young population

9.8   The death rate of Aboriginal and Torres Strait Islander people is how many times that of other Australians?

    a   0.5 times

    b   1.9 times

    c   Three times

    d   Equal to that of other Australians

9.9   Life expectancy for Aboriginal and Torres Strait Islander people is how many years less than that for other Australians?

    a   Ten to 11 years   c   Six to seven years

    b   Five years   d   15 years

9.10   In 2012–13, the rates of morbidity for which condition was five times higher in Aboriginal and Torres Strait Islander people than in other Australians?

    a   Chronic obstructive pulmonary disease

    b   Chronic kidney disease

    c   Cardiovascular disease

    d   Social and emotional wellbeing

9.11   The appalling health of Australia's Aboriginal and Torres Strait Islander people is related to:

    a   The impact of colonisation, racism and oppression

    b   The clustering of health resources in metropolitan areas

    c   Health education

    d   Difficulty in accessing bulk-billing services

9.12 Social determinants of health refer to issues such as:
a Education, employment, housing, income, access to services
b Racism and incarceration
c Political identity
d Both a and b

9.13 What is the Aboriginal and Torres Strait Islander understanding of health?
a Body and mind are separate from culture
b Similar to Western biomedical model
c It is inclusive of the physical, social, emotional and cultural well-being of an individual and the whole community

9.14 What is the aim of the Closing the Gap campaign?
a To raise awareness of the challenges facing Indigenous Australians
b To rectify the disadvantage experienced by Indigenous Australians in health, education, life expectancy, child mortality and employment
c To improve representation for Indigenous Australians in parliament

9.15 The aim of the reflection capability in the Aboriginal and Torres Strait Islander Curriculum Framework is to:
a Identify gaps in knowledge so that they can be targeted in future education
b To recognise the influence of your own culture and identity, your professional (nursing) culture and identity and the culture of the Australian healthcare system on your perceptions of Aboriginal and Torres Strait Islander peoples
c To put yourself in the shoes of your patients, to understand their experience of the healthcare system

9.16 Being critically reflective when caring for Aboriginal and Torres Strait Islander people requires:
a Being prepared to challenge racism
b Being aware of racism and stereotypes, and reporting it after the fact to your supervisor when you see other staff members at fault
c Letting go of associated assumptions and stereotypes
d Both a and c

10 COMMON MANDATORY TRAINING TOPICS

Alister Hodge

In this chapter, you will develop an understanding of:

- infection control:
  - standard precautions
  - hand hygiene
  - personal protective equipment (PPE)
  - sharps management
- fire safety
- work health and safety (WHS)
- waste management
- security
- manual handling:
  - posture rules
  - completion of a manual handling risk assessment.

Mandatory training refers to areas of learning and skills development that you will have to complete successfully as a term of your employment. The topics covered vary between public and private employers, and between states. Mandatory training seeks to target key areas that help to maintain a safe work environment, and safe clinical practices during care delivery. Nurses will generally need refresher training in most topics on a yearly basis to ensure currency. This chapter explores some of the most commonly taught mandatory topics.

INFECTION CONTROL

All healthcare workers have an obligation to take reasonable steps to prevent the spread of infection between staff, patients and the general public. Some simple steps exist that, if undertaken by the clinician, can stop the transmission of disease.

Standard precautions

Standard precautions refer to a series of practices based on the assumption that all blood and body fluids/substances, except for sweat, are potentially infective (NSW Health, 2007). Examples of work practices covered by 'standard precautions' include:

- hand hygiene practices
- appropriate use of gloves
- appropriate use of personal protective equipment (PPE)
- safe use and disposal of sharps
- disinfection, cleaning and sterilisation of non-disposable equipment.

Hand hygiene

Hand hygiene is the most important measure for combatting and controlling infection within the health setting. Hand hygiene refers to the use of alcohol-based hand rub or the washing of hands with water and liquid soap. The Australian Commission on Quality and Safety in Healthcare (ACSQHC) launched a National Hand Hygiene Initiative (NHHI) to decrease the rates of hospital acquired infection via the improvement of clinician hand hygiene practices across the entire country. An organisation called Hand Hygiene Australia was assigned and funded by ACSQHC to implement the NHHI.

Hand Hygiene Australia has identified five moments surrounding clinical care delivery when hand hygiene should be completed. These are:

- before touching a patient
- before a procedure
- after a procedure or body fluid exposure risk
- after touching a patient
- after touching a patient's surroundings.

Clinicians should also wash their hands prior to:

- preparing food
- eating.

And they should wash their hands after:

- using the toilet
- coughing, sneezing or handling tissues/handkerchiefs
- handling waste.

Personal protective equipment

PPE aims to protect health staff from being exposed to infectious agents. Table 10.1 shows appropriate use of gloves/gowns/masks/eye wear (NSW Health, 2007).

Table 10.1 Personal protective equipment

Item	Use
Gloves	Gloves should be worn during food preparation or serving, general cleaning, handling any item or equipment exposed to body fluids, during any direct anticipated contact with a body fluid and when performing invasive procedures, such as cannulation.
Gowns and aprons	Fluid-resistant gowns must be worn when there is an anticipation of splashes or clothing coming into contact with body fluids.
Fluid-repellant masks, protective eye wear	These must be worn while performing any procedure where there is a chance of body fluid splash.

Sharps management

Sharps represent the greatest risk of transmission of blood-borne diseases to the clinician. When working with sharps (syringes/needles/scalpels/razors), obey the following principles:

- Do not pass sharps from hand to hand.
- Do not re-cap needles.

- Do not clean up someone else's sharps.
- Dispose of sharps immediately following use in a sharps bin at the site of care; do not carry in a kidney dish.
- Be wary of potential sharps in soiled linen/linen bags (NSW Health, 2007).

FIRE SAFETY

For a fire to begin, fuel, oxygen and heat must be present in sufficient proportions. Fire prevention seeks to keep fuel and ignition sources separate. Things that you can do to help prevent or stop the spread of fires include keeping corridors and fire doors free of obstruction, ensuring that electrical equipment is tested and tagged, and that fire-fighting equipment is easily accessible.

When faced with a fire, the acronym RACE should be followed:

- R: Remove—remove any person in danger to a place of safety
- A: Alert—alert personnel of the fire via local emergency procedures
- C: Contain—contain if safe to do so, close any doors and windows
- E: Extinguish—extinguish only if safe to do so, if it is a minor fire and you are trained in the use of fire equipment (NSW Health, 2010).

All staff are required to take part in annual training in the use of a fire extinguisher/ fire blanket/and emergency evacuation. Ensure that you are aware of evacuation procedures and location of fire-fighting equipment within your worksite.

There are six classes of fire, based upon the type of fuel involved:

1 Class A—solids, such as paper, textiles, wood, plastics and rubber
2 Class B—flammable liquids, such as petrol, oil and paint
3 Class C—flammable gases, such as propane, butane and methane
4 Class D—metals, such as aluminium, magnesium and titanium
5 Class E—electrically energised equipment
6 Class F—cooking oils and fats.

Check the fire extinguisher to see whether it is appropriate for the type of fire likely to occur. Extinguishers will have a pictograph label to indicate the class of fire for which it is designed. When using an extinguisher, there are four steps to follow:

1 Pull out the pin that prevents accidental depression of the handle.
2 Aim the nozzle at the base of the fire.
3 Squeeze the handle.
4 Sweep the nozzle back and forth as you spray the bottom of the fire.

Fire blankets usually are located in all kitchen areas and at key points throughout a department. The fire blanket is a sheet of fire-retardant material that, when placed over a fire, smothers it of oxygen. Fire blankets are only appropriate for use in the advent of a small fire. If used to extinguish a clothing fire, wrap the victim in the blanket, then roll them on the ground to smother the flames.

If a decision is made to evacuate the building, it is critical that this is completed in a staged and organised fashion that is commensurate with the threat. The steps in an evacuation are:

1 Move people out of the room and to a safe distance from the fire.
2 Move to a different fire compartment—behind next set of fire doors.
3 Move from the building to a pre-organised evacuation point (NSW Health, 2010).

WORK HEALTH AND SAFETY (WHS)

WHS involves promoting and protecting the health, safety and welfare of all people in the workplace. Responsibilities of the employee and employer are articulated in state legislation.

Responsibilities of the employer to make the workplace safe for employees and any person entering the worksite include:

* safe systems of work
* instruction, training and supervision when required
* appropriate equipment
* existence of policies, procedures and safe work practices.

Employees must cooperate with the employer where safety is concerned by:

* not interfering with or misusing safety equipment
* taking reasonable care
* following procedures, policies and safe work practices
* attending training provided.

An important part of WHS is the management of risk. Risk management aims to identify hazards in the worksite that may result in injury or property damage, and subsequently remove or lower the risk of harm. Risk management incorporates four steps:

1 Identify the hazard.
2 Assess risk.
3 Determine the appropriate control of risk.
4 Implement the control.

Methods that may be used to control a risk include, in order of preference:

- Eliminate risk.
- Substitute the risk hazard with something of a lower risk.
- Isolate the hazard.
- Engineering: provide equipment to lower risk.
- Administrative: change a work system to lower risk.
- PPE: equipment is to be worn to protect the employee from the risk (NSW Health, 2013b).

WASTE MANAGEMENT

Waste is separated into different groups to meet the requirements surrounding appropriate disposal of clinical waste, to facilitate recycling and to decrease the cost to the organisation. Most organisations use a colour-coded bin system. Familiarise yourself with the colour-coded system used at your worksite. One common colour-coding system is:

- orange bins: co-mingled recycling—for example, cans/glass/cartons
- blue bins: paper recycling
- green bins: general waste

cytotoxic drugs
Medications that are toxic to cells, targeting rapidly dividing cancer cells.

- yellow bins: clinical waste—for example, items contaminated with body fluids
- purple bins: **cytotoxic drugs**, waste and PPE used during administration of cytotoxic materials
- maroon/burgundy bins: recognisable body parts and metal objects such as prostheses.

SECURITY

Security staff typically are responsible for the protection and safety of staff, visitors and patients at the site where they are based. Security personnel respond to various types of emergencies, including fire alarms, duress alarms/behavioural emergencies and bomb threats. A number of simple measures can be taken to contribute to safety within the worksite:

- Report all suspicious behaviour and people on hospital grounds to security.
- Be aware of and follow local security procedures/policies—for example, use of duress alarms.
- Ensure that your identification badge is visible and worn at all times.

MANUAL HANDLING

Manual handling refers to any activity that requires employees to use any part of their musculoskeletal system to complete their work. Injuries sustained by employees through manual handling cost the organisation through a loss of productive hours, staff replacement and retraining. However, the losses to the employee are worse, with individual costs being a reduction in quality of life, reduction in earning capacity, increased medical expenses and family life implications. Examples of manual handling tasks that may represent increased risk include:

* repetitive actions
* sustained work postures
* pushing, pulling, lowering, lifting, carrying
* holding or restraining a patient
* exposure to vibration (Safe Work Australia, 2017).

Most manual handling injuries are a result of years of poor work practice or posture, leading to cumulative effects of wear and tear. Both the employee and employer have responsibilities towards manual handling in the work place. Employer responsibilities include: undertaking risk management activities for manual handling tasks; consulting with employees and committees; and being proactive in injury prevention through the provision of equipment and training to staff for safe manual handling.

The employee also has responsibilities to comply with safe practices and work policies, to use lifting aids where they are provided, to cooperate with risk management through the reporting of hazards and equipment faults, and to actively participate in training in manual handling.

Posture rules

There are some simple posture rules that should be followed during any tasks requiring manual handling to minimise the risk of injury:

* Keep your ribcage upright.
* Keep your elbows as close to your side as possible when you are performing tasks. Keeping your elbows in this position will reduce the amount of force transmitted through your back.

Manual handling risk assessment

Before completing any manual handling, there are four steps to be taken to reduce the risk of injury.

1 Identify whether the task will place you at risk.
2 Assess what is going to create risk within the task.
3 Control the risk by either elimination or reduction.
4 Evaluate whether your actions will be creating any further risks.

When lifting:

- Assess your load. Determine before you lift whether you will require assistance from another person.
- Keep the load close to your body to decrease strain on your back.
- Maintain correct alignment of your back by avoiding twisting. Use a squat or lunge if picking up an object from below mid-height.
- Lift with your legs rather than your back.
- Tense your abdominal muscles to support your spine.
- Use smooth movements, avoiding jerks or tugging.

Summary

In this chapter, we have examined some common mandatory training topics that nurses need to understand to be able to perform competently. These include infection control, fire safety, work health and safety, waste management, security and safe manual handling. Nurses may need to undertake refresher courses on a yearly basis in these areas to maintain the currency of their knowledge and skills.

Review questions

10.1 Which staff must comply with infection-control policies within the workplace?
    a Only clinical staff
    b Only medical and nursing staff
    c All staff

10.2   Standard precautions must be carried out by all staff to reduce the spread of micro-organisms. Which of the following statements are true in regard to standard precautions?
   a   Standard precautions assume that all body fluids/substances are infectious
   b   Standard precautions are only applicable to patients with high risk of infection
   c   Standard precautions are a method to reduce risk of infection to not only the health worker, but also the patient
   d   Standard precautions involve good hand hygiene, appropriate use of gloves and appropriate use of personal protective equipment such as masks and aprons

10.3   Hand hygiene should be completed:
   a   Before touching a patient
   b   Before completing a procedure
   c   Before touching a patient's surroundings/notes
   d   After a procedure or body fluid exposure risk
   e   After physical contact with a patient
   f   After touching a patient's surroundings

10.4   The chance of needle-stick injury can be reduced by following which of the practices below:
   a   Never re-capping needles
   b   Carrying used sharps in a plastic kidney dish
   c   Disposing of used sharps into a sharps bin directly after use
   d   Not passing sharps between people

10.5   What does RACE stands for?
   a   Remove, Alert, Contain, Extinguish
   b   Raise the Company Emergency Alarm
   c   Retrieve, Alert, Carry, Exit
   d   Remove, Access, Contain, Evacuate

10.6   Place the items below in the appropriate order of evacuation:
   a   Room, building, compartment
   b   Building, room, compartment
   c   Room, compartment, building

10.7 What is the aim of WHS?
   a Protecting employers from litigation when an employee injures themselves at work
   b Reducing the impact of staff injury on sick leave payments
   c Promoting and protecting the health, safety and welfare of all people in the workplace

10.8 An employee has a responsibility, under the WHS Act, to not interfere with or deliberately misuse equipment, to follow policies, procedures and safe work practices, and to attend education provided about safe work practices. True or false?

10.9 A risk to safety has been identified in the workplace. Put the following interventions in order from most effective to least effective for preventing harm.
   a Personal protective equipment
   b Administrative
   c Substitution
   d Engineering
   e Isolation

10.10 An expectation of an employee regarding security at the health worksite includes:
   a Always displaying their photo ID card
   b Stopping a thief or assailant from leaving the premises until the police can arrive
   c Being aware of your local security policies

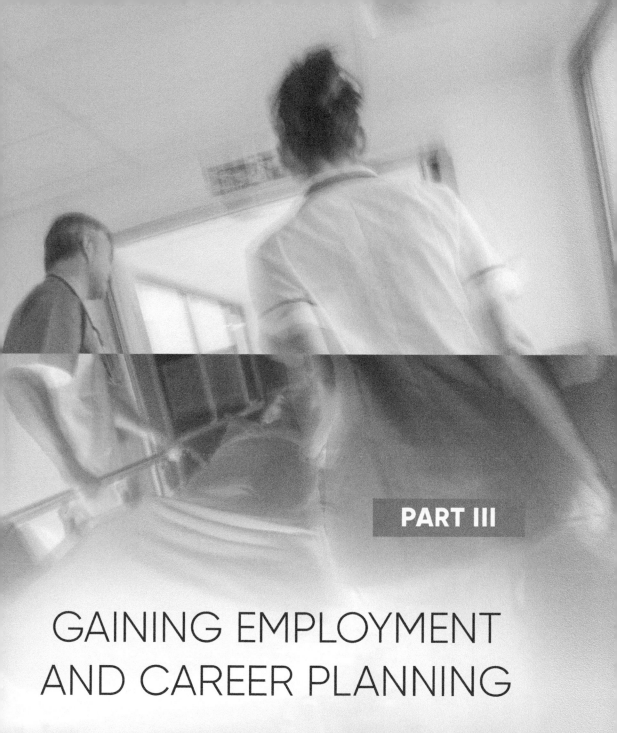

PART III

GAINING EMPLOYMENT AND CAREER PLANNING

11 CAREER PLANNING AND DEVELOPMENT

Wayne Varndell

In this chapter, you will develop an understanding of:

- career planning
- nursing career pathways
- evidence-based practice in nursing
- reflection in clinical practice
- continuing professional development.

Career planning and development are essential activities if nurses are to meet changing community health needs, standards of practice, and professional and organisational expectations. Career planning and development have been fundamental in transforming society's perception of nurses' work as inferior, uneducated and unskilled (Smith, 1982) to a profession comprising autonomous, well-educated and knowledgeable workers practising in a variety of specialised roles and settings (Donner & Wheeler, 2001). Moreover, career development has been a major contributory factor in the advancement of health systems and maintaining high-quality care delivery (International Council of Nurses, 2007). As such, career planning should be an integral part of ongoing personal and professional development.

Career planning is a continuous and iterative process involving self-assessment and goal-setting, which enables the nurse to develop professionally and to grow with change instead of merely reacting to it (Kleinknecht & Hefferin, 1982). Career development is a formal, structured process provided by an organisation for the purpose of increasing employees' awareness, knowledge and capacity to fulfil the needs of the organisation, and is often achieved through workplace education programs (Sonmez & Yildirim, 2009). Despite nurses frequently transitioning between workplaces and assuming different roles throughout their careers, the ways in which nurses plan and develop their careers have received little attention. In response, Donner and Wheeler (2001) proposed a career planning and development model consisting of five phases: scanning; self-assessment and reality check; visioning; planning; and marketing.

Healthcare delivery and nursing do not exist in a vacuum. *Scanning* involves examining the landscape to understand current realities shaping and influencing nursing and healthcare delivery (Donner & Wheeler, 2001). Through networking, reading, attending conferences and discussions, joining professional societies and participating in social media, you can see the world through different perspectives and identify future career opportunities. Further, through the scanning process you can become aware of emerging challenges, gaps in practice, solutions, new ways of working and models of care.

Self-assessment involves evaluating your own experience, knowledge, interests and personal qualities compared with the desired career or identified role (Donner & Wheeler, 2001). The distance between your present readiness and the requirements of the future career or role identifies the directions you need to take in order to be successful. This may include completing further tertiary study (e.g. Master of Nursing in Critical Care) or local courses (e.g. managing change). In order to validate the findings of your self-assessment, seek feedback (or a *reality check*) from a mentor, peer or someone already performing the role in which you are interested. This will expand your understanding of your strengths and limitations, and clarify personal and professional development needs. It will also help you establish whether or not the potential future role or career is realistic or appropriate for the needs of your current work–life balance.

The following example shows a nurse's self-assessment for an advertised clinical nurse position. She uses the selection criteria contained in the job description as the basis for evaluating her current skill level and the areas she needs to develop.

Example: Self-assessment for readiness for clinical nurse position in oncology and haematology

Selection criteria 1: Relevant postgraduate qualification and at least 12 months' experience working within the relevant clinical area of postgraduate qualification

During my appraisal with my Nurse Unit Manager, I was encouraged to work towards becoming a clinical nurse specialist. I have worked in oncology and haematology for over two years since successfully completing my Bachelor of Nursing four years ago. The specialism is challenging and engaging. The local university offers a masters degree in oncology nursing and has an open day in the next two months. I have contacted the course leader to introduce myself and have started to look for a scholarship to assist with costs and have read the hospital's study leave policy. My manager is supportive of me pursuing tertiary qualifications.

Selection criteria 2: Has actively contributed to the development of clinical practice in previous roles

I have completed the mentorship and clinical supervision course, which has enabled me to better support new staff and students in my current role. I have received five evaluations from people I have supervised. I have maintained a record of the people I have mentored and supervised as evidence of my own development as a mentor and clinical supervisor.

Selection criteria 3: Has acted as a resource and mentor for others

Over the past year, I have developed an orientation pack for new starters and students to the ward, which includes contributions from my Nurse Unit Manager, Clinical Educator and past students. The pack outlines the ward philosophy of care, mission statements and core basic knowledge to be developed (e.g. aseptic technique, radiation burn management), and has been externally reviewed. The pack is given to each new starter or student on their first day on the ward. Recently a checklist has been added to indicate areas that new staff/students have completed, which can assist in their development appraisals.

Selection criteria 4: Has actively contributed to own professional development

To optimise care of radiation burns, I have completed a two-day wound-care course. As part of this course, I have evaluated the wound-care products our ward currently stocks and noticed that silver impregnated dressings were rarely used. From a review of the literature, silver impregnated dressings can promote wound/burn healing by reducing colonisation of the wound. I have discussed this observation with the Clinical Educator, who has invited the wound-care nurse specialist to present at our next in-service.

A strategic career plan is your blueprint for change and growth. The career development plan details the areas for development, their associated objectives, goals, actions and resources required (Donner & Wheeler, 2001). The objectives and goals that form the career plan should be considered carefully, preferably in conjunction with your mentor to ensure that the overall plan is successful. Using the SMARTER mnemonic acronym to guide the development of the career plan, and to help you judge each objective and goal, will assist in this process.

SMARTER, an extension of Drucker's (1954) management by objectives concept, is a set of seven criteria to assess the validity of objectives and goals. These are:

1 *Specific:* This first criterion stresses the need for objectives and goals to be clear and unambiguous, rather than broad or general. Use action words (e.g. identify, develop, demonstrate) to describe what you want to achieve.
   - What do you want to accomplish?
   - What is the purpose or benefits of accomplishing the goal?
   - What resources do you need?
   - What are the requirements and constraints?
2 *Measurable:* This second criterion highlights the need to set indicators by which to assess progress. A measurable goal is quantifiable.
   - What is the timeframe to complete the objective?
   - How will you know when an objective or goal is achieved?
3 *Achievable:* This third criterion stresses the importance of objectives and goals of the career plan being realistic and attainable. An attainable goal can be achieved based on your skill, resources and area of practice.
   - How can the objective or goal be achieved within the current resources?
   - Is the planned objective or goal within your scope of practice and/or context of practice?
4 *Relevant:* This fourth criterion stresses the need for choosing objectives or goals that matter and are important. A relevant goal is one that is clearly linked to your key responsibilities and current/future role.
   - Does the objective or goal matter?
   - Is this the right time to undertake this objective/goal?
   - Is this the right time for you?
   - What impact does the objective or goal have on your current lifestyle, work–life balance or free time?
5 *Time-specific:* This fifth criterion focuses on the importance of grounding objectives and goals within a realistic timeframe. This will help motivate you to move forward.

- Can this be achieved adequately within the next four weeks [or other specified period]?
- What can be done within the time that you have available?
- Will the planned outcomes of the objective/goal remain valid?
- How long did a similar objective/goal take to complete fully?

6 *Evaluate:* This sixth criterion stresses the importance of monitoring your progress and documenting your achievements in relation to the specified timeframes for each objective/goal.
- Are you keeping within specified timeframes without compromise?
- Are the objectives and goals still relevant and appropriate?
- Are there any other ways to accomplish the career plan that are now available? If so, in what way should the career plan be changed?

7 *Revise:* This last criterion brings the career plan back full circle and stresses the importance of being flexible in the way you achieve the objectives and goals of the career plan, of being mindful of productivity bias and of re-examining and revising objectives and goals depending upon the results of your evaluation of progress.
- Are you still on track?
- How are the career plan, objectives or goals impacting on you, your motivation and your work–life balance?
- What is the feedback from your mentor or from significant others telling you about your progress to date?
- What lessons have you learned so far from executing the career development plan?

Example: SMARTER goal-setting

Specific: To develop skills in preceptoring to support new graduate nurses transitioning into coronary care.

Measurable: By my next annual appraisal I will have preceptored four new graduate nurses transitioning into coronary care.

Achievable: The hospital currently provides short courses in preceptorship and clinical facilitation that include effective interpersonal and communication skills, teaching and assessment skills, feedback and leadership skills.

Relevant: Coronary care is a highly specialised field of nursing that goes beyond what is taught during pre-registration nurse training. Developing preceptorship skills will be instrumental in supporting nurses new to cardiology nursing to provide safe, high-quality patient care. Developing preceptorship skills will also assist me in moving forward in my career.

Time: To achieve my goal, my objectives will be to:

1   Within the next 2 weeks I will have met with my line manager and nurse educator to discuss preceptorship opportunities within the ward, and negotiate support to attend the hospital preceptorship course.

2   Within 6 months I will have preceptored two new graduate nurses and obtained feedback from my line manager, nurse educator and preceptees regarding my progress in developing as a preceptor.

3   Within 12 months I will have preceptored a total of four new graduate nurses and obtained feedback from my line manager, nurse educator and preceptees regarding my progress in developing as a preceptor.

Evaluate: Feedback from my line manager, the ward nurse educator and preceptees will assist in evaluating and modifying my development as a preceptor.

Revise: I will maintain a reflective journal to record feedback, my thoughts, feelings and decisions to assist in revising my career plan of becoming an effective preceptor.

SELF-MARKETING

Self-marketing involves packaging your personal and professional attributes, qualities and experience to showcase your achievements (Donner & Wheeler, 2001). For nurses, this may take the form of a carefully constructed résumé, but it should grow to include establishing a network, developing quality professional relationships, having a mentor, attending conferences and presenting at conferences, and developing highly complex written and verbal communication skills. A comprehensive self-marketing strategy is a vehicle that you can use to move from planning to the action phase of career development. It is therefore important to understand your strengths and weaknesses and the impression you give to others as a nurse, a professional and a future employee. Conducting a SWOT analysis can assist in identifying areas of expertise as well as areas that require immediate attention to improve your chances of success, matching your strengths to opportunities and to better prepare you for the future. A SWOT analysis consists of four key areas:

1   *Strengths:* Identify your core strengths. List your professional and character attributes and qualities that set you apart from others. Who can you network with to help you achieve greater visibility?

2 *Weaknesses:* Identify your shortcomings, including gaps in training, professional credentials and qualifications. Be realistic and objective.

3 *Opportunities:* List areas where you can add value, such as departmental or organisational projects, mentoring opportunities or performance/quality improvement portfolios.

4 *Threats:* What could you be doing differently to improve your position? What are your biggest roadblocks? What changes do you foresee within your organisation or industry that may impact you directly?

Example: SWOT analysis, preparing for Surgical Clinical Educator role

Strengths: Three years' continuing employment within organisation, familiar with clinical governance and education programs across the surgical specialty. Awarded Nurse of the Year for Clinical Excellence. Supportive co-workers and Nurse Manager strongly supports pursuing qualifications.

Weaknesses: Currently do not hold any educational or assessment-in-the-workplace qualifications. Limited experience, acted as Clinical Educator for two weeks last year. Do not hold any surgical nursing qualification.

Opportunities: Hospital sponsors nurses to undertake the TAFE Certificate IV in workplace assessment. Study leave is available to attend the TAFE course and there are on-site tutors. The next round of scholarship funding is four months away, which could aid in paying to undertake postgraduate study in surgical nursing at the local university.

Threats: The number of staff on sick leave may increase, leading to limited access to study leave or delay my nomination to undertake the hospital-sponsored TAFE IV in workplace assessment. The TAFE Certificate IV workplace assessment course is also held during winter, the busiest time for the surgical unit.

CAREER PLANNING AND DEVELOPMENT PATHWAYS

No two careers in nursing are the same, with so many career options available (Australian Nursing Federation, 2009). Common domains of most career pathways in nursing include clinical knowledge and skills, practice development skills (e.g. research or quality improvement skills), leadership and management skills and experience. Within any given role or clinical setting, domains or attributes may express themselves differently (Table 11.1).

Table 11.1 Summary of common nurse careers, associated qualifications and experience

Career	Qualifications	Clinical experience	Domains	Example
Nurse Practitioner	Bachelor of Nursing Postgraduate qualification in nursing Master of Nursing (Nurse Practitioner) qualification Endorsement by AHPRA	10–12 years post registration	Advanced practice Education Research Clinical leadership	The Nurse Practitioner conducts advanced, comprehensive and holistic health assessment relevant to a specialist field of nursing practice. Demonstrates a high level of confidence and clinical proficiency in carrying out a range of procedures, treatments and interventions that are evidence-based and informed by specialist knowledge. Demonstrates skills in accessing and developing clinical and social knowledge and its application to patient care and the education of others. Recognised as a senior member of the healthcare team and a clinical leader who influences and progresses clinical care and policy. An endorsed Nurse Practitioner has the authority to admit, discharge, order diagnostics and prescribe, and works in a variety of acute, chronic care and community settings.
Clinical Nurse Consultant	Bachelor of Nursing Postgraduate qualification in nursing Master of Nursing qualification	7–10 years post registration	Clinical service and consultancy Leadership Research Education Clinical services planning and management	The Clinical Nurse Consultant has highly advanced specialist knowledge and skills, provides expert clinical advice to patients, carers and members of the healthcare team within a defined specialty. The Clinical Nurse Consultant is a senior role model and leader. Additionally, Clinical Nurse Consultants initiate and lead research, and influence and contribute to the direction of clinical nursing education within the specialty.

Career	Qualifications	Clinical experience	Domains	Example
Clinical Educator/ Clinical Nurse Educator	Bachelor of Nursing Postgraduate study in nursing and education	5–10 years post registration	Education and research Leadership Quality improvement and management Professional Practice and development	The Clinical Educator provides appropriate professional development, support and mentoring to clinical staff. The Clinical Educator also provides clinical training, assesses and demonstrates clinical procedures and formulates and delivers educational programs in line with evidence-based practice and organisational requirements, ensuring clinicians deliver safe, knowledge-based care. Through their leadership and person-centred focus, Clinical Educators aid in developing a patient-focused culture that supports innovative models of care, team nursing and proactive change management. The Clinical Nurse Educator will be responsible for maintaining clinical competency records within the department.
Clinical Nurse Coach	Bachelor of Nursing	5–10 years post registration	Leadership Supervision Facilitation Coaching Practice development	The Clinical Nurse Coach provides point of care, person-centred educational interventions to achieve clinical skills, practice development and stimulate a culture of learning, using a person-centered philosophy and a coaching process. Contributes to the implementation and monitoring of quality and safety standards, service development and the profession by facilitating team participation in life-long learning, research activities and continued development of clinical practice.

continues

Table 11.1 Summary of common nurse careers, associated qualifications and experience *continued*

Career	Qualifications	Clinical experience	Domains	Example
Nurse Manager	Bachelor of Nursing Postgraduate study in nursing and management	5–10 years post registration	Leadership Management Human resource management	The Nurse Manager clinically leads and manages nursing teams to deliver contemporary nursing practice that aligns with patients' needs and organisational goals. Responsible and accountable for the quality of nursing delivered in clinical area. Leads engagement with patients, families and the healthcare team, and is a key decision-maker. Delivers sustainable healthcare and leads quality improvements. Maintains an environment that is safe and culturally appropriate for patients, families and staff. Reports and monitors key performance targets/standards and manages risk, and is a central point of communication between staff, patients and their families.
Associate/ Clinical Nurse Unit Manager	Bachelor of Nursing Postgraduate study	4–6 years post registration	Leadership Management	Specialist knowledge, skills, attributes and abilities within narrower scope of practice related to the clinical area. Supports the Nurse Manager to clinically lead and manage the nursing team to deliver contemporary nursing practice that is aligned with evidence-based practice and organisational goals. Responsible and accountable for the quality of nursing delivered in the clinical area on a shift-by-shift basis. Recognised by the team as an expert resource for others. Decision-maker within scope of practice and role on a shift-by-shift basis. Maintains an environment that is safe and culturally appropriate for patients, families and staff. Supports the Nurse Manager with monitoring and achieving key performance targets/ standards and assists in managing risk.

Career	Qualifications	Clinical experience	Domains	Example
Clinical Nurse Specialist/ Clinical Nurse	Bachelor of Nursing Postgraduate in nursing	2–4 years post registration	Education Leadership Research	Higher level of skill demonstrated in clinical decision-making including problem-solving, and analysis and interpretation of clinical data. Maintains and improves clinical standards. Acts as a resource person, preceptor/ mentor to others in relation to expert clinical practice. Supports and contributes to quality improvement within the area of practice.
Nurse Researcher	Bachelor of Nursing Postgraduate study in research	4-6 years post registration	Communication Leadership Research Education	Nurse researchers work in hospitals, clinics and research laboratories to conduct or assist in research into nursing, healthcare delivery or specific health issues (e.g. childhood obesity, Parkinson's disease). Nurse researchers lead or assist in designing and conducting research, undertake data collection and analysis, and publish results that ultimately shape evidence-based practice, patient outcomes, healthcare policy and delivery.

EVIDENCE-BASED PRACTICE IN NURSING

Healthcare is one of the most dynamic human disciplines. As such, the ever-changing contexts of care, science, policy, technology, treatments and pharmaceuticals impact on nursing practice and the delivery of care to patients. Nurses need to ensure that they can justify the decisions they make with and for patients, and that the care they deliver is evidence-based (ANMC, 2013). The need for clinical decisions and practice to be based in evidence is not only part of professional practice requirements; nurses are morally obligated to demonstrate that decisions and actions are ethical and in the patient's best interests (e.g. beneficence, non-maleficence) (ANMC, 2008b; Beauchamp & Childress, 2012; Benner et al., 2009).

The use of evidence-based practice (EBP) directly relates to better outcomes for patients (Melnyk et al., 2012), and is the gold standard for providing safe and high-quality patient care. However, only a small percentage of nurses utilise EBP on a consistent basis (Committee on Quality of Health Care in America, 2001; Gray et al., 2002; Melnyk et al., 2004; Melnyk et al., 2012). EBP is a problem-solving approach to the delivery of healthcare that draws on and integrates multiple sources of propositional (know-that) and practical (know-how) knowledge, informed by a variety of evidence bases. Types of evidence include research, clinical experience, patient/carer preferences and values, and local context.

Research evidence is knowledge gained from systematic inquiry. While there is agreement that knowledge from research findings generated from rigorous studies constitutes the best type of evidence for informing nurse decision-making and practice, it is important to note its limitations. Research evidence rarely attains absolute certainty, as evidence is dynamic and eclectic. As Upshur (2001) argues, research evidence needs to be viewed as provisional, as it is constantly expanding and evolving.

Clinical experience—that is, knowledge accrued through practice and life experience—is also referred to as practical or know-how knowledge (Titchen & Ersser, 2000). Caring for patients requires nurses to make numerous decisions and undertake complex practices in a highly technical environment, often drawing upon their own clinical experience or that of others to inform and guide their practice (Thompson et al., 2001). Knowing *how* to do something is important but does not equate to competency and therefore proficiency. For example, while a person can learn the steps to insert a urinary catheter, it does not mean that they are able to do so competently without clinical experience and theoretical understanding. As Benner and Wrubel (1989) identify, practical knowledge is not simply confined to the performing of motor skills, but includes non-verbal interpersonal communication skills such as recognising visual cues and gestures within a clinical context. A criticism of practical knowledge is that casually accepting it as justifying decisions and/or actions without reflecting upon the underpinning evidence may lead to suboptimal care being promulgated, and the formation of ritualistic practice—that is, practice based on habits (Acebedo-Urdiales et al., 2014).

Evidence generated from the experiences and preferences of patients is very important from an ethical and moral viewpoint, and is central to understanding the world of the patient. Gathering and incorporating patients' experiences, preferences and values into evidence-based practice and melding this with scientific evidence is a complex task; one individual's experience and preferences may not be the same as those of another individual (Rycroft-Malone et al., 2004). When viewed from an evidence-based perspective, treatment is largely decided by the results of rigorous empirical research and medical practice. Conversely, in terms of designing healthcare and service delivery, increasing importance is given to the involvement of groups or communities as key stakeholders (ACSQHC, 2012).

In addition to evidence obtained from research, clinical and patient experience, the context of care contains sources of evidence. In the course of assessing standards of care, patient satisfaction and identifying areas for improvement, the healthcare team may draw upon:

- audit and performance data
- critical incident findings
- patient stories and complaints/compliments
- local quality improvement project findings
- social and professional communities of practice
- peer feedback
- local and national policy.

This type of evidence source is also referred to as 'internal evidence' (Stetler, 2001). While the importance of locally derived data in driving service redesign and shaping patient care is recognised (ACSQHC, 2012), more needs to be understood about how such data are systematically collected and appraised, how they are integrated with other kinds of evidence, and how they inform individual clinical decision-making.

REFLECTION IN CLINICAL PRACTICE

Nurses are strongly encouraged to be reflective in their practice. Reflection—that is, the examination of personal thoughts and actions—can be used to help you to make sense of work situations and, ultimately, to improve patient care. Further, reflection is a process by which clinicians examine and explore experiences to build upon strengths, identify appropriate future action(s) and align practice with personal and professional standards and research. There are many models of reflection that have been developed by theorists such as Benner and Wrubel (1989), Gibbs (1988), Johns (2000), Driscoll (1994) and, more recently, by Barksby and colleagues (2015). Common to all models of reflection are three key stages: (1) awareness that something is wrong; (2) critically thinking about what is occurring or has occurred in the context of the situation; and (3) developing a course of action to apply in future situations (Thompson & Burns, 2008). The use of a structured model of reflection will improve your understanding and depth of awareness of the issues surrounding an event and its impact on practice and continuing professional development (Platzer et al., 1997). There are three essential forms of reflection: reflection-on-action, reflection-in-action and critical reflection.

Reflection-on-action is the most common form, and involves carefully retracing and examining the events leading up to the situation. While the literature in part focuses on identifying negative personal and/or professional behaviours (Grant & Greene, 2001; Reveans, 1998), positive actions and decisions should also be sought and acknowledged.

Example: Nurse reflection on a spinal cord injury patient

While a spinal cord injury patient was being transferred from his wheelchair to the bed, he suddenly began to shiver, sweat and complain of a headache. Looking at the patient, I noted that he appeared pale. His blood pressure was found to be 220/100. Seeing that his blood pressure was greater than 200 mmHg, I called the treating physician who attended the ward within 5 minutes. After a brief assessment, the physician identified that the patient was experiencing autonomic dysreflexia from a poorly draining suprapubic urinary catheter. He asked me to change it, but first wanted the patient to be administered glycerine trinitrate (GTN) to lower his blood pressure to a safer level. After the GTN was given, the patient's blood pressure dropped to 145/80. Although his blood pressure was still high, the patient was more comfortable. On inspecting the catheter I noticed that it was kinked. On straightening the catheter tubing, urine flowed rapidly into the leg bag. On discussing this with the physician, he advised to monitor the patient's blood pressure and urinary output/flow as the patient may still require a new catheter. On discussing the event with my preceptor, she directed me to the autonomic dysreflexia learning package and policy, to update my knowledge.

Reflection-in-action is concerned with practising critically. For example, as a nurse caring for a patient with a wound, you would be making decisions about the suitability of dressing choices, nutrition, pain relief, positioning and pressure relief, while judging the potential outcome of each choice in relation to optimising wound healing, comfort and wellbeing (Schön, 1995). Reflection-in-action is considered to be the hallmark of an experienced professional.

Critical reflection, while often used interchangeably with 'reflection' in the literature, is different on many levels. Reflection involves the assessment of the assumption implicit in beliefs, including beliefs about how to solve problems, whereas critical reflection is an extension of critical thinking and refers to challenging the *validity* of presuppositions in prior learning, and your assumptions about others, the workplace and yourself. Further, critical reflection asks you to speculate about the future and act; an integral component of professionalism (Leijen et al., 2011).

Example: Engaging in critical reflection

I became frustrated with an elderly patient who kept demanding assistance every time I left the room. No sooner had I attended him, addressed any issues or concerns he had and left the room, he would push the nurse call bell before I stepped out of the door. This behaviour was worse at night. Often the patient would sleep only 2 or 3 hours, but at all other times he would be calling for assistance. On asking him why he kept buzzing, he simple stated that he wanted company. Staff have offered books, puzzles and access to the TV or radio, but none of these things abated his continuing use of the nurse call buzzer. It was 3 am, and the patient had woken after a short sleep of about 2 hours and started calling for assistance again. The other patients had started to become annoyed at the continuing noise of the nurse call system. I approached the patient and delicately explained that his use of the nurse call buzzer was excessive. After he promised to only use the nurse call buzzer if there was an actual need, I left on my tea break.

When I returned, I heard the patient calling out down the corridor. On entering the room, the patient was standing in urine and crying. The nurse call buzzer had been removed. Calming the patient down and assisting him to the shower to clean up, I noticed a sequence of numbers tattooed on his left inner forearm. On asking what they meant, he replied that he had been one of the lucky ones to survive the Nazi concentration camp at Dachau. I asked if the dark worried him, but instead he replied that being alone was far more troubling: 'It's when they came for you.' He went on to explain how he had lost his entire family in Dachau, and that being alone, with no family, the nightmares had returned.

After the patient dressed, we walked back to his room. I reattached the nurse call buzzer and moved a small desk to the corridor outside his room, where I would complete my documentation for the shift. The patient relaxed and went back to sleep, only to occasionally wake to see whether I was still there. I was reminded that hospital is a foreign place, and can be intimidating to those with no support or who are suffering from loss. The patient had no one except the nurse call buzzer and the nursing staff to reorientate himself. He became distressed to the point of urinary incontinence.

The following shift, I asked for the Rabbi to visit, and for social work to identify support groups that could provide social input for the patient. As an interim measure, the hospital arranged for an aged care companion and the pet therapist to visit each day. Social care is just as important as physical care—something that was overlooked on admission.

Several models of critical reflection have been published to facilitate critical reflection, which include Dewey's (1938) model of reflective learning, Habermas's (1978) model of critical reflection and Kolb's (1984) model of reflexive learning. Each model of critical reflection consists of probing questions to systematically guide nurses toward identifying and validating the 'critical' assumptions, beliefs and values that underlie presumed knowledge.

Reflection is individualistic, while in reality nurses operate in and alongside a team of clinicians. Reflection can be done in groups; however, due to impracticalities such as availability of time to assemble the team, cost and team dynamics, clinicians tend to reflect on their own or with a supervisor/mentor. Reflection is assumed to have positive outcomes, yet empirical evidence is limited (Fook et al., 2006). Despite this, reflection is seen as a potent catalyst for professional development, personal growth and practice change across many fields, including medicine (Ménard & Ratnapalan, 2013), psychology (Sifers, 2012), allied health (Chuan-Yuan et al., 2013), social work (Lay & McGuire, 2010; Morley, 2004) and law (Ruyters et al., 2011).

CONTINUING PROFESSIONAL DEVELOPMENT

Nursing is an ever-advancing discipline in an equally progressive and demanding clinical environment. Continuing professional development is the means by which we maintain, improve and broaden our knowledge, expertise and competence, and develop the personal and professional qualities required throughout our professional lives (ANMC, 2008c).

In Australia, since the move to national registration in 2009, continuing professional development (CPD) has become a central element to annual nursing registration. The CPD process of reviewing practice (clinical, academic, administrative), identifying learning needs, planning and participating in relevant learning activities, and reflecting on the value of those learning activities gives focus to what is intended to be a lifelong learning process.

Learning and the activities associated with it have to be related to your context of practice. This refers to the conditions that define and shape an individual's practice, including the type of practice setting (e.g. healthcare, educational organisation or private practice); the location of the practice setting (e.g. rural, urban, remote, mobile); the characteristics of our patients (e.g. health status, age, learning needs or diverse cultures); the nature of the practice or focus (e.g. health promotion, research, management or policy); the complexity of practice; the degree to which practice is autonomous or extended; and the resources that are available, including access to other healthcare professionals.

The Nursing and Midwifery Board of Australia (NMBA) requires Registered Nurses and Registered Midwives to participate in at least 20 hours of CPD annually. Those with dual qualifications in nursing and midwifery are required to undertake 20 hours of both nursing and midwifery CPD annually (NMBA, 2016f). Those wishing to maintain their Nurse Practitioner registration are required to undertake 20 hours of nursing or midwifery CPD, and then a further

10 hours of CPD related to their endorsement (critical care, community, sexual health, etc.), including prescribing and administration of medicines, diagnostic investigations, consultation and referral. Records of CPD hours completed should be kept for at least five years.

What constitutes an hour of CPD?

Active learning refers to the activities undertaken in developing our learning. One hour of CPD may include several different types of active learning (sometimes referred to as effective learning). While there is no specification as to what activities should be chosen, they should be varied (more than three different types of activities should be undertaken) and relevant to your learning needs. The following is a list of examples:

- acting as a preceptor/mentor/tutor
- reflecting on peer feedback, or keeping a practice journal
- undertaking supervised practice for skills development
- active membership of professional groups and committees
- reading professional journals or books
- writing for publication
- presenting or attending conferences, workplace education, in-service or skills workshops
- conducting or contributing to research
- undertaking undergraduate or postgraduate studies specific to your context of practice
- undertaking relevant online or distance education
- developing policy, protocols or guidelines
- writing or reviewing educational materials, journal articles or books.

There are many other types of learning that can also be incorporated into CPD activities.

Demonstrating continuing professional development

While only a small number of those registered with the NMBA will be required to submit their evidence of CPD, dedicating time to regularly document your learning and professional development is essential to consolidate learning (Williams & Jordan, 2007). The depth and extent to which you document or demonstrate your continuing professional development and subsequent learning will vary.

Examples of self-directed learning (individual or small group learning, informal learning) that you could document as evidence of CPD include:

- evaluating your present practice, comparing it with relevant competencies or professional practice standards. An evaluation of present practice may also include providing a reflective account of an issue encountered in your practice.
- identifying and prioritising your learning needs, and from this developing a learning plan
- briefly describing any form of learning you have undertaken, and the number of hours spent in each activity (e.g. reading, reflecting, writing a protocol). You should also demonstrate how this learning links to the points within your learning plan.
- reflecting upon or describing the key things you have learnt and their implications for your practice
- listing examples of directed learning (e.g. courses, conferences, lectures).

With regard to mandatory learning—for example, child protection, fire safety and evacuation training—if it is directly relevant to your area of practice, and it is likely to lead to a change in practice, then it can be included as part of your CPD. However, if the mandatory training does not provide anything new that could contribute to your practice (e.g. reassessment of a skill using existing guidelines that have not changed), it may not count towards your CPD hours.

Professional practice portfolio development

Nurses practise in a continually changing environment, where healthcare delivery is increasingly complex, dynamic and specialised. Despite this, nurses as professionals are ever conscious of the critical need to stay up to date, in order to maintain their competence in delivering safe, judicious and effective care (Williams & Jordan, 2007).

Nurses are highly mobile professionals, accruing experience in a variety of settings and specialties over time (Fukuda-Parr, 2004). The external and internal pressures on all healthcare professionals to make good judgements and decisions have increased considerably in recent years (Johnstone et al., 2004). While nurses readily accept the responsibility for their own personal development, the tools to assist mobile practitioners to collate evidence regarding their individual development, which articulate the link between their professional development and continuing competency, have on occasion been missing.

Nurses need the skills to understand and use evidence to communicate professional responsibilities, commitments, plans, expectations and outcomes. A portfolio is a collection of evidence that demonstrates these skills (Andre & Heartfield, 2007), although the types of evidence will vary. The range of evidence includes:

- *core evidence:* original professional registration or education certificates, and letters of appointment
- *generated evidence:* references, reports, care plans, case or performance reviews, and personal notes, statements or reflections
- *specific evidence:* this can be produced through combining core and generated evidence to focus on a specialist practice standard, domain or competency (Andre & Heartfield, 2007).

A professional practice portfolio puts forward an argument about a level of achievement or the suitability of a nurse for a particular position, and is much more than a résumé—chiefly because a résumé only provides a summary of previous employment and education information. As a broad structured amalgam of materials, a professional portfolio assists in demonstrating:

- a record of employment, education and professional and personal development
- performance based on examination of previous and existing practice
- competency based on examination of previous and current knowledge, skills and experiences
- learning based on knowledge gained and skill development
- future goals and career direction based on consideration and examination of the previous two points
- individual reflective processes.

Demonstrating competence or learning can be a complex task. It may take variable lengths of time to gain competence, depending on the practice context, your education and previous clinical experience; as such, professional portfolios are more than just an ongoing collection of materials in a box. In recent years, numerous 'e-portfolios' or internet-based professional development services have been developed. Many of these have pre-formatted templates to aid in compiling evidence of ongoing learning and development (Figure 11.1). However, nurses need an awareness of what constitutes 'good' evidence, and how this relates to expected practice standards. Multiple tools and checklists are available to assist nurses to assess the quality of evidence (Critical Appraisal Skills Program (CASP), 2014; University of Bern, 2009).

Date 21/10/17	**Describe the learning need/title of learning activity and source/provider** Management of patients using metformin and iodinated contrast agents, implications and common reactions.
CPD hours 4 hours	**Type of learning need** ☒ Clinical knowledge ☐ Non-clinical knowledge ☐ Skill ☐ Attitude ☐ Departmental/Process

Identified learning objectives, links to nursing standards • Contraindications associated with contrast dye, IV and oral. • Risk of contrast-induced nephropathy for patients on metformin. • Role of metformin in regulating blood sugar levels.	**Action plan and resources** • Review of evidence/best-practice literature using CASP management of evidence tools. • Review local guidelines. • Share findings by developing a quick reference guide, update staff orientation guide.

Type of learning activity (time taken)
Literature review (2 hours)
Reflection (1 hour)
Dissemination of findings (1 hour)

Reflection on learning

What? (Event, patient unmet need)
During the morning medication round, the patient was administered their morning dose of metformin as charted. Later in the afternoon, the medical imaging department requested that the patient attend for CT of their left leg. On handing over the patient to the medical imaging department nursing team, they flagged that the patient was for CT with contrast. On review of the patient's medication chart, it was noticed that the morning metformin had been administered, which could potentially result in nephropathy if contrast was administered. The CT scan was re-booked with an explanation and apology given to the patient. On returning to the ward, the nursing team was unaware the request for the patient to have a CT had been made. The medical team was contacted.

So what? (Issues, educational needs)
The nursing team was unaware that a CT with contrast had been arranged for this patient. Further, the medication chart had not been modified to withhold metformin.
The nursing team and I did not know that metformin should be ceased prior to the administration of contrast dye.
The patient was not aware that contrast dye could lead to nephropathy if taking metformin.

Now what? (Key points from learning)
Review of evidence/best practice: *Metformin is used in type 2 diabetes to decrease the amount of glucose produced by the liver, and to increase the body's response to insulin produced by the pancreas. In patients with renal failure (acute or chronic), the renal clearance of metformin is decreased, and there is an associated risk of lactic acidosis, which has a mortality rate of up to 50% (Goergen et al., 2010; Misbin et al., 1998). Some patients who receive intravenous or oral contrast may experience a deterioration of renal function (contrast-induced nephropathy), but this is dependent upon the degree of renal damage and function as measured by eGFR and creatinine level (Baerlocher et al., 2013). In general, metformin should be stopped at the time of contrast administration. It is recommended that metformin be stopped 48 hours before CT for patients with an eGFR of less than 45 mL/min (Stacul et al., 2011). Restarting metformin depends on renal function and the volume of contrast used. Patients who have an eGFR of less than 60 mL/min should restart metformin no sooner than 48 hours after contrast administration and only if renal function remains stable (<25% increase in creatinine above baseline). Patients with an eGFR greater than 60 mL/min who receive a larger amount of intravenous contrast (>100 mL, such as CTs of the abdomen or pelvis, CT angiography of the aorta or lower extremities) should restart metformin no earlier than 48 hours after the procedure (Thomsen et al., 1999).*

Figure 11.1 Example of a CPD template: literature review

If patients with normal renal function who are taking metformin receive less than 100 mL of intravenous contrast (e.g. enhanced CT of the brain), stopping metformin and/or re-checking creatinine levels 48 hours after the procedure may be unnecessary, because the risk of contrast-induced nephropathy in patients with normal renal function is very low (Stacul et al., 2011).

Review of local guidelines: *On reading the local policy 'CT scans and the Administration of Contrast', it is noted that it only discusses withholding metformin for patients receiving intravenous contrast dye. Based upon the review of evidence, the policy needs to be updated to include advice related to administration of oral contrast.*

Action: *Email sent to author of the policy. Within the policy, it outlines the responsibility of the physician ordering any CT involving contrast to withhold the administration of metformin for 48 hours.*

Sharing findings: *From the review of evidence/best practice relating to the administration of metformin and contrast dye, I prepared a short 30-minute education in-service that was delivered four times. There was positive feedback from the staff attending (15 in-service evaluations returned). The key learning points were added to the ward orientation manual. Patient education information leaflets from the medical imaging department are now available on the ward, and are given to patients on metformin.*

Evidence provided

Articles/policies reviewed:

Goergen, S.K., Rumbold, G., Compton, G., et al. 2010. Systematic review of current guidelines, and their evidence base, on risk of lactic acidosis after administration of contrast medium for patients receiving metformin. *Radiology*, 254, 261–9.

Misbin, R.I., Green, L., Stadel, B.V. et al. 1998. Lactic acidosis in patients with diabetes treated with metformin. *New England Journal of Medicine*, 338, 265–6.

Baerlocher, M.O., Asch, M. & Myers, A. 2013. Metformin and intravenous contrast. *Canadian Medical Association Journal*, 185, E78.

Stacul, F., van der Molen, A.J., Reimer, P. et al. 2011. Contrast Media Safety Committee of European Society of Urogenital Radiology (ESUR). Contrast induced nephropathy: updated ESUR Contrast Media Safety Committee guidelines [review]. *European Radiology*, 21, 2527–41.

Thomsen, H.S. & Morcos, S.K. 1999. Contrast media and metformin: Guidelines to diminish the risk of lactic acidosis in non-insulin dependent diabetics after administration of contrast media. *European Radiology*, 9, 738–40.

CT scans and the Administration of Contrast, *St Renin Hospital Policy and Procedures*, 2016.

In-service education/Education materials

Presentation slides, handouts and returned evaluation forms

Patient information leaflets

Update to ward orientation manual

Mentor/peer feedback

- Detailed review highlighting clinical complications of using oral contrast agents in patients prescribed metformin.
- Risks clearly defined and evidenced.
- Appropriate strategies identified to promote team awareness and revision of policy to reduce risk to patients.
- To improve awareness of this issue and response, engage department leadership team and clinical safety officer.

Figure 11.1 Example of a CPD template: literature review *continued*

Date 29/10/17	**Describe the learning need/title of learning activity and source/provider** Paediatric basic life support training.
CPD hours 8 hours	**Type of learning need** [x] Clinical knowledge ☐ Non-clinical knowledge [x] Skill ☐ Attitude ☐ Departmental/Process

Identified learning objectives, links to nursing standards	**Action plan and resources**
• Increase confidence, awareness, skills and ability to respond to basic paediatric emergencies. • Perform basic life support, airway management, cardiac rhythm recognition and defibrillation and recognition of the seriously injured and seriously ill child.	• Completion of recognised paediatric basic life support course for healthcare professionals.

Type of learning activity (time taken)
Face-to-face learning including practice workstations (8 hours)

Reflection on learning

What? (Event, patient unmet need)
Recently commenced working in day surgery which provides services to both adult and paediatric patients such as endoscopy and minor surgery.

So what? (Issues, educational needs)
Previous paediatric life support certification has expired by four years.
20% of cases managed in day surgery are paediatric patients.
As assisting with recovery of paediatric patients, I would be the closest to detect deterioration.

Now what? (Key points from learning)
Promote to staff the need to update/complete their paediatric basic life support training.
Discuss with leadership/education team the possibility of organising paediatric basic life support simulations within the department.

Mentor/peer feedback
• Successful completion of paediatric BLS.
• Opportunities to progress to paediatric advanced life support level and available course dates discussed. Encouraged to follow this up with the Nurse Educator.
• Possibility of incorporating paediatric respiratory and cardiorespiratory arrests as part of department in situ simulations to maintain own and team proficiency discussed. Advised to follow-up with Clinical Nurse Consultant and Director of Medical Education for the department.
• Discussed team debriefing opportunities, identified the valuable role of the Social Worker. Contact details to be added to the in-charge resource folder.

Figure 11.2 Example of a CPD template: training review

Summary

This chapter has focused on the importance of career planning and development for all nurses. We have reviewed how to undertake self-marketing and undertake a SWOT analysis to determine your strengths, weaknesses and how to achieve your career goals. We looked at pathways in nursing and the kinds of experience and qualifications needed for different roles. We considered the importance of evidence-based practice in furthering your nursing career, the role of reflection in clinical practice and the requirement to undertake continuing professional development.

Review questions

11.1 How many hours of continuing professional development are required to annually renew your nursing registration?
   a   10
   b   15
   c   20
   d   30

11.2 Ideally, how many ways of active learning should you demonstrate in your annual continuing professional development portfolio?
   a   1
   b   2
   c   3
   d   4

11.3 Which of the following components should be demonstrated when recording your continuing professional learning activities?
   a   Cost
   b   Number of hours spent learning
   c   Brief description of the learning undertaken
   d   How this learning links with your learning plan

11.4 With regard to forming a professional portfolio, match the following examples to their type of evidence.
   a Core evidence
   b Performance reviews
   c Education certificates
   d Generated evidence
   e Statements demonstrating specialist competency attainment
   f Specific evidence

11.5 Clinical experience can be defined as:
   a Knowledge gained through study
   b Knowledge gained from peer feedback
   c Knowledge gained through practice

11.6 Reflection-on-action can be defined as:
   a Practising critically by judging the outcome of every decision and action
   b Challenging the validity of assumptions about yourself, others and the workplace
   c Retracing decisions, actions and events leading up to a situation

11.7 What is the governing body for nursing and midwifery in Australia?
   a The National Nursing and Midwifery Council
   b The Nursing and Midwifery Board of Australia
   c Australian Nursing & Midwifery Council
   d The Australian Health Practitioner Regulation Agency

11.8 In what year did Australia move to national registration of nurses and midwives?
   a 2001
   b 2004
   c 2009
   d 2015

12 GRADUATE PROGRAMS AND GAINING EMPLOYMENT

Alister Hodge

In this chapter, you will develop an understanding of:

- graduate transition-to-practice programs
- options other than graduate programs
- choosing a department or hospital
- the recruitment process
- what managers are looking for in a potential employee
- how to write a covering letter
- what to include in a résumé
- preparing for interview.

GRADUATE TRANSITION-TO-PRACTICE PROGRAMS

Across Australia, many healthcare facilities provide transition-to-practice programs for new graduate nurses entering the workforce for the first time. The programs may differ in length and format; however, each has been created to provide additional support for new graduate nurses in their first year of practice and to improve retention (Missen et al., 2014). Transition programs can help provide a sense of belonging and improved clinical confidence which, together with educational and clinical support, results in higher job satisfaction (Missen et al., 2014). Research has indicated that graduates who don't take part in a transition-to-practice program tend to experience a more traumatic introduction to the workforce, with higher reported levels of stress (Duchscher, 2009).

As many healthcare providers operate transition programs for nurses entering the workforce, a challenge for you is to identify the program that will provide the support you need. Functional transition programs should have support structures that enable you to develop confidence and clinical competence through the year, while instilling a culture of evidence-based practice and safety.

Research has demonstrated that graduates usually require one year of practice to feel comfortable and confident in their new role as an RN (Missen et al., 2014); therefore, you should consider seeking out transition programs that are at least 12 months in length to provide an appropriate timeframe of support while you adapt to your new role. Hospitals frequently offer three- or four-month rotations to provide a broad experience base through key specialties such as medical, surgical and aged care. Short rotations have been developed for two main reasons: first, an experience that includes medical and surgical nursing provides a solid base for career movement into more specialised areas of nursing; and second, such rotations have been popular with new graduate nurses. However, short rotations exact a price. Anecdotally, it is reported that graduates often don't feel comfortable in a new area until they have worked there for approximately three months. A graduate program consisting of rotations of three to four months followed by a change to a new clinical environment means that you may never feel settled for the entire year. It may be beneficial to search for a graduate program with reduced rotations and longer placements of between six to nine months. Although this may decrease the range of specialties you experience in the transition year, it will allow a greater depth of learning to take place, your confidence to grow and working relationships to develop.

The process for applying for a transition program varies between states. In Victoria, a system called the Graduate Nursing/Midwifery Program Match allows graduates to nominate their top four preferences for employment. Graduates then submit their curriculum vitae (CV), academic transcript, clinical preferences and application form to each of the four preferences. If an interview is secured and completed, the candidates are subsequently ranked by the hospital/health service based on merit post interview. The computer match algorithm then matches the candidate's preferences to the hospital/health service rankings, resulting in a single offer to the graduate. Other states, including Western Australia and South Australia, utilise a streamlined recruitment system whereby the graduate can apply for a graduate position at more than one hospital with the same application.

Ensure that you are aware of the particular process required to apply for a graduate program within the state in which you are seeking work to give yourself the best chance of success.

ALTERNATIVES TO GRADUATE PROGRAMS

Enrolling in a transition-to-practice program, although encouraged, is not compulsory. Moreover, competition for transition programs is often fierce, with more applicants than positions available. If you don't gain entry to a transition program there are other options.

For example, you could consider the private sector, where many hospitals don't participate in the standard graduate match programs, and instead require direct applications. Some advertised positions for RNs, whether in the public or private system, will be suitable for new graduate nurses, and while you may be competing against more experienced nurses, with adequate interview preparation you still have a chance of securing the position.

Keep your options open and be prepared to apply for multiple jobs. Consider fields of nursing that you may not initially have gravitated towards. If you are successful in gaining employment, you may find you unexpectedly enjoy the field. However, if you want to move on, any work experience can be a useful opportunity to consolidate your knowledge, grow as a clinician and make yourself a better applicant for future jobs in a clinical area that holds more interest for you.

While looking for other potential sites of employment outside a graduate program, identify what support structures will be made available to you on entry to the clinical environment. Most wards or nursing services have an orientation program of some sort. In the presence of a nurturing and supportive staff culture towards nursing graduates, there will still be an opportunity to excel.

Check to see whether the following support features are available:

- Is there a structured orientation program to support new staff?
- Is there an education pathway on the ward you are entering to guide your clinical development?
- Are nurse educators available and approachable to ask questions in the clinical environment?
- Is there any formal preceptorship or mentor programs available?
- Do experienced staff oversee new graduate nurses to ensure that there is support if a patient deteriorates or you need to ask a question?
- Are there structures in place to ensure new graduate nurses are given constructive feedback in a timely manner, as well as being given encouragement when they are doing well?

- Are there structures in place to enable the new graduate nurse to be debriefed after a challenging experience?
- Is there evidence of staff cohesion, such as an active social committee?

This information should be freely available from the nurse education unit of the hospital if you send a polite query via email or make a phone call.

Many new graduate nurses apply for a position at a hospital where they gained clinical experience as a student; therefore, while you are on student placement, consider asking the above questions of a supervising senior RN or ward educator.

If these support structures are not available at the site in which you gain employment, ensure you maintain lines of communication with other people who can provide support—for example, new graduate nurses at other sites with whom you studied at university or academic mentors from the university. You should also take advantage of educational opportunities outside of work, whether through the Australian College of Nursing or private education providers.

Nursing agencies provide an option for immediate employment, with some agencies accepting nurse graduates. For those considering this as an option, be aware that working for an agency presents significant challenges for a graduate, and likely a higher degree of stress as you adjust. As an agency nurse, you will be often sent to a different hospital or ward each shift, where you will be expected to cope with a full patient load with little orientation. This can be challenging even for experienced nurses. If possible, see whether the agency can provide you with a line of work (multiple shifts in the same area) in a specialty area in which you have had significant exposure as a student nurse—for example, a medical or surgical ward. This will help to ground you as you start, and allow you to build on pre-existing strengths. It is important to be honest and upfront with the ward staff that you are a new graduate nurse. Be very clear about your own knowledge and scope of practice, and identify who you should contact for help if required during the shift. Keep in mind that each ward in which you work is a potential employer in the future. If you make a good impression, and demonstrate a commitment to your own development combined with safe patient care, your past performance will be recalled during a future interview—so make sure it counts in your favour.

Further study while seeking employment is also an option. Consider adding an Honours year to your Bachelor of Nursing, which can be achieved in one year's full-time study or two years of part-time study. An Honours year combines coursework and research in an area of nursing practice, and aims to extend your research and communication skills, as well as develop your theoretical knowledge to a higher level than that generally expected of a Bachelor level nurse. Honours programs are designed to enhance future career opportunities, and will make you a more attractive candidate for future graduate program intakes. If committing to an Honours year does not appeal, consider completing a Certificate IV in workplace training and assessment, which will be helpful in its own right and may even be a requirement if you pursue a role in education later in your nursing career.

CHOOSING A DEPARTMENT OR HOSPITAL

For the overseas nurse new to Australia, as well as the nursing graduate, there are often both lifestyle and professional factors to be considered when choosing where to apply for a job.

Lifestyle factors

- Where do you want to live: what location will enable you to pursue non-work activities, such as beach, hobbies, family activities, contact with friends? How much will you need to spend on rent and other living expenses within a given suburb?
- How close is the worksite to where you would like to live?
- What distance are you prepared to travel, and how much time are you willing to spend commuting to and from work?
- Will you have a car/motorcycle, or will you be reliant on public transport?

Professional factors

- Will the hospital be able to provide employment within your specialty?
- Are there specific aspects of practice within your specialty of particular interest to you that are not offered at all sites? For example, if your special interest is trauma, you should be aware that not all emergency departments are trauma centres.
- What opportunities will be available for ongoing professional development?
- What day-to-day support structures are present within a department? For example, education, management, ratio of senior to junior staff.
- Are you seeking full-time work or a short contract? Some sites may not accept short contracts.
- What career development opportunities are available?

A good starting point for ascertaining the cost of living in a city/suburb where you think you may want to live is through one of the main Australian real estate websites, such as Domain or Realestate.com. Here you will be able to obtain suburb profiles and identify current rental and property prices.

Information about public hospitals can be found through each state's Department of Health website. These sites contain information about Local Health Networks, hospitals and provided services.

RECRUITMENT PROCESS

Guidance on how to apply for a job and prepare for interview will follow later in this chapter. To help you gain an understanding of the steps through which a department must go to hire a new staff member, the recruitment process itself will be discussed. Many facilities have a standardised recruitment approach. Although differences may apply in specific locations, a common process followed to hire new nursing staff is listed below.

1 A vacancy is identified.
2 The role's position description is reviewed by the employer to ensure it is accurate, up to date and covers minimum details required under state Health Department policy.
3 The selection criteria or 'essential criteria' are reviewed. These must describe the essential requirements of the position and outline the minimum skills, knowledge and experience required to perform the role.
4 The position is advertised. In some instances a person can be interviewed for a role without the position being advertised; however, this only takes place under special circumstances. Some nurses may 'cold call' or approach an employer directly when no position has been advertised. If they are successful in gaining a job, this is usually because there is a state or local shortage of nurses in that particular specialty, allowing the employer to take on new staff without prior advertisement. The advertisement will contain a relevant position description and **selection criteria**. For example, if the selection criteria state that the applicant must have an Advanced Life Support accreditation, you would need to have completed Advanced Life Support training to apply and be eligible for consideration. If you are unable to meet each selection criterion, you will not be granted an interview. A position information package will also be accessible, containing relevant information such as salary range, terms and conditions of employment, code of conduct and so on.

> **selection criteria**
> Features that the applicant must have to be considered for the advertised job.

5 Applications are lodged.

6 Applicants receive acknowledgement of receipt of their application.

7 A selection panel is convened. The selection panel consists of the convenor, and panel members who have knowledge of the position requirements enabling effective assessment of applications. The role of the selection panel is to:
   - determine which of the applicants should proceed to interview
   - further assess the applicants' suitability through an interview
   - conduct necessary verifications—for example, criminal checks, reference checks
   - make a recommendation to the delegated decision-maker regarding making a job offer.

8 The selection panel assesses which applications fulfil the stated selection criteria, ones that do not are culled and not offered an interview.

9 The remaining applicants proceed to interview. The interview is conducted in person where possible; however, it may be conducted over the phone. Following the interview, there is a check of mandatory documentation (**100-point identity check**, nursing registration and so on).

10 The panel analyses the information gained during the interview to determine a list of preferred applicants. For the preferred applicants, two processes will take place:
   - An identity check, criminal record check and internal service check will be undertaken.
   - Referees will be contacted.

11 The panel members will then make a decision about who to recommend for employment.

12 Approval is gained to offer employment.

13 A formal job offer is made (NSW Health, 2015b).

> **100-point identity check** An evaluation of documents to prove who you are. If you have a 100-point document such as a passport, this will suffice as proof. If you use other forms of proof, such as credit card or Medicare card, which are worth fewer points each, they must collectively add up to 100 points to meet the requirement.

What are managers looking for in a potential employee?

Potential employers begin to assess your suitability as a candidate from the moment they look at your CV or cover letter. Panel members start to form an opinion as to whether or not you possess the necessary knowledge, skills and attributes to be an asset to the department as soon as they read your application.

Common examples of desirable attributes that nurse managers within Australia seek include:

- a Registered Nurse with current National Registration
- recent experience in the area of employment
- clinical competence and safety
- professionalism
- evidence of active involvement in your own professional development
- self-awareness
- effective verbal and written communication skills
- the ability to work effectively in a multidisciplinary collaborative team environment
- well-developed time-management/organisational/prioritisation skills
- evidence of problem-solving and decision-making skills
- knowledge of and commitment to continuous quality and practice improvement principles
- computer literacy and competency.

How are desirable attributes demonstrated?

It is important to provide evidence of the above attributes in your cover letter and CV. The positive impression conveyed to the panel via your application can then be developed further in the interview environment.

The following sections will concentrate on how to create your application letter and CV, and how to prepare for the interview to ensure you demonstrate the attributes of a high-quality employee. Upon making it to the interview stage, having a professional portfolio available for interviewers to peruse can help them gain greater insight into you as a clinician, and possibly increase the likelihood of a successful application if they are impressed by what they see. The creation of a professional portfolio was discussed in Chapter 11.

THE COVER LETTER

The cover letter is the first opportunity to make a positive impression on your potential employer, and a personalised letter notifies the reader that you are serious about the application. The cover letter is an introduction to your résumé, intentions, qualifications and abilities. It is a vehicle to showcase key skills and accomplishments that will highlight early on that you are not only competent, but will likely excel within the role.

Cover letter content

When beginning a draft of your cover letter, ensure the following items are included:

- a brief introduction to who you are
- identification of the job for which you are applying, and where you saw the advertisement
- a few words about your background and qualifications or the specialty in which you are interested
- a statement about why you are interested in the role and what qualifies you to successfully complete it
- a mention of the documents you have enclosed—for example, 'I have enclosed my CV, selection criteria and list of referees.'

It takes time and thought to write an effective cover letter. Ensure that you plan the information you want to present in each section, then revisit it and draft once more so that the content is clear and without mistakes. When reading a cover letter, the employer likes to be able to easily grasp the candidate's level of experience, qualifications, enthusiasm and employability. If the employer ascertains from the cover letter that you are likely to hold desirable attributes, will be able to competently fulfil the responsibilities of the job, appear to be professional and enjoy your work, they are much more likely to read your résumé properly, rather than just glancing at it.

Cover letter checklist

Upon completion of the first full draft of your cover letter, compare it with the following list.

Content considerations
- Have you addressed the letter appropriately? Address your application letter to the Nurse Manager responsible for the department. This information can easily be obtained through a brief phone call to the nursing administration unit of the hospital and a polite request for the name of the Nurse Manager, clearly stating that it is for the purpose of writing a job application letter. Ensure you have the spelling and title of the person correct, and avoid addressing the letter 'To whom it may concern'.
- Have you showcased your abilities sufficiently?
- Have you articulated how you will be an asset to the employer?

- Is the letter positive and enthusiastic?
- Have you proofread the document?
- Is your sentence structure clear, understandable and succinct?

Format considerations

- Restrict the letter to one page.
- Ensure the letter is an original printout and not a photocopy.
- Print on good-quality paper.
- Sign the letter with blue or black ink.
- Use a standard letter format. Your address and contact details should be placed at the top right-hand corner of the page, and the details/address of the person to whom you are writing in the top left-hand corner. The first paragraph should provide an introduction to the reason for the letter, the subsequent paragraphs should provide the main information and the final sentence or paragraph should provide a summary of the intent of the letter.
- Do not use more than one typeface. The font size should be easy to read (11 or 12 point).
- Ensure your cover letter is on top of your résumé within the envelope. If possible, use a larger envelope that allows the letter and résumé to remain flat.
- Remember to keep a copy for your own records.

If applying by email, the cover letter content may be placed in the body of the main email, while the résumé, selection criteria and other related documents can be included as attachments.

The cover letter shown in Figure 12.1 succinctly conveys key points to the reader:

- the position being applied for
- where the position was advertised
- currency of registration within Australia
- relevant nursing experience
- demonstrated involvement in and contribution to the applicant's own professional and clinical development
- effective written communication skills
- noted attachments of selection criteria, résumé and referees
- two different means to contact the applicant.

Joe Bloggs RN
Postal address
Email address
Phone number

Date
Nurse Manager
Hospital and Department
Address
City
Job reference number (if available)

Dear Ms Blank,
I would like to apply for the position of a Registered Nurse on the 3 South Orthopaedics Ward, advertised on NSW Health eRecruit.

I am a new Graduate Registered Nurse who has recently completed a Bachelor of Nursing at Wollongong University, where I achieved a Distinction average in my final year. I have relevant experience gained through numerous medical and surgical clinical placements, where I delivered patient-centred care, demonstrated an ability to apply theory to practice, and developed key skills in time management and effective communication.

Although mindful that I am at the beginning of a steep learning curve as I enter the nursing workforce, I am looking forward to this challenge, and am keen to contribute to my own professional development and grow as a clinician. As part of this commitment to lifelong learning to ensure my practice reflects the best available evidence, I recently completed a short course in surgical wound management.

I have current registration to practise within Australia, and would appreciate the opportunity to meet with you, learn more about your department and have the possibility of interviewing for a full-time position.

I can be contacted at the phone number or email address listed above.
Please find attached my résumé, selection criteria and referees.
Thank you for your time in considering my application for a Registered Nurse position within the orthopaedic department, and I look forward to meeting you soon.

Yours sincerely,
Joe Bloggs
[Signature]

Figure 12.1 Example of a cover letter

SELECTION CRITERIA

When an advertised position outlines selection criteria, ensure that you address each of the stated criteria in a separate document. Selection criteria describe the skills, abilities, knowledge and qualifications a candidate must have to be eligible to apply for the position.

Explain clearly and succinctly how you fulfil the criteria with evidence from your clinical practice and/or education. For example, it would not be adequate to merely state you are an effective communicator; provide an example of clinical practice that demonstrates effective communication in action—such as application of the ISBAR framework during clinical handover.

RÉSUMÉ

Your résumé should be a clear and concise document that outlines your education, employment history, areas of knowledge/skills and professional development relevant to the job you are targeting. It is a self-promotional document that clearly conveys to the reader your education, skills, work experience and career achievements. Information should be recorded in point form, avoiding paragraphs. Key information that identifies you as a top applicant must be easily accessible to the reader, not lost in a jumble of sentences. A good résumé helps the potential employer to predict how you may perform in the target position. For an example see Figure 12.2.

Common areas that nursing résumés address include the following:

- *Applicant contact details:* These should be in point form, stating name, postal address, contact phone number and email address.
- *Summary statement:* This is a statement that conveys to the reader what type of clinician you are, where your passions lie and the key positive attributes that enable you to deliver quality patient care.
- *Registration:* Provide evidence of currency of Australian nursing registration to practise.
- *Education history:* Record here only significant courses related to your desired area of employment (e.g. healthcare related undergraduate degree, postgraduate certificate/diploma/degrees or equivalent pre-Bachelor courses). Education within this section should have been delivered by a recognised higher education provider, such as a university or nursing college. List qualifications in chronological order with the most recent listed first. State the year

Résumé
Joe Bloggs
21 Dene Lane
Geelong VIC 3125
Mobile: 0400 000 000
Email: joebloggs@email.com

SUMMARY
I am a new Graduate Registered Nurse who is dedicated to providing evidence-based care. I have a strong work ethic, and enjoy contributing to patient care within a collaborative, team environment. I have a strong desire to build on the knowledge and skills acquired during my undergraduate training, and look forward to embracing the challenges and development opportunities of your New Graduate Transition to Practice Program.

REGISTRATION:
Registered Nurse   Reg No: NMW0001111

EDUCATION:
Bachelor of Nursing (2016)
La Trobe University, Melbourne

EMPLOYMENT HISTORY
January 2014 to 2015:
Assistant in Nursing
The Alfred Hospital, Surgical Ward, VIC

UNDERGRADUATE CLINICAL PLACEMENTS
3rd Year: [*Insert type—for example, 'critical care', and key areas of development achieved during the placement*]
2nd Year:
1st Year:

CAREER ACHIEVEMENTS
Dean's list for academic achievement (2016)

REFEREES
Jane Brown—Nurse Manager, Surgical Ward   Professor Alice Jenkins
The Alfred Hospital   La Trobe University
Phone: Phone:
Email: Email:

Figure 12.2 Example of a résumé

of completion, course name and education provider. If there is a particular achievement linked to one of the courses that may set you apart from other candidates with the same qualification, consider including a brief statement— for example, 'Average mark: Distinction'.

- *Employment history:* List in chronological order with the most recent first. State dates of service, institution, specialty/department worked in and role. For previous employment that may provide an indication of areas of knowledge, skills and experience that will be valuable in the job being sought, state in point form key related information and achievements that represent the quality, development and extent of clinical practice you attained within the role. Be wary of only listing responsibilities. Your future employer will know what they expect the base functioning nurse to be capable of—this is not what they are seeking, so include items that depict you as a high performer. If you are a new graduate nurse, consider listing clinical placements undertaken during your Bachelor of Nursing.

- *Short courses:* Record only short courses attended within the previous five years that are relevant to the job being applied for. Courses delivered outside a five-year window may not reflect current best practice. State the year accessed, the name of the course and the CPD hours attained. For Australian applicants, it may be relevant to include only short courses that are Royal College of Nursing Australia (RCNA) accredited to contribute to CPD hours for registration. A statement can be made that a clear record of your participation in continuing educational development is accessible in your professional practice portfolio.

- *Conference presentations/posters:* If you have presented or contributed to a conference presentation or poster, state the year, conference and title of the presentation. If an award was gained through your contribution, include it here.

- *Publications:* If you have authored or contributed to a publication, list in chronological order, with the most recent first.

- *Career achievements:* Note highlights that indicate you are a high-achieving clinician—for example, university awards.

- *References:* Include at least two referees, one of whom must be a manager from your most recent job. The second referee cannot be a peer: it must be either another manager or a person holding a senior position, such as an educator or nurse consultant, who can provide critical appraisal of your previous performance. As a new graduate applying for your first job, use one of your clinical supervisors as the clinical reference and a lecturer/academic who can provide suitable appraisal. For each referee, where possible, include an email address as well as a phone number. This is particularly important to assist contact being made if your referee resides in another country and time zone.

Things not to include

When identifying whether or not you should include a piece of information in your résumé, remove anything that is not relevant to the position for which you are applying or your ability to adequately perform the job. Personal details should be limited to name and contact information.

When reviewing your résumé draft, consider the following:

- Is this information relevant?
- Could this sentence or statement be perceived negatively?
- Can I word this in a positive way?

Try to gain feedback, but if you are in doubt about whether to include something, remove it.

INTERVIEW PREPARATION

Once you have secured an interview, you need to prepare for it. The educated, competent and articulate professional portrayed in your cover letter and résumé must correlate with the impression generated in the interview room if you are to be successful. So how do you prepare for an interview and give yourself the best chance of success?

Complete background research on the department

Familiarise yourself with information about the department that you wish to join, its organisational structure, stated goals and values, key personnel and patient base. Having a basic understanding of the department may help you to frame some of your interview answers. Rudimentary information about many public hospitals and their departments can often be located on the state/territory Department of Health website. However, if possible, make contact with the manager and see whether you can organise a personal visit to the department prior to your interview. This is a chance to meet some of the staff, become more familiar with the organisation you are trying to join and ask any questions that you have about patients, models of care, education opportunities and so on.

Preparing good interview answers

Developing answers for a variety of questions, and then practising the delivery of your answers, is crucial for achieving a polished performance during the interview. If you have already prepared a response for a given type of question, you are much less likely to stumble through a lacklustre answer.

It is usually possible to identify most areas that a set of interview questions may seek to explore, as each member of the interview panel usually is allowed no more than two questions to probe your abilities. Therefore, the questions asked will focus on elucidating your ability to fulfil the role's scope of practice and essential criteria.

Planning your response to common essential criteria required for RN roles is a good idea, as these skills and experience will be required regardless of the job for which you apply.

Common essential criteria are:

- recent experience in the position's area of employment
- clinical competence and safety
- professionalism
- evidence of active involvement in your own professional development
- self-awareness
- effective verbal and written communication skills
- the ability to work effectively within a multidisciplinary collaborative team environment
- well-developed time-management/organisational/prioritisation skills
- evidence of problem-solving and decision-making skills
- knowledge of and commitment to continuous quality and practice improvement principles
- computer skills.

The interviewer will be framing questions that seek to identify evidence of your skills in the above areas. Some examples of such questions are provided below:

- Please detail your experience, knowledge and skills that you think will assist you to work within our department.
- What methods do you utilise to ensure your practice is evidence-based and current?
- If we were to talk to your colleagues in the staffroom, what do you think would be their impression of you as a clinician?

- What is an area of your practice that you consider you do well, and what is an area that you would like to improve upon?
- Please outline some short-term and long-term goals for your educational and professional development.

Clinical scenario questions aim to identify what process you utilise for assessment, and how this informs your decision-making and problem-solving skills. Often the interviewer is trying to find evidence that you are working through a structured format of assessment that will allow you to prioritise interventions—for example, primary survey, head-to-toe or systems assessment. The clinical scenario question is also a useful tool to gauge how you manage difficult communication encounters between fellow staff members. Examples of this type of question are provided below.

- A nurse criticises the care you have delivered to a patient while in the clinical area and in front of other staff. How would you react and manage this situation?
- A patient is brought to the emergency department after sustaining a head injury from a physical assault at the pub. Witnesses report a loss of consciousness at the scene. The patient is initially alert and orientated on arrival; however, they later become agitated and confused, refuse treatment and try to leave the department. How would you manage this situation and what are your priorities?
- You walk into your patient's room and find your patient pale, **apnoeic** and unresponsive. What would you do? Please detail any relevant algorithm to help you prioritise your assessment and interventions, and list the medications, equipment and staff with which you may need to work.

  apnoeic Not breathing.

- You have pricked your finger while re-capping a sharp after use with a patient. What would you do next?
- You have been asked by a doctor to deliver a medication order of 25 mg IVI midazolam to an elderly patient in a side room who has become agitated, the aim being to help sedate and reduce his agitation. How would you proceed with this order? (NB: midazolam is a benzodiazepine sedative, and 25 mg is a dangerously high dose for this medication.)
- You note that an intervention a doctor wants to complete with a patient is inappropriate for the clinical situation, and may actually place the patient at further risk. How would you resolve this situation?

If you are an experienced nurse from overseas, you may be looking to apply for more senior nursing roles soon after entering the Australian health system. Interview questions for higher grades of nursing (e.g. Clinical Nurse Specialist,

Nurse Unit Manager, Nurse Educator, Clinical Nurse Consultant) will probe for a deeper level of knowledge—both clinical and of the role sought—and the ability to articulate assessment methods, prioritisation, interpretation of findings and the identification of issues that may affect care and how these could be resolved.

Examples of questions that may be asked during such an interview (dependent on role) may include:

- What skills and qualities would you bring that would make you successful in this position?
- How do you see the role of [title of role] enhancing quality both within your clinical environment and in the hospital environment in general?
- What strategies have you used to reflect on and measure your own performance? How do you know you are doing a good job?
- What strategies have you used in the past to implement change? What was the outcome?
- How would you be able to promote advancement of clinical practice within the specialty?
- Can you tell us about two major quality improvement/practice development activities or projects with which you have been involved? In particular, can you describe what difference these activities made in improving patient care outcomes and nursing development?
- Clinical education and planning are central aspects of the Clinical Nurse Consultant role. How would you fulfil this requirement?
- How would you identify what the education priorities are in your workforce?
- Please explain some of the contemporary challenges/issues facing [specialty area] within this state.
- What is competence and how would you demonstrate it within this role?
- How have you been involved in research and how has it been applied to your clinical area?
- If you were successful in being appointed to this role, describe the research opportunities that you would take advantage of.
- How have you previously demonstrated clinical leadership and how would you incorporate this into your new role?
- What is your understanding of the role?
- If successful, you will be working within a pressurised, multidisciplinary environment, where there will be differences of opinion regarding patient management. How will you deal with these situations to ensure that the patient receives best-practice care?

- Clinical service planning is part of your role. How would you identify areas within your service that would require development? How would you implement the change process?
- If we talked to a colleague of yours and asked them to describe an element of practice requiring improvement, and an area of practice that was completed at a high level, what do you think they would say about you?
- How do you think staff regard you in your current role as a senior clinician and why?
- What methods of communication aid interaction with medical colleagues?

Try to keep your answers brief and concise, and avoid rambling, as you run the risk of losing your train of thought halfway through the answer while under stress. Once you have written your answers, consider having them reviewed by your clinical mentor to confirm their appropriateness. Practise delivering your answers out loud while on your own. Once your confidence with them increases, get a family member or housemate to question you. Ask whether they understood your responses, and what impression you created. It may be worth watching yourself in the mirror or videoing yourself answering the questions. This allows you to see yourself from the interviewer's perspective, and may prompt you to work on aspects of unconscious body language or posture that affect the impression created.

In summary, the key to good preparation for interview questions—whatever the role—is to identify the essential criteria of the job being advertised as well as the objectives of the role, and prepare a few questions for each one.

CREATE THE RIGHT IMPRESSION

Appropriate attire is important for making the correct impression as a competent professional. A safe option is smart casual, but avoid jeans or revealing clothes. Also avoid overpowering perfume. Do not chew gum and avoid smoking immediately prior to entering the interview. Shake hands firmly but not aggressively. When answering questions, be sure to look at each panel member, but direct most of your attention to the person asking the specific question. Avoid fidgeting, as this will only distract and potentially irritate the interviewers.

Have a list of questions to ask the employer

At the conclusion of most interviews, the interviewee will be given an opportunity to ask the panel any question that they may have about the prospective employment. Having one or two insightful questions is another opportunity to set yourself apart from the other candidates.

Bring the correct documentation

It is a good idea to take along an extra copy of your résumé, references and any letters of recommendation that you have. Ensure you have a copy of your nursing registration and 100 points of identification. Typically, the easiest way to provide 100 points of ID is through your passport; otherwise, bring your driver's licence and a few other items such as a Medicare card or credit card.

Job interview scenario

A new graduate Registered Nurse, Jane Smith, arrives for her interview with at least 10 minutes to spare prior to her allotted interview time. She has a copy of her cover letter, essential criteria, résumé, references, nurse's registration and 100 points of ID. Arriving early provides ample time for her to sit in the waiting area, take some slow deep breaths and focus on the coming interview.

Jane is invited into the interview room and introduced to a panel of three interviewers. She returns their greeting with a smile and briefly shakes hands with each member, helping to establish rapport and demonstrating an ability to interact with strangers in a new environment.

Each interviewer asks two questions. For each question, Jane focuses on the question being asked. The interview questions are based around the essential criteria advertised for the job, and although they are not the exact questions that Jane has prepared, they are along similar lines. The time she has invested in preparing answers allows her to deliver considered answers without becoming flustered. At one point, she realises that her mind has wandered during a question. Instead of rambling and hoping she gets the answer right, Jane clarifies what the question was before proceeding. During her answers, she aims to speak clearly and avoid rushing, while maintaining an open posture.

Below are examples of two questions asked, and Jane's responses during her interview:

---

1 Please detail your experience, knowledge and skills that you think will assist you to work within our department?

'As a New Graduate RN, I am aware that I'm at the start of a steep learning curve in the coming year—a challenge that I'm looking forward to embracing. That being said, my undergraduate degree has prepared me to a safe level of beginner practice, and I have completed rotations through similar clinical areas to those offered in this hospital's Graduate Transition Program. Key areas of knowledge and skills gained from my training and placements that I think will help my future work include competent physical assessment, time management and functional communication techniques such as utilising an ISBAR framework during handover or escalation of patient issues, along with a willingness to contribute to my own development.'

Jane's answer demonstrates that she has insight about her beginner scope of practice, and the challenges awaiting her if she is successful in gaining employment. However, she is also able to clearly articulate key skills that will allow her to function as part of a multidisciplinary team while maintaining safe patient care. This demonstrates maturity and self-awareness that will be valued in the potential team member.

2 You walk into your patient's room and find the male patient pale, apnoeic and unresponsive. What would you do in this situation?

'I recognise that this scene fits the picture of a clinical emergency, and therefore I would use a DRABC basic life support algorithm to guide my actions. I would check for danger in the room, then seek a response from the patient by first speaking loudly in his ear, then via a pain response such as a trapezius pinch if he didn't respond to my voice. If there was no response I would then ensure I had help coming by pressing the emergency buzzer to initiate a team response before moving on to check the patient's airway.' [Jane completes walk through of basic life support.]

Through her answer, Jane has demonstrated that she is able to recognise a clinical emergency, and that she has the presence of mind to immediately apply the appropriate algorithm for prioritising assessment and interventions on such an occasion. She is thus able to demonstrate a key base quality for safe practice in the clinical setting.

At the conclusion of the interview, Jane thanks the panel for the opportunity to be interviewed, and makes her professional practice portfolio available for the panel to read through if they wish.

After leaving, while the interview is still fresh in her mind, she finds a quiet place and jots down the questions that she was asked, and areas that she feels she could improve upon in her responses. She also mentally notes the areas where she felt she answered well. By using the interview as a learning opportunity, no matter what the outcome may be, Jane ensures that the interview experience will help to improve her performance in future similar situations.

Summary

In this chapter, we have looked at getting ready for employment after graduation. Graduate nurse transition programs have been described and the benefits they offer considered. Advice has been provided on choosing the right working environment for you and the recruitment process has been outlined. Finally, we have looked at how to create the best impression possible when applying for a job, from writing an effective covering letter and producing a résumé to preparing for a job interview.

GLOSSARY

100-point identity check An evaluation of documents to prove who you are. If you have a 100-point document such as a passport, this will suffice as proof. If you use other forms of proof, such as credit card or Medicare card, which are worth fewer points each, they must collectively add up to 100 points to meet the requirement.

acuity Relates to the intensity of nursing care required by the patient.

adventitious airway noise An abnormal sound heard from a patient's lungs or airways, e.g. wheeze.

apnoeic Not breathing.

assault A threat of bodily harm coupled with an apparent, present ability to cause the harm.

association A linear and predictive relationship between two variables that move in relation to each other.

battery The actual infliction of unlawful force or offensive contact with the 'person' of another—for example, touching a person's body.

benign Not harmful in effect.

capnography Measures the amount of CO_2 in an exhaled breath, known as 'end-tidal CO_2', or '$ETCO_2$' with a normal range of 35–45 mmHg. Capnography is used to help assess the adequacy of ventilation, i.e. the movement of air in and out of the lung.

coercion or duress Refers to a situation whereby an individual performs an act as a result of violence, threat or other pressure against them.

cognitive This term relates to the conscious processes of perception, imagining, memory, judgement, reasoning and communication. Cognitive impairment may be related to infections (e.g. sepsis), vitamin deficiency, medications or dementia.

complementary roles When different health professions complete different aspects of management that together work towards the same over-arching goal of holistic patient care.

consensuality Pupils should have a consensual response to light—for example, when light is shone into one eye, the opposite pupil should contract at the same time.

crepitus A grating sensation on palpation caused by the ends of fractured bone rubbing against each other.

cytotoxic drugs Generally used during the treatment of cancer. Cytotoxic drugs are medications that are toxic to cells, targeting rapidly dividing cancer cells.

dangerous drug cupboard This is a separate locked cupboard securely attached to the wall or floor, purely dedicated for the storage of S4D and S8 medications or additional accountable medication as determined by local policy. All medication stored in the cupboard must accounted for in a dangerous drug register.

dangerous drug register A dedicated register in which all transactions, administrations or discarding of restricted medications is recorded.

denomination A distinct religious body that is defined by its doctrine, a set of beliefs/ teachings, and church authority (for example, the Bible).

didactic teaching A situation where information is presented by a teacher to a student with little interaction—for example, a teacher presenting a topic from the front of the classroom.

differential diagnosis A list of possible diagnoses that could account for the patient presentation.

diluent A substance used to reduce the concentration of (i.e. dilute) an injectable medication, such as normal saline (0.9% sodium chloride) or water, for injection.

escalation Refers to a situation where the clinician notes information that must be acted upon immediately. 'Escalation' involves bringing this information to the notice of appropriate staff to enact needed change—for example, for a deteriorating patient, this would be the senior treating doctor to make a decision regarding changes to the clinical management plan, and the Nurse Unit Manager, who may need to reprioritise nursing resources to assist in managing the patient.

evidence-based practice The process of making conscientious and judicious clinical decisions based upon proven evidence, combined with clinical experience and patient expectations.

falls risk screen Refers to a brief process to estimate the level of falls risk of a patient.

fiduciary A person who holds a legal or ethical relationship of trust with one or more individuals, such as a nurse and a patient in their care.

haemodynamic compromise Haemodynamics is the study of blood movement. Compromise of blood flow is manifested in a drop of blood pressure and tissue perfusion.

healthcare-associated infection (HAI) An infection that occurs as a result of a healthcare intervention.

iatrogenic Refers to an illness, injury or negative patient outcome caused by clinician activity or treatment.

implied consent Consent that is not expressly granted by a person, but rather implicitly granted by their actions or inactions.

independent check This check should be made with no assistance from another party— the person responsible completes the entire check, including any calculations, from the original documentation and their own observations.

involuntary client Refers to treatment or action undertaken against someone's will, to ensure their safety and that of others.

iterative process A process of reaching a decision by means of a repeated and converging cycle of operations.

left lateral position Also known as recovery position. Decreases the chance that an unconscious person will aspirate in the event of vomiting.

livor mortis A deep reddish-purple colour that forms on the sides of the face, earlobes, neck and posterior surfaces of the body because of blood pooling in the dependent regions of the body; usually starts 30 minutes after death.

Medication Management Plan A national, standardised chart used by nursing, medical, pharmacy and allied health staff to improve the accuracy of medication documentation and administration.

mitigate To lessen or make less severe.

morbidity Refers to how often a disease occurs within a population.

mortality Refers to the incidence of death in a population.

non-punitive environment Healthcare is an extremely complicated environment with the potential for many things to go wrong. A non-punitive approach recognises that clinicians rarely make a mistake deliberately. Instead of punishing the person who made a mistake, the focus is directed towards understanding what contributed to the mistake in the first place (e.g. communication error, a lack of guidelines or education) so that this can be rectified and future occurrences prevented.

Nurse Navigators Registered nurses who have an in-depth understanding of the health system, including disease-specific knowledge, who engage, guide and support patients with complex health conditions that require a high degree of comprehensive, clinical care.

patent airway An airway that is open and clear of obstruction, allowing inhalation of oxygen and exhalation of carbon dioxide.

preceptor A nurse who provides support and guidance to the graduate as they transition to a new clinical area.

provider number A unique number that medical or endorsed nurse practitioners can acquire. It allows the clinician to make referrals for specialist services, requests for pathology or diagnostic imaging services, and their patients to claim Medicare rebates for the services provided.

rigor mortis The progressive stiffening of muscles after death.

selection criteria Features that the applicant must have to be considered for the advertised job.

skin colour/perfusion When assessing breathing, assessing skin colour can give an indication of oxygen saturation of haemoglobin. With adequate oxygen saturation of haemoglobin, the patient's skin will have colour. Poor oxygen saturation will be evidenced by pale skin, progressing to blue/cyanosed skin as oxygen saturation decreases. In relation to circulation assessment, a patient with normal blood pressure should be well perfused—that is, have colour to their skin. If they have low blood pressure, this will be evidenced by poor perfusion, pale skin and a capillary refill time of greater than 2 seconds.

social media Refers to the online and mobile technologies that allow the creating and sharing (i.e. posting) of information, ideas, opinions, photos, videos and other forms of expression via virtual communities and networks, such as social networking sites, personal websites and blogs.

stridor An abnormal airway sound caused by turbulent airflow in the upper airway, high pitched in sound.

subcutaneous emphysema Describes the presence of air trapped within the tissue below the skin, and has the sensation of rice paper under your fingers on palpation.

tachypnoea Describes abnormal fast respiratory rate.

tracheal deviation The trachea should be midline as it descends past the supra-sternal notch. Movement of the trachea to left or right, i.e. deviation, is evidence of possible tension pneumothorax.

tracheal tug Caused by upper airway obstruction, it is an abnormal downward movement of the trachea during inspiration.

vital signs Refers to clinical measurements that reflect the essential body functions; includes body temperature (T), heart rate (HR), respiratory rate (RR), peripheral oxygen saturation (SpO_2), blood pressure (BP) and pain.

voluntary client An individual who voluntarily complies with treatment or action.

warfarin An anticoagulant that limits the blood's ability to form clots.

Appendix 1

COMMON MEDICAL ACRONYMS AND ABBREVIATIONS

Acronyms and abbreviations are part of everyday clinical oral and written communication, and have evolved from the need to communicate quickly and accurately. However, they are frequently the major cause of mistakes, and drug and procedure errors (Dunn & Wolfe, 2001; Garbutt et al., 2005; ISMP, 2005; JCAHO, 2001). In addition, acronyms and abbreviations vary across health organisations and between specialties (e.g. AKA, 'above knee amputation' in orthopaedics, stands for 'also known as' in clerical administration), and importantly, exclude or confuse patients. Health organisations may have their own approved list of recognised acronyms and abbreviations (e.g. ACSQHC, 2011), which you should become familiar with. The following is a list of commonly used acronyms and abbreviations.

Abbreviation	Description (meaning)
AAA	abdominal aortic aneurysm
abdo.	abdomen
ABG	arterial blood gas
addit.	addendum, added to
adduct.	adduction
ADH	antidiuretic hormone
ADL	activities of daily living
ADR	adverse drug reaction
AF	atrial fibrillation
AHNM	After Hours Nurse Manager
AICD	automatic implantation cardioverter defibrillator
AM	morning
AMO	Admitting Medical Officer
appt.	appointment
ARDS	acute respiratory distress syndrome
ARF	acute renal failure
ausc.	auscultation
Ax	assessment
BBB	bundle branch block
BCC	basal cell carcinoma

Abbreviation	Description (meaning)
bd	given twice a day
BG	background
BGL	blood glucose level
BIBA	brought in by ambulance
BLS	basic life support
BMI	body mass index
BNO	bowels not open
BO	bowels open
BP	blood pressure
BPM/bpm	beats per minute
BTF	Between the Flags
BW	birth weight
Bx	biopsy
C & S	culture and sensitivity
C (1–7)	cervical (1–7), e.g. C5 quadriplegic
c/o	complained of
CAPD	continuous ambulatory peritoneal dialysis
capsule, cap(s)	capsule
CCF	congestive cardiac failure
CERS	Clinical Emergency Response System
CHD	congenital heart disease
CKD	chronic kidney disease
cm	centimetre
CN (1–12)	cranial nerve
CNC	Clinical Nurse Consultant
CNE	Clinical Nurse Educator
CNS	central nervous system
CNS	Clinical Nurse Specialist
COAD	chronic obstructive airway disease
CPR	cardiopulmonary resuscitation
CRF	chronic renal failure
CSF	cerebrospinal fluid
CSU	catheter specimen of urine
CT	computerised axial tomography, e.g. CT head (scan)
CVAD	central venous access device
CVC	central venous catheter
CVD	cardiovascular disease
CVP	central venous pressure
CXR	chest X-ray
D & V	diarrhoea and vomiting
D/W	discussed with
Dept	department
DIC	disseminated intravascular coagulopathy
DOA	dead on arrival
DOB	date of birth
DoCS	Department of Community Services
DON	Director of Nursing Services
Dr	Doctor
Dx	diagnosis

Abbreviation	Description (meaning)
EBV	Epstein-Barr virus
ECG	electrocardiogram
Echo.	echocardiogram
ECMO	extracorporeal membrane oxygenation
ECT	electroconvulsive therapy
ED	emergency department
EEG	electro-encephalogram
EEN	Endorsed Enrolled Nurse
EN	Enrolled Nurse
ENT	ear, nose and throat
EPAP	expiratory positive airway pressure
ETT	endotracheal tube
EUC	electrolytes, urea, creatinine
EVD	external ventricular drain
F/U	follow up
FBC	full blood count
FEV^1	forced expiratory volume over 1 second
FFP	fresh frozen plasma
FH, FHx	family history
FiO$_2$	fraction inspired oxygen
#	fracture
FROM	full range of movement
FVC	forced vital capacity
FWB	full weight bearing
g	gram
G & H	blood group and hold serum
G (*number*)	Gravida, e.g. G1
GA	general anaesthetic
GCS	Glasgow Coma Scale
GFR	glomerular filtration rate
GI	gastrointestinal
GIT	gastrointestinal tract
GM Stain	gram stain
GP	general practitioner
HAI	healthcare-associated infection
Hb	haemoglobin
HBV	hepatitis B virus
HC	head circumference
HCCC	Health Care Complaints Commission
HIV	human immune deficiency virus
HPC	history of presenting complaint
HPV	human papilloma virus
HR	heart rate
HSDNM	heart sounds dual and no murmur
Ht	height
Hx	history
ICC	intercostal catheter
ICD	intercostal drain
ICP	intracranial pressure

Abbreviation	Description (meaning)
ID	identification
IDC	indwelling catheter
IG	intragastric
IM	intramuscular
indep.	independent(ly)
inj.	injection
IOL	intraocular lens
IOP	intraocular pressure
IPAP	inspiratory positive airway pressure
IPPV	intermittent positive-pressure ventilation
IV	intravenous—avoid IVI as it could be mistaken for IV 1
IVAD	implantable venous access device
IVC	inferior vena cava
IVT	intravenous therapy
JMO	Junior Medical Officer
JVP	jugular venous pressure
kCal	kilocalorie
kg	kilogram
kJ	kilojoule
KUB (scan)	kidney urinary bladder (scan)
K-wire	Kirschner wire
L	litre
L (1 to 5)	lumbar, e.g. L2 fracture
LA	local anaesthetic
lat.	lateral
left, (L)	left
LFT	liver function tests
LIF	left iliac fossa
LIH	left inguinal hernia
LLL	left lower lobe
LLQ	left lower quadrant
LOC	loss of consciousness
LOS	length of stay
LP	lumbar puncture
LRTI	left respiratory tract infection
LSCS	lower segment caesarean section
LUL	left upper lobe
LUQ	left upper quadrant
mane, morning	to be given in the morning
MAP	mean arterial pressure
max	maximum
MC&S	microscopy, culture and sensitivities
MDI	metered dose inhaler
MET	Medical Emergency Team
mets	metastases
mg	milligram
mg/L	milligram per litre
microgram, MICROg	microgram—avoid µg as it could be mistaken for mg, which is 1000 times larger

Abbreviation	Description (meaning)
midday	to be given at midday
min	minimum
mL	millilitre
mm	millimetre
Mmol, mmol	millimole
MMSE	Mini-Mental State Exam
MO	Medical Officer
mob.	mobility/mobilisation
MRE	multiple-resistant enterobacter
MRI	magnetic resonance imaging
MRO	multi-resistant organism
MRSA	methicillin resistant *Staphylococcus aureus*
MSU	mid-stream specimen of urine
MVA	motor vehicle accident
NAI	non-accidental injury
NBM	nil by mouth
NE	Nurse Educator
NEB, neb	nebulised
NG	nasogastric
NIDDM	non-insulin dependent diabetes mellitus
night, nocte	to be given at night
NIM	nurse-initiated medication
NIV	non-invasive ventilation
No.	number
NOF	neck of femur
NP	Nurse Practitioner
NUM	Nurse Unit Manager
NWB	non-weight bearing
O&G	obstetrics and gynaecology
O/A	on admission *or* on arrival
O/E	on examination
O2 Sat	oxygen saturation
Obs., obs.	observation
OD	overdose
OG	orogastric
Oint	ointment
OPD	outpatients department
ORIF	open reduction internal fixation
OT	operating theatre *or* occupational therapy
P *(number)*	parity, e.g. P1
PCA	patient-controlled analgesia
pCO_2	partial pressure of carbon dioxide
PE	pulmonary embolism
PERL	pupils equal, reacting to light
PEARL	pupils equal, accommodating and reactive to light
PEEP	positive end-expiratory pressure
PEG	percutaneous enteral gastrostomy
Pess.	pessary
PFT	pulmonary function test

Abbreviation	Description (meaning)
pH	degree of acidity or alkalinity
physio	physiotherapist
%	per cent
PICC	peripherally inserted central catheter
PIP	peak inspiratory pressure
PIVC	peripherally inserted venous catheter
PKU	phenylketonuria
PM	after midday
PMHx	past medical history
PO	oral, by mouth, orally
POP	plaster of paris
post-op	post-operative
PPE	personal protective equipment
PR	per rectum
prem.	premature
pre-med.	pre-operative medication
pre-op	pre-operative
prn	given when required
PROM	passive range of motion
Pt.	patient
PU	passed urine
PUO	pyrexia of unknown origin
PV	per vagina
PWB	partial weight bearing
qid	four times daily—avoid qd as it could be mistaken for every day/daily
R/O	removal of
R/V	review
Reg	Registrar (Medical Officer)
resp.	respiratory, e.g. resp rate
Rh	rhesus factor (Rh –ve or Rh +ve)
RIF	right iliac fossa
right, (R)	right
RIH	right inguinal hernia
RLL	right lower lobe (lung)
RLQ	right lower quadrant
RM	Registered Midwife
RML	right middle lobe (lung)
RMO	Resident Medical Officer
RN	Registered Nurse
ROM	range of movement
RR	respiratory rate
RSV	respiratory syncytial virus
RUL	right upper lobe
RUL	right upper lobe (lung)
RUQ	right upper quadrant
RVOT	right ventricular outflow tract
Rx	treatment
S (1–5)	sacral vertebrae
S/B	seen by

Abbreviation	Description (meaning)
SAE	serious adverse event
SAH	subarachnoid haemorrhage
SDH	subdural haematoma
SG	specific gravity
SLR	straight leg raise
SMO	Senior Medical Officer
SOAP	subjective objective assessment plan
SOB	short of breath
SOBOE	shortness of breath on exertion
SP	speech pathologist
SpO$_2$	saturation of peripheral oxygen
Spont.	spontaneous
stat	given immediately
Subcut	subcutaneous—avoid SC as it could be mistaken for SL (sublingual)
Subling	sublingual, under the tongue
Supp	suppository
SVC	superior vena cava
SVT	supraventricular tachycardia
SW	social worker
T (1–12)	thoracic, e.g. T2 fracture
t/f, T/F	transfer
T2DM	type 2 diabetes mellitus
tab	tablet
TB	tuberculosis
TBA	to be arranged
TBI	traumatic brain injury
tds	given three times a day—avoid TID as it could be mistaken for bd (twice daily)
temp.	temperature
TENS	transcutaneous electrical nerve stimulation
TKVO	to keep vein open
Top.	topical
TPN	total parenteral nutrition
TPR	temperature, pulse, respiration
U/A	urinalysis
U/O	urine output
U/S	ultrasound
URTI	upper respiratory tract infection
UTI	urinary tract infection
UWSD	under water seal drain
VBG	venous blood gas
VEB	ventricular ectopic beats
VF	ventricular fibrillation
VMO	Visiting Medical Officer
VQ scan	ventilation perfusion scan
WBAT	weight bearing as tolerated
WBC	white blood cells
WCC	white cell count
Wt	weight

Appendix 2

COMPARATIVE NAMES OF COMMON MEDICATIONS

Australian approved name[1,2]	Previous name[1,2]	US adopted name [3]	Common international brand names[1,2,3]
ANALGESICS			
fentanyl		fentanil	Sublimaze, Duragesic
hydromorphone			Dilaudid
morphine			Avinza, Kadian, Sevredol
oxycodone			Endone, Oxycontin
paracetamol		acetaminophen	Panadol, Tylenol
pizotifen			Sandomigran
rizatriptan			Maxalt, Rizatriptan
sumatriptan			Imitrex, Sumavel
ANTIBIOTICS			
amoxicillin	amoxycillin		Amoxil
cefalexin	cephalexin	cephalexin	Keflex, Keftab
cefazolin	cephazolin		Ancef, Kefzol, Cefazolin
cefotaxime			Claforan, Cefotaxime
cefuroxime			Kefurox, Zinacef, Zinnat
clarithromycin			Biaxin, Clarac, Clarithro
norfloxacin			Noroxin, Nufloxib, Roxin
phenoxymethylpenicillin		penicillin-V	Beepen, Betapen, V-Cillin K
procaine benzylpenicillin	procaine penicillin		Bicillin C-R
roxithromycin			Rulide
trimethoprim			Primsol
vancomycin			Vancocin
ANTICOAGULANTS			
dabigatran			Pradaxa
enoxaparin			Lovenox, Clexane

Notes
[1] Department of Health (2016).
[2] Medicines.org.au (2017).
[3] MedlinePlus (2015).

Australian approved name[1,2]	Previous name[1,2]	US adopted name [3]	Common international brand names[1,2,3]
rivaroxaban			Xarelto
warfarin			Coumadin
ANTIEMETICS			
metoclopramide			Reglan
ondansetron			Zofran
prochlorperazine			Stemitil, Compazine
ANTIEPILEPTICS			
carbamazepine			Tegratol, Epitol, Carbatrol
clonazepam			Klonopin
gabapentin			Neurontin
lamotrigine			Lamictal
levetiracetam			Keppra
phenytoin			Dilantin
retigabine		ezogabine	Potiga, Trobalt
sodium valproate			Epilim
ANTIHISTAMINES			
cetirizine			Zyrtec, Zodac,
fexofenadine			Allegra, Fexotabs, Telfast
loratadine			Claratyne, Claritin
promethazine			Phenergan
ANTI-INFLAMMATORIES			
diclofenac			Voltaren
ibuprofen			Motrin, Advil, Nurofen
indometacin	indomethacin		Indocin, Indocid
mefenamic acid			Ponstan, Ponstel
meloxicam			Mobic, Movalis
penicillamine			D-Penamine
piroxicam			Mobilis, Feldene
ANTILIPEDEMIC			
atorvastatin			Lipitor, Caduet, Liptruzet
rosuvastatin			Crestor
ANTIPARKINSONS			
benzatropine			Cogentin
levodopa and decarboxylase inhibitor		levodopa and carbidopa	Sinemet, Duopa
rasagiline			Azilect
ANTIPSYCHOTICS			
chlorpromazine			Promapar, Largactil
citalopram			Celexa, Celapram
escitalopram			Lexapro

Australian approved name[1,2]	Previous name[1,2]	US adopted name[3]	Common international brand names[1,2,3]
ANTIPSYCHOTICS			
continued			
fluoxetine			Prozac, Lovan
fluvoxamine			Luvox, Faverin
haloperidol			Serenace, Haldol
lithium			Lithicarb, Eskalith
midazolam			Hypnovel, Versed
quetiapine			Seroquel
zopiclone		eszopiclone	Imovane, Lunesta
ANTIVIRALS			
abacavir			Triumeq
famciclovir			Famvir
lamivudine			Epivir
nevirapine			Viramune
ritonavir			Norvir
valaciclovir		valacyclovir	Valtrex
CARDIAC THERAPY			
ambrisentan			Letairis
amiodarone			Cordarone, Pacerone
amlodipine			Norvasc, Amvaz
bisoprolol			Zebeta
clonidine			Catapres
digoxin			Lanoxin, Cardoxin
epinephrine	adrenaline		Adrenalin
felodipine			Plendil
flecainide			Tambocor
glyceryl trinitrate		nitroglycerin	Nitrostat, Nitro-Dur, Nitrolingual
labetalol			Normodyne,
lercanidipine			Zanidip
lidocaine	lignocaine		Xylocaine
methyldopa			Aldoril, Aldomet, Dopamet
metoprolol			Lopressor, Toprol, Betaloc
nicorandil			Ikorel, Ikotab
nifedipine			Adalat, Procardia,
perindopril			Idaprex, Aceon
pindolol			Visken, Barbloc
prazosin			Minipress
propranolol			Inderal, Deralin
verapamil			Tarka, Isoptin

Australian approved name[1,2]	Previous name[1,2]	US adopted name [3]	Common international brand names[1,2,3]
DIABETES			
acarbose			Glucobay, Precose
glibenclamide		glyburide	Daonil, Diabeta
gliclazide			Glyade, Diamicron
glimepiride			Amaryl
linagliptin			Tradjenta
metformin			Fortamet, Glucophage, Diabex, Formet
DIURETICS			
furosemide	frusemide		Lasix, Frusemide
hydrochlorothiazide			Esidrix
indapamide			Lozol, Natrilix
spironolactone			Aldactone, Spiractin
GASTROINTESTINAL DISORDERS			
bisacodyl			Ducolax, Bisalax
butylscopolamine		hyoscine butylbromide	Transderm Scop, Buscopan
cimetidine			Magicul, Tagamet
docusate sodium			Coloxyl
esomeprazole			Vimovo, Nexium
lactulose			Lac-Dol, Actilax, Enulose
lansoprazole			Zopral, Prevacid
pantoprazole			Somac, Protonix
ranitidine			Zantac
IMMUNO-SUPPRESSANTS			
azathioprine			Imuran
ciclosporin	cyclosporin	cyclosporine	Neoral, Gengraf
tacrolimus			Prograf, Pacrolim
RESPIRATORY DISEASE			
beclometasone	beclomethasone		Qvar, Beclovent
fluticasone			Flixotide, Flovent
ipratropium bromide			Atrovent
salbutamol		albuterol	Ventolin
salmeterol			Seretide, Serevent

Source: Based on Department of Health (2015).

ANSWERS TO REVIEW QUESTIONS

Chapter 1
1.1 True
1.2 D
1.3 C
1.4 A, C, D, E
1.5 False
1.6 New graduate peers, clinical mentors such as educator or a senior nurse.
1.7 Professional identity is linked to yet different from your overall self-concept as an individual (who you think you are). It is a sense of self that is acquired from the role and work you complete as a nurse, and is influenced by interactions with others as well as your position in society.
1.8 A, D, E
1.9 E

Chapter 2
2.1 True
2.2 B
2.3 B
2.4 A
2.5 True
2.6 False
2.7 A
2.8 True
2.9 False
2.10 True
2.11 D
2.12 B

Chapter 3
3.1 False
3.2 A
3.3 B
3.4 True
3.5 A, C
3.6 A, B, D
3.7 True
3.8 B, C
3.9 C, A, B, D
3.10 B

Chapter 4
4.1 A
4.2 D
4.3 A
4.4 A
4.5 D
4.6 A, B, C, D
4.7 A

Chapter 5
5.1 E
5.2 E
5.3 A and C
5.4 False
5.5 False
5.6 D
5.7 B
5.8 A
5.9 A, B, D, E and F
5.10 B
5.11 C

Chapter 6
6.1 True
6.2 Introduction, Situation, Background, Request/recommendation
6.3 C
6.4 A, B, C, D
6.5 A, C, D

6.6	B
6.7	False
6.8	True
6.9	A, C
6.10	A, B, C
6.11	A, B, C, E

Chapter 7

7.1	D
7.2	True
7.3	B
7.4	C
7.5	True
7.6	C
7.7	A
7.8	A
7.9	B
7.10	True
7.11	A, B, C, D, F
7.12	A
7.13	False
7.14	A, B, C, E, F

Chapter 8

8.1	A
8.2	C
8.3	A
8.4	C
8.5	D
8.6	C
8.7	A
8.8	B

Chapter 9

9.1	A
9.2	B
9.3	C
9.4	D
9.5	B
9.6	A
9.7	C
9.8	B
9.9	A
9.10	D
9.11	A
9.12	D
9.13	C
9.14	B
9.15	B
9.16	D

Chapter 10

10.1	C
10.2	A, C, D
10.3	A, B, D, E, F
10.4	A, C, D
10.5	A
10.6	C
10.7	C
10.8	True
10.9	C, E, D, B, A
10.10	A, C

Chapter 11

11.1	B
11.2	C
11.3	B, C and D
11.4	A + C, B + D and E + F
11.5	C
11.6	C
11.7	B
11.8	C

REFERENCES

Aboriginal Health Council of South Australia 2016. Aboriginal health worker role. Retrieved from http://ahcsa.org.au/our-programs/aboriginal-health-worker-role.

Acebedo-Urdiales, M., Medina-Noya, J. & Ferre-Grau, C. 2014. Practical knowledge of experienced nurses in critical care: A qualitative study of their narratives. *BMC Medical Education*, 14, 1–15.

ACEM, ANZCA & JFICM 2003. Minimum standards for transport of critically ill patients. *Emergency Medicine Australasia*, 15, 197–201.

Agency for Clinical Innovation 2013. *Understanding the process to develop a model of care: An ACI framework* (version 1.0). Retrieved from www.aci.health.nsw.gov.au/__data/assets/pdf_file/0009/181935/HS13-034_Framework-DevelopMoC_D7.pdf.

Allen, B., Holland, P. & Reynolds, R. 2014. The effect of bullying on burnout in nurses: The moderating role of psychological detachment. *Journal of Advanced Nursing*, 71, 381–90.

Allen, C. & Stevens, S. 2007. Health service integration: A case study in change management. *Australian Health Review*, 31, 267–75.

Altmiller, G. 2011. Teaching clinical nurse specialist students to resolve conflict. *Clinical Nurse Specialist*, 25, 260–2.

Andre, K. & Heartfield, M. 2007. *Professional portfolios: Evidence of competency for nurses and midwives*. Sydney: Elsevier.

Andrews, J. 2013. *Cultural, ethnic and religious reference manual for health care providers*. Kernersville, NC: Jamarda Resources.

Andrews, M. & Boyle, J. 2012. *Transcultural concepts in nursing care*. Philadelphia, PA: Lippincott.

Arnetz, J., Winbald, U., Höglund, A., Lindahl, B., Spångberg, K., Wellentin, L., Wang, Y., Ager, J. & Arnetz, B. 2010. Is patient involvement during hospitalization for acute myocardial infarction associated with post-discharge treatment outcome? *Health Expectations: An International Journal of Public Participation in Health Care and Health Policy*, 13, 298–311.

Atkins, S. & Williams, A. 1995. Registered nurses' experiences of mentoring undergraduate nursing students. *Journal of Advanced Nursing*, 21, 1006–15.

Australian Association of Social Workers (AASW) 2017. What is social work? Retrieved from www.aasw.asn.au/information-for-the-community/what-is-social-work.

Australian Bureau of Statistics (ABS) 2007. *National survey of mental health and wellbeing: Summary of results*. Cat. no. 4326. Retrieved from www.ausstats.abs.gov.au/ausstats/subscriber.nsf/0/6AE6DA447F985FC2CA2574EA00122BD6/$File/43260_2007.pdf.

—— 2011. 2011 census QuickStats: all people; usual residents. Retrieved from www.censusdata.abs.gov.au/census_services/getproduct/census/2011/quickstat/0.

—— 2015. *Australian demographic statistics*. Cat. no. 3101.0. Retrieved from www.abs.gov.au/ausstats/abs@.nsf/mf/3101.0.

—— 2017a. *Australia, migration 2015–16*. Cat no. 3412.0. Canberra: ABS.

—— 2017b. Census reveals a fast changing, culturally diverse nation. Media Release, 27 June. Retrieved from www.abs.gov.au/ausstats/abs@.nsf/lookup/Media%20Release3.

—— 2017c. Religion in Australia: 2016 Census data summary. In *Census of Population and Housing: Reflecting Australia*. Cat no. 2071.0.0. Canberra: ABS.

Australian College of Nursing 2015. ACN policy. Retrieved from www.acn.edu.au/policy.

Australian Commission on Safety and Quality in Health Care (ACSQHC) 2004. *Summary rationale for a national medication chart.* Retrieved from www.safetyandquality.gov.au/wp-content/uploads/2012/02/chration.pdf.

—— 2005. *Complaints management handbook for healthcare services.* Sydney: Australian Council for Safety and Quality in Healthcare.

—— 2007. *The Australian Charter of Healthcare Rights.* Retrieved from www.safetyandquality.gov.au/national-priorities/charter-of-healthcare-rights/.

—— 2009. *Developing a safety and quality framework for Australia.* Sydney: ACSQHC.

—— 2011. *Recommendations for Terminology, Abbreviations and Symbols used in Prescribing and Administration of Medicines.* Sydney: ACSQHC.

—— 2012. *National Safety and Quality Health Service Standards.* Sydney: ACSQHC.

—— 2013a. *National medication management plan user guide.* Retrieved from www.safetyandquality.gov.au/wp-content/uploads/2010/01/Medication-Management-Plan-User-Guide.pdf.

—— 2013b. *Australian Open Disclosure Framework.* Retrieved from www.safetyandquality.gov.au/wp-content/uploads/2013/03/Australian-Open-Disclosure-Framework-Feb-2014.pdf.

—— 2014. *Australian Commission on Safety and Quality in Healthcare Strategic Plan 2014–2019.* Sydney: ACSQHC.

—— 2015. Governance. Retrieved from www.safetyandquality.gov.au/about-us/governance.

—— 2017. *National Safety and Quality Health Service Standards* (2nd edn). Sydney: ACSQHC.

Australian Council on Healthcare Standards (ACHS) 2013. *Risk management and quality improvement handbook.* Retrieved from www.achs.org.au/media/69305/risk_management_and_quality_improvement_handbook_july_2013.pdf.

Australian Government 2017. *Poisons Standard.* Retrieved from https://www.legislation.gov.au/Details/F2017L00057.

Australian Health Ministers' Advisory Council 2004. *Cultural respect framework for Aboriginal and Torres Strait Islander health, 2004–2009.* Adelaide: Department of Health.

Australian Health Practitioner Regulation Agency (AHPRA) 2014. Social media policy. Retrieved from www.nursingmidwiferyboard.gov.au/Codes-Guidelines-Statements/Policies/Social-media-policy.aspx.

—— 2016. *Annual report 2015/16.* Retrieved from www.ahpra.gov.au/annualreport/2016/downloads.html, p. 38.

Australian Indigenous HealthInfoNet 2013. Overview of Australian Indigenous health status, 2013. Retrieved from www.healthinfonet.ecu.edu.au/health-facts/overviews.

Australian Institute of Health and Welfare (AIHW) 2014a. Australia's health system. Retrieved from www.aihw.gov.au/australias-health/2014/health-system.

—— 2014b. Preventing and treating ill health. Retrieved from www.aihw.gov.au/australias-health/2014/preventing-ill-health/#t3.

—— 2015a. Emergency department care 2014–15: Australian hospital statistics. Health services series no. 65. Cat. no. HSE 168. Canberra: AIHW.

—— 2015b. *The health and welfare of Australia's Aboriginal and Torres Strait Islander peoples.* Cat. no. AIHW 147. Retrieved from www.aihw.gov.au/WorkArea/DownloadAsset.aspx?id=60129551281.

—— 2016. *Australia's Health 2016.* Australia's health series no. 15. Cat. no. AUS 199. Canberra: AIHW.

Australian Medical Association 2016. AMA career advice hub: becoming a doctor. Retrieved from https://ama.com.au/careers/becoming-a-doctor.

Australian Nurse Teachers' Society (ANTS) 2010. *Australian Nurse Teacher Professional Practice Standards.* New South Wales, Australia: ANTS. Retrieved from www.ants.org.au/ants/mod/resource/view.php?id=600.

Australian Nursing & Midwifery Accreditation Council (ANMAC) 2010. *Standards for Assessment of Nurses and Midwives for Migration Purposes*. Retrieved from https://www.anmac.org.au/skilled-migration-services.

—— 2012. *Registered Nurse Accreditation Standards, 2012*. Retrieved from www.anmac.org.au/sites/default/files/documents/ANMAC_RN_Accreditation_Standards_2012.pdf.

—— 2013. *Revised Standards for Assessment of Nurses and Midwives for Migration Purposes*. Retrieved from www.anmac.org.au/sites/default/files/documents/Revised_Standards_for_Assessment_of_Nurses_and_Midwives_for_Migration_Puposes.pdf.

—— 2014. *Midwife Accreditation Standards, 2014*. Retrieved from www.anmac.org.au/sites/default/files/documents/ANMAC_Midwife_Accreditation_Standards_2014.pdf.

Australian Nursing Federation 2009. *Fact sheet 3: A snapshot of nursing careers, qualifications and experience*. Retrieved from http://anf.org.au/documents/reports/Fact_Sheet_Snap_Shot_Nursing_Career_Paths.pdf.

Australian Nursing and Midwifery Federation (ANMF) 2013a. *ANMF Strategic Framework, 2013–2017*. Retrieved from www.anmf.org.au/documents/ANMF_Strategic_Framework.pdf.

—— 2013b. Child abuse and neglect [Position Statement]. Retrieved from http://anmf.org.au/documents/policies/PS_Child_abuse_and_neglect.pdf.

—— 2014. Compulsory reporting of abuse in aged care settings for nurses and assistants in nursing [Position Statement]. Retrieved from http://anf.org.au/documents/policies/PS_Compulsory_reporting.pdf.

—— 2015. About the Australian Nursing and Midwifery Federation. Retrieved from http://anmf.org.au/pages/about-the-anmf.

Australian Physiotherapy Association 2017. Physiotherapy in Australia. Retrieved from www.physiotherapy.asn.au.

Australian Politics 2015. Scott Morrison encourages states to let private sector run schools and hospitals. *The Guardian*, 3 October. Retrieved from https://www.theguardian.com/australia-news/2015/oct/03/scott-morrison-encourages-states-to-let-private-sector-run-schools-and-hospitals.

Australian Red Cross 2017. Our service. Retrieved from www.donateblood.com.au/about.

Australian Resuscitation Council & New Zealand Resuscitation Council (ANZCOR) 2016. ANZCOR Guideline 8: Cardiopulmonary resuscitation. Retrieved from https://resus.org.au/download/section_8/anzcor-guideline-8-cpr-jan16.pdf.

Avery, G. 2017. *Law and ethics in nursing healthcare: An introduction* (2nd edn). Thousand Oaks, CA: Sage.

Bailey, S.C., Fang, G., Annis, I.E., O'Conor, R., Paasche-Orlow, M.K. & Wolf, M.S. 2015. Health literacy and 30-day hospital readmission after acute myocardial infarction. *BMJ Open*, 5, e006975. Retrieved from http://doi.org/10.1136/bmjopen-2014-006975.

Ball, C. & Dunn L. 1995. *Non-governmental organisations: Guidelines for good policy and practice*. London: The Commonwealth Foundation.

Ball, J., Murrells, T., Rafferty, A., Morrow, E. & Griffiths, P. 2013. 'Care left undone' during nursing shifts: Associations with workload and perceived quality of care. *BMJ Quality and Safety*, 23(2), 116–25.

Barksby, J., Butcher, N. & Whysall, A. 2015. A new model of reflection for clinical practice. *Nursing Times*, 111, 21–3.

Barritt, E. 1973. Florence Nightingale's values and modern nursing education. *Nursing Forum*, 12, 472–6.

Batalden, M., Batalden, P., Margolis, P., Seid, M., Armstrong, G., Opipari-Arrigan, L. & Hartung, H. 2016. Coproduction of healthcare service. *BMJ Quality & Safety*, 25, 509.

Bate, P. & Robert, G. 2006. Experience-based design: From redesigning the system around the patient to co-designing services with the patient. *Quality and Safety in Healthcare*, 15, 307–10.

Batey, M. & Lewis, F. 1982. Clarifying autonomy and accountability in nursing service: Part 1. *Journal of Nursing Administration*, 12, 13–18.

Beauchamp, T. & Childress, J. 2012. *Principles of biomedical ethics*. Oxford: Oxford University Press.

Beaumont, K. 2008. Deterioration in hospital patients: Early signs and appropriate actions. *Nursing Standard*, 23, 43–8.

Beck, S., Weiss, M., Ryan-Wenger, N., Donaldson, N., Aydin, C., Towsley, G. & Gardner, W. 2013. Measuring nurses' impact on health care quality: Progress, challenges, and future directions. *Medical Care*, 51, S15–22.

Benjamin, A. 2008. Audit: how to do it in practice. *BMJ*, 336, 1241.

Benner, P. 2001. *From novice to expert: Excellence and power in clinical nursing practice*. Upper Saddle River, NJ: Prentice Hall.

Benner, P. & Tanner, C. 1987. Clinical judgment: How expert nurses use intuition. *American Journal of Nursing*, 87(1), 23–31.

Benner, P., Tanner, C. & Chesla, C. 2009. *Expertise in nursing practice: Caring, clinical judgement, and ethics*. New York: Springer.

Benner, P. & Wrubel, J. 1989. *The primacy of caring*. Menlo Park, CA: Addison-Wesley.

Berkman, N.D., Sheridan, S.L., Donahue, K.E., Halpern, D.J., Viera, A., Crotty, K. et al. 2011. Health literacy interventions and outcomes: An updated systematic review. *Evidence Report/Technology Assessment* (Full Rep), 199, 1–941.

Berry-Millett, R. & Bodenheimer, T.S. 2009. *Care management of patients with complex health care needs*. Research Synthesis Report No. 19, Princeton, NJ: The Synthesis Project.

Bertram, M., Norman, R., Kemp, L. & Vos, T. 2011. Review of the long-term disability associated with hip fractures. *Injury Prevention*, 17, 365–70.

Bigby, J. & Ashley, S. 2008. Disparities in surgical care strategies for enhancing provider–patient communication. *World Journal of Surgery*, 32, 529–32.

Billingsley, S., Collins, A. & Miller, M. 2007. Healthy student, healthy nurse: A stress management workshop. *Nurse Educator*, 32, 49–51.

Bittner, N. & Gravlin, G. 2009. Critical thinking, delegation, and missed care in nursing practice. *Journal of Nursing Administration*, 39, 142–6.

Blanchfield, K.C. & Biordi, D.L. 1996. Power in practice: A study of nursing authority and autonomy. *Nursing Administration Quarterly*, 20, 42–9.

Blass, F. & Ferris, G. 2007. Leader reputation: the role of mentoring, political skill, contextual learning, and adaptation. *Human Resource Management*, 46, 5–19.

Bohmer, R. 2010. Fixing health care on the front lines. *Harvard Business Review*, 88, 62–9.

Bolger, G. & Moss, R. 2015. Reducing errors in blood transfusion with barcodes. *Nursing Times*, 111, 18–19.

Bonnet, M.H. & Arand, D.L. 2017. Treatment of insomnia in adults. UpToDate. Retrieved from www.uptodate.com/contents/treatment-of-insomnia-in-adults.

Bonura, D.F., Roesler, M. & Pacquiao, D. 2001. Culturally congruent end-of-life care for Jewish patients and their families. *Journal of Transcultural Nursing*, 12, 211–20.

Boulding, W., Glickman, S., Manary, M., Schulman, K. & Staelin, R. 2011. Relationship between patient satisfaction with inpatient care and hospital readmission within 30 days. *American Journal of Managed Care*, 17, 41–8.

Boursnell, M. & Prosser, S. 2010. Increasing identification of domestic violence in emergency departments: A collaborative contribution to increasing the quality of practice of emergency nurses. *Contemporary Nurse*, 35, 35–46.

Bove, L. & Jesse, H. 2010. Worklists: Helping to transform nursing care. *ANIA-Caring Newsletter*, 25, 1–7.

Boyett, J. 2016. *12 major world religions: The beliefs, rituals, and traditions of humanity's most influential faiths.* Berkeley, CA: Zephyros Press.

Bradley, C. 2012. *Hospitalisations due to falls by older people, Australia 2008–09.* Canberra: AIHW.

——2014. *Hospitalisations due to falls by older people, Australia, 2009–10.* Injury Research and Statistics Series 70. Cat. no. INJCAT 146. Canberra: AIHW.

Brady, R., Fraser, S., Dunlop, M., King, P., Paterson-Brown, S. & Gibb, A. 2007. Bacterial contamination of mobile communication devices in the operative environment. *Journal of Hospital Infection*, 66, 397–8.

Brennan, N. & Flynn, M. 2013. Differentiating clinical governance, clinical management and clinical practice. *Clinical Governance: An International Journal*, 18, 114–31.

Brewer, C.S., Kovner, C.T., Djukic, M., Fatehi, F., Greene, W., Chacko, T.P. & Yang, Y. 2016. Impact of transformational leadership on nurse work outcomes. *Journal of Advanced Nursing*, 72, 2879–93.

Brunero, S., Cowan, D., Grochulski, A. & Garvey, A. 2006. *Stress management for nurses.* Retrieved from www.health.nsw.gov.au/nursing/Publications/stress-mngt.pdf.

Burkhardt, M. & Nathaniel, A. 2013. *Ethics and issues in contemporary nursing.* Clifton Park, NY: Thompson Delmar Learning.

Butterworth, T., Faugier, J. & Burnard, P. 1998. *Clinical supervision and mentorship in nursing.* Cheltenham: Stanley Thornes.

Callaly, T. & Arya, D. 2005. Organizational change management in mental health. *Australian Psychiatry*, 13, 120–3.

Cameron, P. & O'Reilly, G. 2010. Trauma. In P. Cameron, G. Jelinek, A. Kelly, L. Murray & A. Brown (eds), *Textbook of adult emergency medicine.* Sydney: Churchill Livingstone Elsevier.

Cancer Council NSW 2013. The role of NGOs. *The state of cancer control in Australia 1987–2007.* Retrieved from www.cancercouncil.com.au/reports-and-publications/state-of-cancer-control-in-australia-1987-2007/cancer-control/role-of-ngos/.

Card, A.J., Ward, J.R. & Clarkson, P.J. 2014. Rebalancing risk management—part 1: The process for active risk control (PARC). *Journal of Healthcare Risk Management*, 34, 21–30.

Carroll, P. & Shiraishi, C. 1995. The Catholic patient in the emergency department. *Journal of Emergency Nursing*, 21, 513–14.

Cashin, A., Carery, M., Watson, N., Clark, G., Newman, C. & Waters, C. 2009. Ultimate doctor liability: a myth of ignorance or myth of control? *Collegian*, 16, 125–129.

Cashin, A., Stasa, H., Gullick, J., Conway, R., Cunich, M. & Buckley, T. 2015. Clarifying clinical nurse consultant work in Australia: A phenomenological study. *Collegian*, 22, 405–12.

Cass, A., Lowell, A., Christie, M., Snelling, P., Flack, M., Marrnganyin, B. & Brown, I. 2002. Sharing the true stories: Improving communication between Aboriginal patients and health-care workers. *Medical Journal of Australia*, 176, 466–70.

Central Coast Local Health Network & Northern Sydney Local Health Network 2011. *International medical graduates: orientation handbook* (2nd edn). Retrieved from www.cclhd.health.nsw.gov.au/careers/Documents/IMGOrientationHandbook.pdf.

Chaloner, C. 2007. Ethics in nursing: The way forward. *Nursing Standard*, 21, 40–1.

Chang, E. & Hancock, K. 2003. Role stress and role ambiguity in new nursing graduates in Australia. *Nurse and Health Sciences*, 5, 155–63.

Cheragi, M.A., Manoocheri, H., Mohammadnejad, E. & Ehsani, S.R. 2013. Types and causes of medication errors from nurse's viewpoint. *Iranian Journal of Nursing and Midwifery Research*, 18, 228–31.

Chuan-Yuan, C., Ying-Tai, W., Ming-Hsia, H. & Jia-Te, L. 2013. Reflective learning in physical therapy students: Related factors and facilitative effects of a short introduction. *Procedia: Social and Behavioral Sciences*, 93, 1362–7.

Churpek, M.M., Yuen, T.C. & Edelson, D.P. 2013. Risk stratification of hospitalized patients on the wards. *Chest,* 143, 1758–65.

Cipriano, P.F., Bowles, K., Dailey, M., Dykes, P., Lamb, G. & Naylor, M. 2013. The importance of health information technology in care coordination and transitional care. *Nursing Outlook,* 61, 475–89.

Comerford, M. 2004. Issues in patient education. *Journal of Midwifery & Women's Health,* 49, 203–9.

—— 2010. Issues in patient education: Principles of patient education. Retrieved from www. medscape.com/viewarticle/478283_3.

Committee on Identifying and Preventing Medication Errors 2007. *Preventing medication errors: Quality chasm series.* Washington DC: The National Academies Press.

Committee on Quality of Health Care in America 2001. *Crossing the quality chasm: A new health system for the 21st century.* Washington, DC: Institute of Medicine.

Congress of Aboriginal and Torres Strait Islander Nurses and Midwives (CATSINaM) 2015a. CEO's welcome. Retrieved from http://catsinam.org.au/about-us/ceos-welcome.

—— 2015b. What we do. Retrieved from http://catsinam.org.au/about-us/what-we-do.

Constantino, T. 2015. IMS Health Study: Patient options expand as mobile healthcare apps address wellness and chronic disease treatment needs. QuintilesIMS. Retrieved from www. imshealth.com/en/about-us/news/ims-health-study:-patient-options-expand-as-mobile-health-care-apps-address-wellness-and-chronic-disease-treatment-needs.

Cook, M. & Leathard, H. 2004. Learning for clinical leadership. *Journal of Nursing Management,* 12, 436–44.

Coroner's Court (New South Wales) 2015a. What happens when the Coroner is involved? Retrieved from www.coroners.justice.nsw.gov.au/Pages/what_happens_process/what_happens_process. aspx.

—— 2015b. The Coroner's role. Retrieved from www.coroners.justice.nsw.gov.au/Pages/coroner_role/coroner_role.aspx.

Council of Australian Governments (COAG) 2009. *Closing the gap in Indigenous disadvantage.* Retrieved from www.coag.gov.au/closing_the_gap_indigenous_disadvantage.

—— 2010. Council of Australian Governments meeting, 19 and 20 April 2010, Canberra communiqué. Retrieved from www.coag.gov.au/sites/default/files/communique/2010-20-04.pdf.

—— 2014. *Closing the gap in Indigenous disadvantage* (6th annual report). Retrieved from www.coag. gov.au/closing_the_gap_indigenous_disadvantage.

Cowin, L., Johnson, M., Wilson, I. & Borgese, K. 2013. The psychometric properties of five professional identity measures in a sample of nursing students. *Nurse Education Today,* 33, 608–13.

Crawford, M. J., Rutter, D., Manley, C., Weaver, T., Bhui, K., Fulop, N. & Tyrer, P. 2002. Systematic review of involving patients in the planning and development of healthcare. *BMJ,* 325, 1263.

Creasia, J. & Parker, B. 2001. *Conceptual foundations: The bridge to professional nursing practice.* Toronto: Mosby.

Critical Appraisal Skills Program 2014. CASP checklists. Retrieved from www.casp-uk.net/ #!checklists/cb36.

Croskerry, P. 2009. A universal model of diagnostic reasoning. *Academic Medicine,* 84, 1022–8.

Curtis, A., Tzannes, A. & Rudge, T. 2011. How to talk to doctors: A guide for effective communication. *International Nursing Review,* 58, 13–20.

Cushin, A., Carey, M., Watson, N., Clark, G., Newman, C. & Waters, C. 2009. Ultimate doctor liability: A myth of ignorance or myth of control? *Collegian,* 16, 125–9.

Cuthbertson, B.H., Boroujerdi, M., Mckie, L., Aucott, L. & Prescott, G. 2007. Can physiological variables and early warning scoring systems allow early recognition of the deteriorating surgical patient? *Critical Care Medicine,* 35, 402–9.

Davidson, P., Elliott, D. & Daly, J. 2006. Clinical leadership in contemporary clinical practice: Implications for nursing in Australia. *Journal of Nursing Management*, 14, 180–7.

Davidson, S. 2005. The management of violence in general psychiatry. *Advances in Psychiatric Treatment*, 11, 362–70.

Davies, N. 2009. Build an effective team. *Nursing Standard*, 23, 72.

Demir, S., Demir, S.G., Bulut, H. & Hisar, F. 2014. Effect of mentoring program on ways of coping with stress and locus of control for nursing students. *Asian Nursing Research*, 8, 254–60.

Department of Health 2012. *Mental Health Statement of Rights and Responsibilities*. Retrieved from www.health.gov.au/internet/main/publishing.nsf/content/mental-pubs-m-rights2.

—— 2013a. *National Primary Health Care Strategic Framework*. Retrieved from www.health.gov.au/internet/main/publishing.nsf/content/6084A04118674329CA257BF0001A349E/$File/NPHCframe.pdf.

—— 2013b. *National Aboriginal and Torres Strait Islander Health Plan, 2013–2023*. Retrieved from www.health.gov.au/internet/main/publishing.nsf/content/B92E980680486C3BCA257BF0001BAF01/$File/health-plan.pdf.

—— 2014. *Aboriginal and Torres Strait Islander Health Curriculum Framework*. Retrieved from www.health.gov.au/internet/main/publishing.nsf/Content/72C7E23E1BD5E9CFCA257F640082CD48/$File/Health%20Curriculum%20Framework.pdf.

—— 2015. Australian Statistics on Medicines 2015. The Pharmaceutical Benefits Scheme. Retrieved from www.pbs.gov.au/info/statistics/asm/asm-2015.

—— 2016. Updating medicine ingredient names: List of affected ingredients. Therapeutic Goods Administration. Retrieved from www.tga.gov.au/updating-medicine-ingredient-names-list-affected-ingredients.

Department of Health (UK) 2001. *The Report of the Public Inquiry into Children's Heart Surgery at the Bristol Royal Infirmary 1984-1995: Learning From Bristol*. Retrieved from www.bristol-inquiry.org.uk/final_report/index.htm.

Department of Health and Human Services Tasmania. 2010. Local Hospital Networks: fact sheet. Retrieved from www.dhhs.tas.gov.au/__data/assets/pdf_file/0013/61015/Local_hospital_networks_-_fact_sheet.pdf.

Department of Social Services 2003. *Multicultural Australia: United in diversity*. Canberra: Commonwealth of Australia.

Dewey, J. 1938. *Experience and education*. New York: Touchstone.

Dietitians Association of Australia 2017. Dietitian or nutritionist? Retrieved from https://daa.asn.au/what-dietitans-do/dietitian-or-nutritionist/.

Dohmann, E. 2009. *Accountability in nursing: Six strategies to build and maintain a culture of commitment*. Marblehead: HCPro.

Dolan, B. 2012. Survey: 71 percent of US nurses use smartphones. Retrieved from http://mobihealthnews.com/17172/survey-71-percent-of-us-nurses-use-smartphones.

Donner, G. & Wheeler, M. 2001. Career planning and development for nurses: The time has come. *International Nursing Review*, 48, 79–85.

Doswell, W., Braxter, B., Devito Dabbs, A., Nilsen, W. & Klem, M. 2013. mHealth: Technology for nursing practice, education, and research. *Journal of Nursing Education and Practice*, 3, 99–109.

Douglas, K. 2014. Nurses eat their own: Bullying and horizontal violence takes its toll. *Australian Nursing and Midwifery Journal*, 21, 20–4.

Doyle, C., Lennox, L. & Bell, D. 2013. A systematic review of evidence on the links between patient experience and clinical safety and effectiveness. *BMJ Open*, 3, doi: 10.1136/bmjopen-2012-001570.

Doyle, J. 2008. Barriers and facilitators of multidisciplinary team working: A review. *Paediatric Nursing*, 20, 26–9.

Driscoll, J. 1994. Reflective practice for practice. *Senior Nurse*, 13, 47–50.

Drucker, P. 1954. *The practice of management*. New York: HarperCollins.

Duchscher, J. 2009. Transition shock: The initial stage of role adaptation for newly graduated registered nurses. *Journal of Advanced Nursing*, 65, 1103–13.

Duckett, S. 2005. Living in the parallel universe in Australia: Public Medicare and private hospitals. *Canadian Medical Association Journal*, 173, 745–7.

Duckett, S. & Willcox, S. 2015. *The Australian health care system*. Melbourne: Oxford University Press.

Dudgeon, P., Rickwood, D., Garvey, D. & Gridley, H. 2014. A history of Indigenous psychology. In P. Dudgeon, H. Milroy & R. Walker (eds), *Working together: Aboriginal and Torres Strait Islander mental health and wellbeing principles and practice* (2nd edn). Canberra: Commonwealth of Australia.

Duerden, M.G. & Hughes, D.A. 2010. Generic and therapeutic substitutions in the UK: Are they a good thing? *British Journal of Clinical Pharmacology*, 70, 335–41.

Duffield, C.M., Roche, M.A., Blay, N. & Stasa, H. 2011. Nursing unit managers, staff retention and the work environment. *Journal of Clinical Nursing*, 20, 23–33.

Duffy, J. 2013. *Quality caring in nursing and health systems: Implications for clinicians, educators, and leaders*, New York: Springer.

Duignan, P. 2007. *Educational leadership: Key challenges and ethical tensions*. Cambridge: Cambridge University Press.

Dunn, E. & Wolfe, J. 2001. Let go of Latin! *Veterinary and Human Toxicology*, 43, 235–6.

Dutton, P. 2014. *Rebuilding primary care*. Media release. Retrieved from www.health.gov.au/internet/budget/publishing.nsf/content/4F6FF55008B6AF6FCA257CD5007FF4A0/$File/Rebuilding%20Primary%20Care.pdf.

Dyess, S. & Sherman, R. 2009. The first year of practice: New graduate nurses' transition and learning needs. *Journal of Continuing Education in Nursing*, 40, 403–10.

Eager, K. 2001. *Health planning: Australian perspectives*. Sydney: Allen & Unwin.

Elder, R., Evans, K. & Nizette, D. (eds). 2009. *Psychiatric and mental health nursing*. Sydney: Mosby.

Eley, R., Soar, J., Buikstra, E., Fallon, T. & Hegney, D. 2009. Attitudes of Australian nurses to information technology in the workplace. *Computers, Informatics, Nursing*, 27, 114–21.

Ellershaw, J. & Ward, C. 2003. Care of the dying patient: The last hours or days of life. *British Medical Journal*, 326, 30–4.

Elliott, J., McNeil, H., Ashbourne, J., Huson, K., Boscart, V. & Stolee, P. 2016. Engaging older adults in healthcare decision-making: A realist synthesis. *Patient*, 9, 383–93.

Emmerton, L., Rizk, M., Bedford, G. & Lalor, D. 2015. Systematic derivation of an Australian standard for Tall Man lettering to distinguish similar drug names. *Journal of Evaluation in Clinical Practice*, 21, 85–90.

Evans, D., Hodgkinson, B., Lambert, L. & Wood, J. 2001. Falls risk factors in the hospital setting: A systematic review. *International Journal of Nursing Practice*, 7, 38–45.

Faithfull-Byrne, A., Thompson, L., Schafer, K.W., Elks, M., Jaspers, J., Welch, A., Williamson, M., Cross, W. & Moss, C. 2017. Clinical coaches in nursing and midwifery practice: Facilitating point of care workplace learning and development. *Collegian*, 24, 403–10.

Faugier, J. & Woolnough, H. 2003. Lessons from LEO. *Nursing Management*, 10, 22–5.

Fischer, S.A. 2016. Transformational leadership in nursing: A concept analysis. *Journal of Advanced Nursing*, 72, 2644–53.

Fook, J., White, S. & Gardner, F. 2006. Critical reflections: a review of contemporary literature and understandings. In S. White, J. Fook & F. Gardener (eds), *Critical reflection in health and social care*. Maidenhead: Open University Press.

Forrester, K. & Griffiths, D. 2014. *Essentials of law for health professionals*. Sydney: Elsevier.

Foster-Turner, J. 2006. *Coaching and mentoring in health and social care*. Oxford: Radcliffe Publishing.

Francis, R. 2013. *Report of the Mid Staffordshire NHS Foundation Trust Public Inquiry: Executive summary*. Retrieved from www.midstaffspublicinquiry.com.

Franklin, N. & Chadwick, S. 2013. The impact of workplace bullying in nursing. *Australian Nursing Journal*, 21, 31.

Fry, S.T. 2008. *Ethics in nursing practice: A guide to ethical decision making*. Oxford: Wiley-Blackwell.

Fukuda-Parr, S. (ed.) 2004. *Human development report, 2004: Cultural liberty in today's diverse world*. Retrieved from http://hdr.undp.org/sites/default/files/reports/265/hdr_2004_complete.pdf.

Garbutt, J., Milligan, P., McNaughton, C., Waterman, B., Clairborne Dunagan, W. & Fraser, V. 2005. A practical approach to measure the quality of handwritten medication orders. *Journal of Patient Safety*, 1: 195–200.

Garcia, B.H., Elenjord, R., Bjornstad, C., Halvorsen, K.H., Hortemo, S. & Madsen, S. 2017. Safety and efficiency of a new generic package labelling: A before and after study in a simulated setting. *BMJ Quality and Safety*, 26, 817–23.

Gellis, Z. 2001. Social work perceptions of transformational and transactional leadership in health care. *Social Work Research*, 25, 17–25.

Gibbs, G. 1988. *Learning by doing: A guide to teaching and learning methods*. Oxford: Oxford Further Education Unit.

Gill, C.J. & Gill, G.C. 2005. Nightingale in Scutari: Her legacy reexamined. *Clinical Infectious Diseases*, 40, 1799–805.

Girard, N. 2007. Multitasking: How much is too much? *AORN Journal*, 85, 505–6.

Goodall, A. 2011. Physician-leaders and hospital performance: Is there an association? *Social Science & Medicine*, 73, 535–9.

Government of South Australia 2014. Workplace bullying. Retrieved from www.eoc.sa.gov.au/eo-you/workers/work/workplace-bullying.

Government of Western Australia 2014. *WA high risk medication policy*. Department of Health, Western Australia. Retrieved from www.health.wa.gov.au/circularsnew/attachments/947.pdf.

Grant, A. & Greene, J. 2001. *Coach yourself: Make a real change in your life*. London: Momentum Press.

Gray, D. 2006. *Health sociology: An Australian perspective*. Sydney: Pearson Education.

Gray, G. 1998. Access to medical care under strain: New pressures in Canada and Australia. *Journal of Health Politics, Policy and Law*, 23, 905–46.

Gray, M., Bliss, D.Z., Bookout, K., Colwell, J., Dutcher, J.A., Engberg, S., Evans, E., Jacobson, T. & Scemons, D. 2002. Evidence-based nursing practice: A primer for the WOC nurse. *Journal of Wound Ostomy & Continence Nursing*, 29, 283–6.

Green, L., Allard, S. & Cardigan, R. 2015. Modern banking, collection, compatibility testing and storage of blood and blood components. *Anaesthesia*, 70: 3–e2.

Greenleaf, R. 1977. *Servant leadership: A journey into the nature of legitimate power and greatness*. New York: Paulist Press.

Griffen, M. 2004. Teaching cognitive rehearsal as a shield for lateral violence: An intervention for newly licensed nurses. *Journal of Continuing Education for Nurses*, 35, 257–63.

Grimmer, K., Kennedy, K., Fulton, A., Guerin, M., Uy, J., Wiles, L. & Carroll, P. 2015. *Evidence check: Does comprehensive care lead to improved patients' outcomes in acute care settings?* Sydney: Sax Institute, ACSQHC.

Groves, P., Finfgeld-Connett, D. & Wakefield, B. 2014. It's always something: Hospital nurses managing risk. *Clinical Nursing Research*, 23, 296–313.

Habermas, J. 1978. *Knowledge of human interests*. London: Heinemann.

Haddad, M., Moxham, L. & Broadbent, M. 2013. Graduate registered nurse practice readiness in the Australian context: An issue worthy of discussion. *Collegian*, 20, 233–8.

Haffey, F., Brady, R. & Maxwell, S. 2013. A comparison of the reliability of smartphone apps for opioid conversion. *Drug Safety*, 36, 111–17.

Hamrosi, K., Taylor, S. & Aslani, P. 2006. Issues with prescribed medications in Aboriginal communities: Aboriginal health workers' perspectives. *Rural and Remote Health*, 6. Retrieved from www.rrh.org.au/articles/subviewnew.asp?ArticleID=557.

Hanssen, T.A., Nordrehaug, J.E., Eide, G.E. & Hanestad, B.R. 2007. Improving outcomes after myocardial infarction: A randomized controlled trial evaluating effects of a telephone follow-up intervention. *European Journal of Cardiovascular Prevention and Rehabilitation*, 14, 429–37.

Harper, E. 2012. Engineering a learning healthcare system: Using health information technology to develop an objective nurse staffing tool. In *NI 2012: Proceedings of the 11th International Congress on Nursing Informatics*.

Harris, N. 2001. Management of work-related stress in nursing. *Nursing Standard*, 16, 47–52.

Hassoun, A., Vellozzi, E. & Smith, M. 2004. Colonisation of personal digital assistants carried by healthcare professionals. *Infection Control and Hospital Epidemiology*, 25, 1000–1.

Headspace 2017. Who are we? Retrieved from www.headspace.org.au/about-us/who-we-are/.

Health Education and Training Institute (HETI) 2012. *The superguide: A handbook for supervising allied health professionals*. Sydney: HETI. Retrieved from www.heti.nsw.gov.au/Global/allied-health/The-Superguide.pdf.

—— 2014. *NSW Health: Respecting the difference*. Retrieved from www.nswhealth.seertechsolutions.com.au.

Health Workforce Australia 2013. *Australia's health workforce: Nurses in focus*. Adelaide: HWA.

Heineken, J. 1982. Power: Conflicting views. *Journal of Nursing Administration*, 15, 36–9.

Henley, A. & Clayton, J. 1982. The five signs of Sikhism. *Health and Social Service Journal*, 92, 943–5.

Herbert, A. 2001. *Protocols and customs at the time of Maori death*. Retrieved from www.whakawhetu.co.nz/sites/default/files/Protocols%20%26%20Customs%20at%20the%20Time%20of%20a%20Maori%20Death.pdf.

Higgins, R. 2011. *Tangihanga: Death customs*. Retrieved from www.TeAra.govt.nz/en/tangihanga-death-customs/page-1.

Hills, M. & Albarran, J.W. 2010a. After death 2: Exploring the procedures for laying out and preparing the body for viewing. *Nursing Times*, 106, 22–4.

—— 2010b. After death 1: Caring for bereaved relatives and being aware of cultural differences. *Nursing Times*, 106, 19–20.

Hodge, A. & Marshall, A. 2007. Violence and aggression in the emergency department: A critical care perspective. *Australian Critical Care*, 20, 61–7.

Hodge, A., Perry, L., Daly, B., Hagness, C. & Tracy, D. 2011. Revision and evaluation of an 'advanced' nursing role in an Australian emergency department. *Australasian Emergency Nursing Journal*, 14, 120–8.

Holliday, K. & Pearce, A. 2007. Stabilisation and transfer. In K. Curtis, C. Ramsden, & J. Friendship (eds), *Emergency and trauma nursing*. Sydney: Mosby Elsevier.

Hooker, L., Ward, B. & Verrinder, G. 2012. Domestic violence screening in maternal and child health nursing practice: A scoping review. *Contemporary Nurse*, 43, 198–215.

Hope, M. 2011. *Multicultural care at the time of death and dying*. Retrieved from www.alfredicu.org.au/assets/Documents/ICU-Guidelines/DeathAndDying/CaldmulticulturalCareDeathDying.pdf.

Horton, D. 2015. *Unity and diversity: The history and culture of Aboriginal Australia*. Retrieved from www.gov.au/Ausstats/abs@.nsf/Previousproducts/1301.0Feature%20Article31994?opendocument&tabname=Summary&prodno=1301.0&issue=1994&num=&view=.

Horvath, J. 2014. *Review of Medicare Locals: Report to the minister for health and minister for sport*. Retrieved from www.health.gov.au/internet/main/publishing.nsf/content/A69978FAABB1225 ECA257CD3001810B7/$File/Review-of-Medicare-Locals-may2014.pdf.

Hsieh, C., Yun, D., Bhatia, A., Hsu, J. & Ruiz De Luzuriaga, A. 2015. Patient perceptions on the usage of smartphones for medical photography and for reference in dermatology. *Dermatologic Surgery*, 41, 149–54.

Hudson, P. & Marshall, A. 2008. Extending the nursing role in emergency departments: Challenges for Australia. *Australasian Emergency Nursing Journal*, 11, 39–48.

Hudspeth, R. 2007. Understanding delegation is a critical competency for nurses in the new millennium. *Nursing Administration Quarterly*, 31, 183–4.

Hurley, M. 2007. Managing stress in the workplace. *Nursing Management*, 14, 16–18.

Hutchinson, M. 2009. Restorative approaches to workplace bullying: Educating nurses towards shared responsibility. *Contemporary Nurse*, 32, 147–55.

Hutchinson, M., Wilkes, L., Jackson, D. & Vickers, M. 2010. Integrating individual, work group and organizational factors: Testing a multidimensional model of bullying in the nursing workplace. *Journal of Nursing Management*, 18, 173–81.

Institute for Safe Medication Practices (ISMP) 2005. ISMP's list of error-prone abbreviations, symbols, and dose designations. Retrieved from www.ismp.org/Tools/errorproneabbreviations. pdf.

Institute of Medicine 2011. *The future of nursing: Leading the change, advancing health*. Washington, DC: National Academies Press.

International Council of Nurses 2007. *Career development in nursing* [Position Statement]. Retrieved from www.icn.ch/images/stories/documents/publications/position_statements/C02_Career_ Development_Nsg.pdf.

—— 2012. *The ICN code of ethics for nurses*. Retrieved from www.icn.ch/images/stories/documents/ about/icncode_english.pdf.

Jackson, D. & Daly, J. 2004. Current challenges and issues facing nursing in Australia. *Nursing Science Quarterly*, 17, 352–5.

Jacques, T., Fisher, M., Hillman, K. & Fraser, K. (eds) 2009. *DETECT manual: Detecting deterioration, evaluation, treatment, escalation and communicating in teams*. Sydney: Department of Health.

Jacques, T., Harrison, G., Mclaws, M. & Kilborn, G. 2006. Combinations of early signs of critical illness predict in-hospital death: The SOCCER Study [signs of critical conditions and emergency responses]. *Resuscitation*, 71, 327–34.

Johns, C. 2000. *Becoming a reflective practitioner*. Oxford: Blackwell.

Johnson, M., Cowin, L., Wilson, I. & Young, H. 2012. Professional identity and nursing: Contemporary theoretical developments and future research challenges. *International Nursing Review*, 59, 562–9.

Johnstone, M.-J. 2011. Nursing and justice as a basic human need. *Nursing Philosophy*, 12, 34–44.

Johnstone, M.-J., Da Costa, C. & Turale, S. 2004. Registered and enrolled nurses: Experiences of ethical issues in nursing practice. *Australian Journal of Advanced Nursing*, 22, 24–30.

Johnstone, M.-J., Kanitsaki, O. & Currie, T. 2008. The nature and implications of support in graduate nurse transition programs: An Australian study. *Journal of Professional Nursing*, 24, 46–53.

Jones, D. 2010. The medical emergency team. In P. Cameron, G. Jelinek, A. Kelly, L. Murray & A. Brown (eds), *Textbook of adult emergency medicine* (3rd edn). Sydney: Churchill Livingstone.

Jonsen, A., Siegler, M. & Winslade, W. 2006. *Clinical ethics: A practical approach to ethical decisions in clinical medicine*. New York: McGraw-Hill.

Jooste, K. 2004. Leadership: A new perspective. *Journal of Nursing Management*, 12, 217–23.

Jorm, C.M., White, S. & Kaneen, T. 2009. Clinical handover: Critical communications. *Medical Journal of Australia*, 190, 108–9.

Kangasniemi, M., Pakkanen, P. & Korhonen, A. 2015. Professional ethics in nursing: An integrative review. *Journal of Advanced Nursing*, 71, 1744–57.

Keast, K. 2015. Australia's Chief Nurse Dr Rosemary Bryant: My career as a nurse leader. Retrieved from https://healthtimes.com.au/hub/nursing-careers/6/guidance/kk1/australias-chief-nurse-dr-rosemary-bryant-my-career-as-a-nurse-leader/461.

Kendall-Raynor, P. 2012. New delegation standards could strengthen nurses' accountability. *Nursing Standard*, 26, 5.

Kennedy, C., Brooks-Young, P., Brunton Gray, C., Larkin, P., Connolly, M., Wilde-Larsson, B., Larsson, M., Smith, T. & Chater, S. 2014. Diagnosing dying: An integrative literature review. *BMJ Supportive & Palliative Care*, 4, 263–70.

Kerridge, I., Lowe, M. & McPhee, J. 2005. *Ethics and law for the health professions*. Sydney: Federation Press.

Kilner, E. & Sheppard, L. 2010. The role of teamwork and communication in the emergency department: A systematic review. *International Emergency Nursing*, 18, 127–37.

Kiser, K. 2011. 25 ways to use your smartphone: Physicians share their favorite uses and apps. *Minnesota Medicine*, 94, 22–9.

Kitson, A., Marshall, A., Bassett, K. & Zeitz, K. 2013. What are the core elements of patient-centred care? A narrative review and synthesis of the literature from health policy, medicine and nursing. *Journal of Advanced Nursing*, 69, 4–15.

Kleinknecht, M.K. & Hefferin, E.A. 1982. Assisting nurses toward professional growth: A career development model. *Journal of Nursing Administration*, 12, 30–6.

Kolb, D. 1984. *Experiential learning: Experience as the source of learning and development*. London: Prentice Hall.

Kotter, J. & Rathgeber, H. 2016. *That's not how we do it here! A story about how organizations rise, fall—and can rise again*: London: Portfolio Penguin.

Kurrle, S. 2004. Elder abuse. *Australian Family Physician*, 33, 807–12.

Lamb, B., Taylor, C., Lamb, J., Strickland, S., Vincent, C., Green, J. & Sevdalis, N. 2013. Facilitators and barriers to teamworking and patient centeredness in multidisciplinary cancer teams: Findings of a national study. *Annals of Surgical Oncology*, 20, 1408–16.

Lamond, D. & Thompson, C. 2000. Intuition and analysis in decision making and choice. *Journal of Nursing Scholarship*, 32, 411–14.

Lane, A. & Cheek, J. 1997. Health policy and the nursing profession: A deafening silence. *International Journal of Nursing Practice*, 3, 2–9.

Larson, A., Gillies, M., Howard, P. & Coffin, J. 2007. It's enough to make you sick: The impact of racism on the health of Aboriginal Australians. *Australian and New Zealand Journal of Public Health*, 31, 322–9.

Laschinger, H., Grau, A., Finegan, J. & Wilk, P. 2010. New graduate nurses' experiences of bullying and burnout in hospital settings. *Journal of Advanced Nursing*, 66, 2732–42.

Laschinger, H.K., Wong, C.A. & Grau, A.L. 2013. Authentic leadership, empowerment and burnout: A comparison in new graduates and experienced nurses. *Journal of Nursing Management*, 21, 541–52.

Lay, K. & McGuire, L. 2010. Building a lens for critical reflection and reflexivity in social work education. *Social Work Education: The International Journal*, 29, 539–50.

LeBlanc, E., Hillier, T., Pedula, K., Rizzo, J., Cawthon, P. & Fink, H. 2011. Hip fracture and increased short-term but not long-term mortality in healthy older women. *Archives of Internal Medicine*, 171, 1831–7.

Leijen, A., Valtna, K., Leijen, D. & Pedaste, M. 2011. How to determine the quality of students' reflections? *Studies in Higher Education*, 37, 203–17.

Lenthall, S., Wakerman, J., Opie, T., Dunn, S., Macleod, M., Dollard, M., Rickard, G. & Knight, S. 2011. Nursing workforce in very remote Australia: Characteristics and key issues. *Australian Journal of Rural Health*, 19, 32–7.

Levett-Jones, T. & Fitzgerald, M. 2005. A review of graduate nurse transition programs in Australia. *Australian Journal of Advanced Nursing*, 23, 40–5.

Levine, C., Halper, D., Peist, A. & Gould, D.A. 2010. Bridging troubled waters: Family caregivers, transitions, and long-term care. *Health Affairs*, 29, 116–24.

Lewis, C. 2011. From the editor's perspective: Suggestions to regain a healthy work–life balance. *Journal of Vascular Nursing*, 29, 133–4.

Lewis, J. 2005. Being around and knowing the players: Networks of influence in health policy. *Social Science & Medicine*, 65, 2125–36.

Lu, C.Y., MacNeill, P., Williams, K. & Day, R. 2008. Access to high cost medicines in Australia: Ethical perspectives. *Australia and New Zealand Health Policy*, 5, 4.

McAllister, M., John, T. & Gray, M. 2009. In my day: Using lessons from history, ritual and our elders to build professional identity. *Nurse Education in Practice*, 9, 277–83.

McComb, S. & Hebdon, M. 2013. Enhancing patient outcomes in healthcare systems through multidisciplinary teamwork. *Clinical Journal of Oncology Nursing*, 7, 669–72.

McMurray, A., Chaboyer, W., Wallis, M. & Fetherston, C. 2010. Implementing bedside handover: Strategies for change management. *Journal of Clinical Nursing*, 19, 2580–9.

Madsen, W., McAllester, M., Godden, J., Greenhill, J. & Reed, R. 2009. Nursing's orphans: How the system of nursing education in Australia is undermining professional identity. *Contemporary Nurse*, 32, 9–18.

Maher, P. 1999. A review of 'traditional' Aboriginal health beliefs. *Australian Journal of Rural Health*, 7, 229–36.

Malloy, T. & Penprase, B. 2010. Nursing leadership style and psychosocial work environment. *Journal of Nursing Management*, 18, 715–25.

Manthey, M. 2009. The 40th anniversary of primary nursing: Setting the record straight. *Creative Nursing*, 15, 36–8.

Mantzoukas, S. & Watkinson, S. 2006. Review of advanced nursing practice: The international literature and developing the generic features. *Journal of Clinical Nursing*, 16, 28–37.

Marquis, K. & Huston, C. 2009. *Leadership roles and management functions in nursing: Theory and application*. Philadelphia, PA: Lippincott, Williams & Wilkins.

Martin, K. 2003. Ways of knowing, being and doing: A theoretical framework and methods for Indigenous and Indigenist research. In K. McWilliam, P. Stephenson & G. Thompson (eds), *Voicing dissent*. Brisbane: University of Queensland Press.

Mathews, B., Walsh, K. & Fraser, J. 2006. Mandatory reporting by nurses of child abuse and neglect. *Journal of Law and Medicine*, 13, 505–17.

Mathukia, C., Fan, W., Vadyak, K., Biege, C. & Krishnamurthy, M. 2015. Modified Early Warning System improves patient safety and clinical outcomes in an academic community hospital. *Journal of Community Hospital Internal Medicine Perspectives*, 5(2), doi: 10.3402/jchimp.v5.26716.

Medicines.org.au 2017. Retrieved from www.medicines.org.au/index.cfm.

MedlinePlus 2015. Bethesda, MD: National Library of Medicine (US). Retrieved from https://medlineplus.gov/druginformation.html.

Melnyk, B.M., Fineout-Overholt, E., Fischbeck Feinstein, N., Li, H., Small, L., Wilcox, L. & Kraus, R. 2004. Nurses' perceived knowledge, beliefs, skills, and needs regarding evidence-based practice: Implications for accelerating the paradigm shift. *Worldviews on Evidence-Based Nursing*, 1, 185–93.

Melnyk, B.M., Fineout-Overholt, E., Gallagher-Ford, L. & Kaplan, L. 2012. The state of evidence-based practice in US nurses: Critical implications for nurse leaders and educators. *Journal of Nursing Administration*, 42, 410–17.

Ménard, L. & Ratnapalan, S. 2013. Reflection in medicine: models and application. *Canadian Family Physician*, 59, 105–7.

Mercy Hospital 2016. Tikaka best practice guidelines. Retrieved from www.mercyhospital.org.nz/about-us/mercy-hospital/tikaka-best-practice-guidelines.

Merriam-Webster 2007. *Merriam-Webster's medical desk dictionary*. Springfield, IL: Thomson Delmar Learning.

Mickan, S. & Rodger, S. 2000. Characteristics of effective teams: a literature review. *Australian Health Review*, 23, 201–8.

Mills, J., Francis, K., Birks, M., Coyle, M., Henderson, S. & Jones, J. 2010. Registered nurses as members of interprofessional primary health care teams in remote or isolated areas of Queensland: Collaboration, communication and partnerships in practice. *Journal of Interprofessional Care*, 24, 587–96.

Milton, C.L. 2004. The ethics of personal integrity in leadership and mentorship: A nursing theoretical perspective. *Nursing Science Quarterly*, 17, 116–20.

Missen, K., McKenna, L. & Beauchamp, A. 2014. Satisfaction of newly graduated nurses enrolled in transition-to-practice programmes in their first year of employment: A systematic review. *Journal of Advanced Nursing*, 70, 2419–33.

Mitchell, P.H. 2008. Defining patient safety and quality care. In R.G. Hughes (ed.), *Patient Safety and Quality: An evidence-based handbook for nurses*. Rockville, MD: Agency for Healthcare Research and Quality (US).

Mooney, N. 2013. Introduction to Indigenous Australia. Retrieved from http://australianmuseum.net.au/Indigenous-Australia-Introduction.

Morley, C. 2004. Critical reflection in social work: A response to globalisation? *International Journal of Social Welfare*, 13, 297–303.

Moroney, N. & Knowles, C. 2006. Innovation and teamwork: Introducing multidisciplinary team ward rounds. *Nursing Management*, 13, 28–31.

Moylan, C.A., Herrenkohl, T.I., Sousa, C., Tajima, E.A., Herrenkohl, R.C. & Russo, M.J. 2010. The effects of child abuse and exposure to domestic violence on adolescent internalizing and externalizing behavior problems. *Journal of Family Violence*, 25, 53–63.

Mullen, J. 2015. Patient education and communication. In K. Curtis & C. Ramsden (eds), *Emergency and trauma care*. Sydney: Elsevier.

Murphy, L. 2005. Transformational leadership: A cascading chain reaction. *Journal of Nursing Management*, 13, 128–36.

Nagpal, K., Arora, S., Abboudi, M., Vats, A., Wong, H.W., Manchanda, C., Vincent, C. & Moorthy, K. 2010. Postoperative handover: Problems, pitfalls and prevention of error. *Annals of Surgery*, 252, 171–6.

Nakata, M. 2007. The cultural interface. *Australian Journal of Aboriginal and Torres Strait Islander Education*, 36, 7–14.

Nakata, M., Nakata, V., Keech, S. & Bolt, R. 2012. Decolonial goals and pedagogies for Indigenous studies. *Decolonization: Indigeneity, Education & Society*, 1, 120–40.

National Aboriginal Community Controlled Health Organisation (NACCHO) 2017. About the National Aboriginal Community Controlled Health Organisation. Retrieved from www.naccho.org.au/about/.

National Aboriginal Health Strategy Working Party 1989. *A National Aboriginal Health Strategy: Report*. Canberra: AGPS.

National Aboriginal and Torres Strait Islander Health Worker Association (NATSIHWA) 2016. History. Retrieved from www.natsihwa.org.au.

National Patient Safety Agency 2004. *Safe handover: Safe patients,* London: British Medical Association.

Naylor, M.D., Hirschman, K.B., O'Connor, M., Barg, R. & Pauly, M.V. 2013. Engaging older adults in their transitional care: What more needs to be done? *Journal of Comparative Effectiveness Research,* 2, 457–68.

Nguyen, K.-H., Chaboyer, W. & Whitty, J. 2015. Pressure injury in Australian public hospitals: A cost-of-illness study. *Australian Health Review,* 39, 329–36.

Nicholson Thomas, E., Edwards, L. & McArdle, P. 2017. Knowledge is power: A quality improvement project to increase patient understanding of their hospital stay. *BMJ Quality Improvement Reports,* 6. Retrieved from http://bmjopenquality.bmj.com/content/6/1/u207103.w3042.full.

Northern Territory Government 2017. Restricted Schedule 4 Medicines PHC Remote Guideline. Retrieved from http://remotehealthatlas.nt.gov.au/restricted_schedule_4_medicines.pdf.

Northouse, P. 2015. *Leadership: Theory and practice.* Thousand Oaks, CA: Sage.

NSW Government 2011. Public Health System Nurses' and Midwives' (State) Award.

NSW Health 2005a. *Patient Safety and Clinical Quality Program.* Policy Directive PD2005_608. Retrieved from www1.health.nsw.gov.au/pds/ActivePDSDocuments/PD2005_608.pdf.

—— 2005b. *Consent to medical treatment: Patient information.* Policy Directive PD2005_406. Retrieved from www1.health.nsw.gov.au/pds/ActivePDSDocuments/PD2005_406.pdf.

—— 2007. *Infection Control Policy.* Policy Directive PD2007_036. Retrieved from www1.health.nsw.gov.au/pds/ActivePDSDocuments/PD2007_036.pdf.

—— 2010. *Fire safety in health care facilities.* Policy Directive PD2010_024. Retrieved from www1.health.nsw.gov.au/pds/ActivePDSDocuments/PD2010_024.pdf.

—— 2011a. *Domestic Violence Routine Screening Program.* Snapshot Report 9. Retrieved from www.health.nsw.gov.au/publications/Publications/Domestic_Violence_Screening.pdf.

—— 2011b. *Bullying: Prevention and management of workplace bullying in NSW Health.* Retrieved from www1.health.nsw.gov.au/pds/ActivePDSDocuments/PD2011_018.pdf.

—— 2013a. *Violence prevention and management: Promoting acceptable behaviour in the workplace.* Retrieved from www.heti.nsw.gov.au/Courses/Violence-Prevention---Promoting-Acceptable-Behaviour-in-the-Workplace.

—— 2013b. *Work health and safety: Better practice procedures.* Retrieved from www1.health.nsw.gov.au/pds/ActivePDSDocuments/PD2013_050.pdf.

—— 2014. *NSW Health Team Framework.* Retrieved from www.heti.nsw.gov.au/Global/Multimedia/leadership/NSW-Health-Team-Framework.pdf.

—— 2015a. *Incident management, complaints, public interest disclosures and disciplinary/grievance procedures.* Retrieved from www.health.nsw.gov.au/legislation/Pages/incident-management-complaints.aspx.

—— 2015b. *Recruitment and selection of staff to the NSW Health Service.* Retrieved from www1.health.nsw.gov.au/pds/ActivePDSDocuments/PD2015_026.pdf.

NSW JMO Forum 2016. *The doctor's compass.* Sydney: Health Education and Training Institute.

NSWNMA. 2017. Why join? Retrieved from www.nswnma.asn.au/nswnmamembers/benefits.

Nursing and Midwifery Board of Australia (NMBA) 2006. *Midwifery Competency Standards.* Retrieved from www.nursingmidwiferyboard.gov.au/documents/default.aspx?record=WD10%2f1350&dbid=AP&chksum=Yp0233q3xmE5YVjiy%2fy0mA%3d%3d.

—— 2010. *A National Framework for the Development of Decision-making Tools for Nursing and Midwifery Practice.* Melbourne: NMBA.

—— 2013a. *Code of Ethics for Nurses in Australia,* Melbourne: NMBA.

—— 2013b. *Code of Ethics for Midwives in Australia,* Melbourne: NMBA.

—— 2014. *Nurse Practitioner Standards for Practice.* Retrieved from www.nursingmidwiferyboard. gov.au/Registration-and-Endorsement/Endorsements-Notations.aspx#nurse.

—— 2015a. Internationally qualified nurses and midwives. Retrieved from www.nursingmidwifery board.gov.au/Registration-and-Endorsement/International.aspx.

—— 2015b. *Registration standard: English language skills.* Melbourne: NMBA.

—— 2016a. *Standards for Practice: Enrolled Nurses.* Melbourne: NMBA.

—— 2016b. *Fact sheet: Enrolled nurses and medication administration.* Melbourne: NMBA.

—— 2016c. *National Competency Standards for the Registered Nurse.* Melbourne: NMBA.

—— 2016d. *Registration Standard: Recency of Practice.* Melbourne: NMBA.

—— 2016e. *Fact sheet: Registered Nurse standards for practice.* Melbourne: NMBA.

—— 2016f. *Continuing Professional Development: Fact sheet.* Retrieved from www.nursingmidwifery board.gov.au/Codes-Guidelines-Statements/FAQ/CPD-FAQ-for-nurses-and-midwives.aspx.

—— 2018a. *Code of Professional Conduct for Nurses in Australia.* Melbourne: NMBA.

—— 2018b. *Code of Professional Conduct for Midwives in Australia.* Melbourne: NMBA.

Oberle K. & Allen, M. 2001. The nature of advanced practice nursing. *Nursing Outlook,* 49, 148–53.

Occupational Therapy Australia 2017. About occupational therapy. Retrieved from www.otaus. com.au/about.

O'Daniel, M. & Rosenstein, A. 2008. Professional communication and team collaboration. In R. Hughes (ed.), *Patient safety and quality: An evidence-based handbook for nurses.* Rockville, MD: Agency for Healthcare Research and Quality.

O'Leary, K., Ritter, C., Wheeler, H., Szekendi, M., Brinton, T. & Williams, M. 2010. Teamwork on inpatient medical units: Assessing attitudes and barriers. *Quality and Safety in Health Care,* 19, 117–21.

Omeri, A. & Raymond, L. 2009. Diversity in the context of multicultural Australia: Implications for nursing practice. In J. Daly, S. Speedy & D. Jackson (eds), *Contexts of nursing: An introduction* (3rd edn). Sydney: Elsevier Churchill Livingstone.

Paans, W., Sermeus, W., Neiweg, R. & Van Der Schans, C. 2010. Determinants of the accuracy of nursing diagnoses: Influence of ready knowledge, knowledge sources, disposition toward critical thinking, and reasoning skills. *Journal of Professional Nursing,* 26, 232–41.

Palmer, G. & Short, S. 2007. *Health care and public policy: An Australian analysis.* Melbourne: Macmillan.

Paradies, Y., Harris, R. & Anderson, I. 2008. *The impact of racism on Indigenous health in Australia and Aotearoa: Towards a research agenda.* Darwin: Cooperative Research Centre for Aboriginal Health.

Parkes, C., Laungani, P. & Young, B. 2015. *Death and bereavement across cultures.* London: Routledge.

Pascoe, H., Gill, S.D., Hughes, A. & McCall-White, M. 2014. Clinical handover: An audit from Australia. *The Australasian Medical Journal,* 7, 363–71.

Paton, J.Y., Ranmal, R. & Dudley, J. 2015. Clinical audit: Still an important tool for improving healthcare. *Archives of Disease in Childhood—Education & Practice Edition,* 100, 83–8.

Pattinson, N. 2008. Caring for patients after death. *Nursing Standard,* 22, 48–56.

Pavlish, C., Brown-Saltzman, K., Hersh, M., Shirk, M. & Rounkle, A.M. 2011. Nursing priorities, actions, and regrets for ethical situations in clinical practice. *Journal of Nursing Scholarship,* 43, 385–95.

Pavlish, C., Brown-Saltzman, K., Jakel, P. & Rounkle, A. 2012. Nurses' responses to ethical challenges in oncology practice: An ethnographic study. *Clinical Journal of Oncology Nursing,* 16, 592–600.

Pharmaceutical Society of Australia 2017. What pharmacists do and where they work. Retrieved from www.psa.org.au/about/pharmacy-as-a-career/what-pharmacists-do-and-where-they-work.

Phillips, C., Hall, S., Pearce, C., Travaglia, J., De Lusignan, S., Love, T. & Kljakovic, M. 2010. *Improving quality through clinical governance in primary health care.* Canberra: Australian Primary Healthcare Research Institute.

Phillips, C., Kenny, A., Esterman, A. & Smith, C. 2014. A secondary data analysis examining the needs of graduate nurses in their transition to a new role. *Nurse Education in Practice*, 14, 106–11.

Pigott, H. 2001. Facing reality: The transition from student to graduate nurse. *Australian Nursing Journal*, 8, 24–6.

Piscotty, R. & Kalisch, B. 2014. Lost opportunities ... the challenges of 'missing nursing care'. *Nursing Management*, 45, 40–4.

Platzer, H., Snelling, J. & Blake, D. 1997. Promoting reflective practitioners in nursing: A review of theoretical models and research into the use of diaries and journals to facilitate reflection. *Teaching in Higher Education*, 2, 103–21.

Pomey, M.-P., Ghadiri, D. P., Karazivan, P., Fernandez, N. & Clavel, N. 2015. Patients as partners: A qualitative study of patients' engagement in their healthcare. *PLoS ONE*, 10, e0122499.

Potter, P., Deshields, T. & Kuhrik, M. 2010. Delegation practices between registered nurses and nursing assistive personnel. *Journal of Nursing Management*, 18, 157–65.

Powell, S. 2005. To multitask or not to multitask: That is the question. *Lippincott's Case Management*, 10, 221–2.

Power, P. 1999. Community treatment orders: The Australian experience. *Journal of Forensic Psychiatry*, 10, 91.

Powley, D. 2013. Reducing violence and aggression in the emergency department. *Emergency Nurse*, 21, 26–9.

Private Health Insurance Ombudsman 2017a. *Lifetime health cover.* Retrieved from www.privatehealth.gov.au/healthinsurance/incentivessurcharges/lifetimehealthcover.htm.

—— 2017b. *How Health Funds Work.* Retrieved from www.privatehealth.gov.au/healthfunds/howhealthfundswork.

Queensland Government 2017. Work-related bullying. Retrieved from www.worksafe.qld.gov.au/injury-prevention-safety/mental-health-at-work/tools-and-resources/workplace-bullying.

Queensland Health 2011. *Health Care Providers' Handbook on Hindu Patients.* Brisbane: Division of the Chief Health Officer, Queensland Health.

—— 2015. *Sad news, sorry business: Guidelines for caring for Aboriginal and Torres Strait Islander people through death and dying.* Retrieved from www.health.qld.gov.au/__data/assets/pdf_file/0023/151736/sorry_business.pdf.

Quested, B. & Rudge, T. 2003. Nursing care of dead bodies: A discursive analysis of last offices. *Journal of Advanced Nursing*, 41, 553–60.

Rafferty, A. 1993. *Leading questions: A discussion paper on the issues of nurse leadership.* London: King's Fund.

Ramsden, I. 1992. *Kawa whakaruruhau: Guidelines for nursing and midwifery education.* Wellington: Nursing Council of New Zealand.

Rathert, C., Wyrwich, M.D. & Boren, S.A. 2013. Patient-centered care and outcomes: A systematic review of the literature. *Medical Care Research and Review*, 70, 351–79.

Reveans, R. 1998. *ABC of action learning.* London: Lemos and Crane.

Reynolds, J. & Rogers, A. 2003. Leadership styles and situations. *Nursing and Management*, 9, 27–30.

Rigney, L.I. 1997. Internationalisation of an Indigenous anti-colonial cultural critique of research methodologies: A guide to Indigenist research methodology and its principles. *Journal of Native American Studies*, 14(2), 109–21.

Riley, W. 2009. High reliability and implications for nursing leaders. *Journal of Nursing Management*, 17, 238–46.

Ritter, B. 2003. An analysis of expert nurse practitioners' diagnostic reasoning. *Journal of the American Academy of Nurse Practitioners*, 15, 137–41.

Robbins, B. & Davidhizar, R. 2007. Transformational leadership in health care today. *Health Care Manager*, 26, 234–9.

Roman, C., Poole, S., Walker, C., Smit, D.V. & Dooley, M.J. 2016. A 'time and motion' evaluation of automated dispensing machines in the emergency department. *Australasian Emergency Nursing Journal*, 19, 112–17.

Roughead, E.E., Semple, S.J. & Rosenfeld, E. 2016. The extent of medication errors and adverse drug reactions throughout the patient journey in acute care in Australia. *International Journal of Evidence-Based Healthcare*, 14, 113–22.

Rumbold, G. 1999. *Ethics in nursing practice*. London: Baillière-Tindall.

Russo, P., Cheng, A., Richards, M., Graves, N. & Hall, L. 2015. Healthcare-associated infections in Australia: Time for national surveillance. *Australian Health Review*, 39, 37–43.

Ruyters, M., Douglas, K. & Law, S. 2011. Blended learning using role-plays, wikis and blogs. *Journal of Learning Design*, 4, 45–55.

Rycroft-Malone, J., Seers, K., Titchen, A., Harvey, G., Kitson, A. & McCormack, B. 2004. What counts as evidence in evidence-based practice? *Nursing and Health Care Management and Policy*, 47, 81–90.

Saccomano, S. & Pinto-Zipp, G. 2011. Registered nurse leadership style and confidence in delegation. *Journal of Nursing Management*, 19, 522–33.

Safe Work Australia 2017. *Lifting, pushing and pulling*. Retrieved from www.safeworkaustralia.gov.au/manual-handling.

Salanova, M., Lorente, L., Chambel, M.J. & Martinez, I.M. 2011. Linking transformational leadership to nurses' extra-role performance: The mediating role of self-efficacy and work engagement. *Journal of Advanced Nursing*, 67, 2256–66.

Scally, G. & Donaldson, L.J. 1998. The NHS's 50th anniversary: Clinical governance and the drive for quality improvement in the new NHS in England. *BMJ*, 317, 61–5.

Schön, D. 1995. *The reflective practitioner: How professionals think in action*. Aldershot: Arena.

Seago, J. 2008. Professional communication. In R. Hughes (ed.), *Patient safety and quality: An evidence-based handbook for nurses*. Rockville, MD: Agency for Healthcare Research and Quality.

Sharp, A. 2010. A poor state of health: NSW hospitals the worst in the country. *Sydney Morning Herald*, 28 January. Retrieved from www.smh.com.au/national/a-poor-state-of-health-nsw-hospitals-the-worst-in-the-country-20100128-n1ry.html.

Sifers, S. 2012. Reflecting on teaching through reflective service-learning: A pedagogical journey. *Reflective Practice: International and Multidisciplinary Perspectives*, 13, 651–61.

Simmons, S. 2012. Striving for work–life balance. *Nursing*, 42, 25–6.

Simpson, J. 2014. Mandatory reporting of child abuse and neglect. *Queensland Nurse*, 33(2), 32–3.

Sinclair, R. 2004. Aboriginal social work education in Canada: Decolonizing pedagogy for the seventh generation. *First Peoples Child & Family Review*, 1, 49–61.

Skår, R. 2010. The meaning of autonomy in nursing practice. *Journal of Clinical Nursing*, 19, 2226–34.

Smith, M.A. 2011. Are you a transformational leader? *Nursing Management*, 42, 44–50.

Smith, M.E., Chiovaro, J.C., O'Neil, M., Kansagara, D., Quinones, A.R., Freeman, M., Motu'apuaka, M.L. & Slatore, C.G. 2014. Early warning system scores for clinical deterioration in hospitalized patients: A systematic review. *Annals of the American Thoracic Society*, 11, 1454–65.

Smith, M.M. 1982. Career development in nursing: An individual and professional responsibility. *Nursing Outlook*, 30, 128–31.

Sockolow, P., Laio, C., Chittams, J. & Bowles, K. 2012. Evaluating the impact of electronic health records on nurse clinical process at two community health sites. In *NI 2012: Proceedings of the 11th International Congress on Nursing Informatics*.

Sonmez, B. & Yildirim, A. 2009. What are the career planning and development practices for nurses in hospitals? Is there a difference between private and public hospitals? *Journal of Clinical Nursing*, 18, 3461–71.

Spears, L.C. 2010. Character and servant leadership: Ten characteristics of effective, caring leaders. *The Journal of Virtues and Leadership*, 1, 25–30.

Speech Pathology Australia 2017. What is a speech pathologist? Retrieved from www.speechpathologyaustralia.org.au/SPAweb/General_Information/SPAweb/General_Information/What_is_a_Speech_Pathologist/What_is_a_Speech_Pathologist.aspx

Spiegelhalter, D.J. 1999. Surgical audit: Statistical lessons from Nightingale and Codman. *Journal of the Royal Statistical Society: Series A (Statistics in Society)*, 162, 45–58.

Standing Council on Health 2013. *National Primary Healthcare Strategic Framework*. Canberra: Commonwealth Government.

Stanley, D. 2006a. In command of care: Clinical leadership in uncertain times. *Journal of Research in Nursing*, 2, 30–9.

—— 2006b. In command of care: Toward the theory of congruent leadership. *Journal of Research in Nursing*, 2, 132–44.

—— 2006c. Role conflict: Leaders and managers. *Nursing Management*, 13, 31–7.

—— 2007. Lights in the shadows: Florence Nightingale and others who made their mark. *Contemporary Nurse*, 24, 45–51.

—— 2008. Congruent leadership: Values in action. *Journal of Nursing Management*, 16, 519–24.

Starr, L. 2010. Preparing those caring for older adults to report elder abuse. *Journal of Continuing Education in Nursing*, 41, 231–5.

State Government of Victoria 2006. *PUPPS 3: Pressure ulcer point prevalence survey. Statewide report*. Melbourne: State Government of Victoria.

Statistics New Zealand 2013. *2013 Census QuickStats about Māori*. Retrieved from www.stats.govt.nz/Census/2013-census/profile-and-summary-reports/quickstats-about-maori-english.aspx.

Staunton, P. & Chiarella, M. 2013. *Law for nurses and midwives*. Sydney: Churchill Livingstone.

Stephenson, J. 1999. *Corporate capability: Implications for the style and direction of work-based learning*. Working Paper 99-14. Retrieved from http://pandora.nla.gov.au/pan/22468/20021106-0000/www.uts.edu.au/fac/edu/rcvet/working%20papers/9914Stephenson.pdf.

Stetler, C. 2001. Updating the Stetler model of research utilization to facilitate evidence based practice. *Nursing Outlook*, 49, 272–8.

Stevenson, J.E., Nilsson, G.C., Petersson, G.I. & Johansson, P.E. 2010. Nurses' experience of using electronic patient records in everyday practice in acute/inpatient ward settings: A literature review. *Health Informatics Journal*, 16, 63–72.

Stewart, B.M. & Krueger, L.E. 1996. An evolutionary concept analysis of mentoring in nursing. *Journal of Professional Nursing*, 12, 311–21.

Stone, A.G., Russell, R.F. & Patterson, K. 2004. Transformational versus servant leadership: A difference in leader focus. *Leadership & Organization Development Journal*, 25, 349–61.

Strategic Relations and Communications 2012. *Healthcare records—documentation and management*. Sydney: Department of Health.

Strauss, S., Johnson, M., Marquez, C. & Feldman, M. 2013. Characteristics of successful and failed mentoring relationships: A qualitative study across two academic health centres. *Academic Medicine*, 88, 82–9.

Sullivan, E., Hegney, D. & Francis, K. 2013. An action research approach to practice, service and legislative change. *Nurse Researcher*, 21, 8–13.

Sun, N., Wang, L., Zhou, J., Qiang, Y., Zhang, Z., Li, Y., Liang, M., Cheng, L., Gao, G. & Cui, X. 2011. International comparative analyses of healthcare risk management. *Journal of Evidence-Based Medicine*, 4, 22–31.

Sveinsdóttir H., Ragnarsdóttir E.D. & Blöndal K. 2016. Praise matters: The influence of nurse unit managers' praise on nurses' practice, work environment and job satisfaction: A questionnaire study. *Journal of Advanced Nursing*, 72, 558–68.

Tasmanian Government 2014. Schedule 8 and Declared Schedule 4 Medicines Management Policy. Department of Health and Human Services, Tasmania. Retrieved from www.catag.org.au/wp-content/uploads/2014/06/SPP-MSR-Policy-Schedule-8-and-Declared-Schedule-4-Management-20140804.pdf.

Tasmanian Government 2016. *How to prevent and respond to workplace bullying: A psychosocial hazard*. http://worksafe.tas.gov.au/__data/assets/pdf_file/0008/355724/Bullying_Guide.pdf.

Thomas, M.J.W., Schultz, T.J., Hannaford, N. & Runciman, W.B. 2013. Failures in transition: Learning from incidents relating to clinical handover in acute care. *Journal for Healthcare Quality*, 35, 49–56.

Thompson, C., McCaughan, D., Cullum, N., Sheldon, T., Thompson, D. & Mulhall, A. 2001. The accessibility of research-based knowledge for nurses in United Kingdom acute care settings. *Journal of Advanced Nursing*, 36, 11–22.

Thompson, D. & Burns, H. 2008. Reflection: An essential element of evidence-based practice. *Journal of Emergency Nursing*, 34, 246–8.

Titchen, A. & Ersser, S. 2000. Explicating, creating and validating professional craft knowledge. In J. Higgs & A. Titchen (eds), *Practice knowledge and expertise in the health professions*. Oxford: Butterworth Heinemann.

Toropov, B. & Buckles, L. 2011. *The complete idiot's guide to the world's religions*. New York: Alpha Books.

Townsend, R. 2007. Nursing and the law. In K. Curtis, C. Ramsden & J. Friendship (eds), *Emergency & trauma nursing*. Sydney: Mosby Elsevier.

Towsley, G., Beck, S. & Pepper, G. 2013. Predictors of quality in rural nursing homes using standard and novel methods. *Research in Gerontological Nursing*, 6, 116–26.

Tracey, C. & Nicholl, H. 2006. Mentoring and networking. *Nursing Management*, 12, 28–32.

Travaglia, J., Debono, D., Spigelman, A. & Braithwaite, J. 2011. Clinical governance: A review of key concepts in the literature. *Clinical Governance: An International Journal*, 16, 62–77.

Treanor, J. 2014. How to develop better practice in response to patients' complaints. *Nursing Management*, 21, 22–7.

Tremaine, R., Dorrian, J., Paterson, J., Neall, A., Piggott, E., Grech, C. & Pincombe, J. 2011. Actigraph estimates of the sleep of Australian midwives: The impact of shift work. *Biological Research for Nursing*, 15, 191–9.

Ulrich, C.M., Taylor, C., Soeken, K., O'Donnell, P., Farrar, A., Danis, M. & Grady, C. 2010. Everyday ethics: Ethical issues and stress in nursing practice. *Journal of Advanced Nursing*, 66, 2510–19.

United Nations 1948. *Universal Declaration of Human Rights*. Retrieved from www.ohchr.org/EN/UDHR/Documents/UDHR_Translations/eng.pdf.

—— 1966. *International Covenant on Economic, Social and Cultural Rights*. Retrieved from www.ohchr.org/Documents/ProfessionalInterest/cescr.pdf.

University of Bern 2009. STROBE checklists. Retrieved from www.strobe-statement.org/index.php?id=available-checklists.

Upshur, R. 2001. The status of qualitative research as evidence. In J. Morse, J. Swanson & A. Kuzal (eds), *The nature of qualitative evidence.* Thousand Oaks, CA: Sage.

van Dierendonck, D. 2011. Servant leadership: A review and synthesis. *Journal of Management,* 37, 1228–61.

Victoria State Government 2017. Defining bullying. Retrieved from www2.health.vic.gov.au/health-workforce/working-in-health/promoting-safety-in-the-workplace/workplace-bullying/defining-bullying.

Walker, A., Earl, C. & Cuddihy, L. 2013. Graduate nurses' transition and integration into the workplace: A qualitative comparison of graduate nurses' and nurse unit managers' perspectives. *Nurse Education Today,* 33, 291–6.

Walker, A., Yong, M., Pang, L., Fullarton, C., Costa, Z.B. & Dunning, T. 2013. Work readiness of graduate health professionals. *Nurse Education Today,* 33, 116–22.

Walker, R., Schultz, C. & Sonn, C. 2015. Cultural competence: Transforming policy, services, programs and practice. In P. Dudgeon, H. Milroy & R. Walker (eds), *Working together: Aboriginal and Torres Strait Islander mental health and wellbeing principles and practice* (2nd edn). Canberra: Commonwealth of Australia.

Wallace, M. 2014. *Health care and the law.* Sydney: Thomson Reuters.

Walter, S., Li, L., Dunsmuir, M. & Westbrook, J. 2014. Managing competing demands through task-switching and multitasking: A multi-setting observational study of 200 clinicians over 1000 hours. *BMJ Quality & Safety,* 23, 231–41.

Warren, J., Fromm, R., Orr, R., Rotello, L. & Horst, H. 2004. Guidelines for the inter- and intra-hospital transport of critically ill patients. *Critical Care Medicine,* 32, 256–62.

Waterman, H. 2011. Principles of 'servant leadership' and how they can enhance practice. *Nursing Management,* 17, 24–6.

Waterworth, S. 2003. Time management strategies in nursing practice. *Journal of Advanced Nursing,* 43, 432–40.

Watts, D. 2015. A brief Aboriginal history. Retrieved from www.aboriginalheritage.org/history/history.

Weller, J., Boyd, M. & Cumin, D. 2014. Teams, tribes and patient safety: Overcoming barriers to effective teamwork in healthcare. *Postgraduate Medical Journal,* 90, 149–54.

West, R. 2014. *Rising to the challenge of our time: Better health and wellbeing for our nation's first people.* Retrieved from www.acn.edu.au/sites/default/files/publications/Oration_Booklet_2014_C7_Rising%20to%20the%20challenge%20of%20our%20time.pdf.

West, R., Usher, K. & Foster, K. 2010. Increased numbers of Australian Indigenous nurses would make a significant contribution to 'closing the gap' in Indigenous health: What is getting in the way? *Contemporary Nurse,* 36, 121–30.

West, S., Ahern, M., Byrnes, M. & Kwanten, L. 2007. New graduate nurses' adaptation to shift work: Can we help? *Collegian,* 14, 23–30.

Westbrook, J., Woods, A., Rob, M., Dunsmuir, W. & Day, R. 2010. Association of interruptions with an increased risk and severity of medication administration errors. *Archives of Internal Medicine,* 170, 683–90.

Westrick, S. 2013. *Essentials of nursing law and ethics.* Burlington, MA: Jones & Bartlett.

Westwood, C. 2010. How to achieve a work–life balance. *Nursing Management,* 17, 20–1.

Wharton, T. & Ford, B. 2014. What is known about dementia care recipient violence and aggression against caregivers? *Journal of Gerontology Social Work,* 57, 460–77.

Wilkes, G. 2010. Abdominal trauma. In P. Cameron, G. Jelinek, A. Kelly, L. Murray & A. Brown (eds), *Textbook of adult emergency medicine* (3rd edn). Sydney: Churchill Livingstone.

Willetts, G. & Clarke, D. 2014. Constructing nurses' professional identity through social identity theory. *International Journal of Nursing Practice,* 20, 164–9.

Williams, M. & Jordan, K. 2007. The nursing professional portfolio: A pathway to career development. *Journal for Nurses in Staff Development*, 23, 125–31.

Winch, S. 2007. Nursing and clinical ethics. In K. Curtis, C. Ramsden & J. Friendship (eds), *Emergency and trauma nursing*. Sydney: Elsevier.

Winterstein, T. 2012. Nurses' experiences of the encounter with elderly neglect. *Journal of Nursing Scholarship*, 44, 55–62.

Wong, C.A. & Cummings, G.G. 2007. The relationship between nursing leadership and patient outcomes: A systematic review. *Journal of Nursing Management*, 15, 508–21.

Wong, C.A., Cummings, G.G. & Ducharme, L. 2013. The relationship between nursing leadership and patient outcomes: A systematic review update. *Journal of Nursing Management*, 21, 709–24.

Wong M.C., Yee, K.C. & Turner P. 2008. A structured evidence-based literature review regarding the effectiveness of improvement interventions in clinical handover. *Clinical Handover Literature Review*. eHealth Services Research Group, University of Tasmania.

Woodrow, P. 2005. Recognising and managing stress. *Nursing Older People*, 17, 31–2.

World Health Organization (WHO) 1946. *Constitution of the World Health Organization*. Retrieved from http://apps.who.int/gb/bd/PDF/bd47/EN/constitution-en.pdf?ua=1.

—— 2007. Patient Identification. Retrieved from www.who.int/patientsafety/solutions/patientsafety/PS-Solution2.pdf.

—— 2017. Health and Human Rights Publication Series. Retrieved from www.who.int/gender-equity-rights/knowledge/hhr-publication-series/en.

Wu, R., Rossos, P., Quan, S., Reeves, S., Lo, V., Wong, B., Cheung, M. & Morra, D. 2011. An evaluation of the use of smartphones to communicate between clinicians: A mixed-methods study. *Journal of Medical Internet Research*, 13, 1–15.

Zunkel, G., Cesarotti, E., Rosdahl, D. & McGrath, J. 2004. Enhancing diagnostic reasoning skills in nurse practitioner students. *Nurse Educator*, 29, 161–5.

INDEX

Printed and bound by CPI Group (UK) Ltd, Croydon, CR0 4YY

23/10/2024

01777692-0001